NEUROTOXICOLOGY: A CLINICAL SOURCE BOOK

By

PETER G. BERNAD
M.D., M.P.H., F.A.C.P.

LEXIS® LAW PUBLISHING
CHARLOTTESVILLE, VIRGINIA

Library of Congress Catalog Card No. 98-85162
ISBN 0-327-00132-1

6606710

DEDICATION

This book is dedicated to my patients over the last fifteen years. They have opened my eyes, filled my heart, and stimulated my mind about neurotoxicological illnesses. I'm indebted as well to my children, Daniel M. Bernad, David A. Bernad, and Jonathan M. Bernad, who have helped by sacrificing their time to allow me to complete this work. Special thanks also to my wife, Dr. Martha Bernad, who has supported me over the years and helped me to achieve my dreams.

SUMMARY OF CONTENTS

TABLE OF CONTENTS

CHAPTER 1

NEUROTOXIC EXPOSURE

CHAPTER 2

MEDICAL HISTORY

CHAPTER 3

PHYSICAL AND NEUROLOGIC EXAMINATIONS

CHAPTER 4

LABORATORY ANALYSIS

CHAPTER 5

PSYCHOMETRICS; NEUROPSYCHOLOGICAL ASSESSMENT

CHAPTER 6

IMAGING AND NEUROPHYSIOLOGIC STUDIES

CHAPTER 7

VOLATILE SOLVENTS

CHAPTER 8

METALS

CHAPTER 9

ORGANOPHOSPHATE INSECTICIDES

CHAPTER 12

OTHER TOXIC AGENTS

PREFACE

There are in fact two things, science and opinion; the former begets knowledge, the latter ignorance.

—Hippocrates (c. 460-377 BCE), *Law*, Book I.

There are many reasons to write a book. The sheer joy of expressing one's thoughts on paper can be excuse enough. In this book, the objective is to bring together under one cover some of the current scientific thinking on environmentally induced illnesses caused by neurotoxins. It is well known that chemicals can affect health. Since our exposure to them is on the rise, environmental neurotoxicology is a subject with serious claims to our attention. In this book, I attempt to assess the neurological damage that results from toxic environmental effects. This involves the evaluation of occupational risks and nutritional factors, among other contributors to the damage. Deficiencies of certain nutrients in the diet, for instance, can lead to certain illnesses, as can an overabundance of other types of nutrients.

Over the last fifteen years, I have striven to understand the relationship between chemicals and the environment, and the impact of chemicals on the human nervous system. Chemicals are known to have caused alterations in brain, nerve, and muscle function and to have had adverse effects on the autonomic nervous system. Time-honored scientific approaches are available to assess causation in these instances. When phenomena affecting populations are studied, for example, epidemiologic methodologies are used. The quest for data and their interpretation often require a team approach where industrial hygienists, engineers, and practitioners of other critical disciplines collaborate in assessing risks and evaluating findings.

In my work as a consultant, I am frequently asked to study individuals rather than populations. Consequently, this book addresses primarily the problems of individuals who have developed the symptoms found in neurotoxicological disease. In attempting to assess the neurological damage done by environmental toxins, I base my approach on science and the scientific method, using a clinical approach that involves careful scrutiny of data obtained from patient histories, from physical and neurological examinations, and from laboratory tests. I then form opinions based on my analysis of these data. The results must be well understood and analyzed in order to be clearly and effectively communicated later.

Not infrequently in contemporary society, the issues raised by the presence of toxic chemicals are addressed in the legal arena rather than in the laboratory. In the last decade of the twentieth century, more problems are settled in courtrooms and judges' chambers than in laboratories and classrooms. There has been an explosive growth in tort litigation relating to either real or alleged toxic chemical injuries. This book is a methodological overview of a fast-growing field. Its aim is to serve as an information source for those who need an educated introductory grasp of neurotoxicology — what it includes and how it is practiced. Here they will learn that the nervous system can at times suffer toxic damage from specific chemicals. Just as important, readers will become acquainted with the characteristics of nutrients essential to the maintenance of health.

It is undeniable that today, health and wholeness are energetically sought through alternative treatment modalities which are becoming part of orthodox therapies. Acupuncture, herbal medicine, holistic remedies, and nutritional supplementation are increasingly among the array of methods being promoted as legitimate treatments. Rigorous scientific evaluation must precede the acceptance of these practices, of course, even as the idea that we can usefully draw from many traditions daily gains ground. This primer of neurotoxicology will hopefully find many uses as the diversity continues to grow.

I offer this book as a contribution to this vast and engrossing process.

Peter G. Bernad
Washington, D.C.
April 1998

Chapter 1

NEUROTOXIC EXPOSURE

For the first time in the history of the world, every human being is now subjected to contact with dangerous chemicals, from the moment of conception until death.

—Rachel Carson, *Silent Spring* (1962).

§ 1-1. Overview of Toxicity.

We live in a world of chemicals. The quantum leaps in science and technology that have occurred since the Industrial Revolution have been made possible through the use of myriad potentially toxic substances, natural and synthetic. Since humankind learned how to make and use fire, we have become willing to accept the interrelated risks of environmental damage and toxicity involved in the use of dangerous forces and substances as the price for the overall benefits they provide. Nevertheless, it is now universally recognized that workers have a right to be protected from toxic chemicals and that the population at large has a right to an environment that is protected and reasonably safe to enjoy.

The concept of "occupational disease" was known long before it was recognized as a scientific discipline. One of the earliest and classic treatises was *De Morbis Artificum Diatriba* by Bernardino Rammazzini (1633-1714), published in English in 1703 under the title, *Diseases of Workers*. In the United States, Dr. Alice Hamilton (1869-1970) was an early advocate of industrial medicine. She advocated and defended the rights of workers to be protected from toxic exposure in a prolific output of books, articles and speeches.

Public awareness of environmental issues increased dramatically with the publication of Rachel Carson's *Silent Spring* in 1962. A series of toxic environmental disasters in the 1950s through the 1970s also increased demand for governmental intervention and for greater responsibility on the part of industry. In 1953 and 1960, there were outbreaks of methylmercury poisoning in the Minamata Bay area of Japan and elsewhere (Takeuchi, 1977). The resulting disease was quickly named "Minamata disease." Methylmercury, a known toxic substance, was a waste product of industries along the bay. Fish contaminated with the mercury compound were the actual source of the poisoning. The disease produced a wide range of symptoms and was particularly devastating for fetuses. Many children were born with severe defects, including mental retardation and paralysis. Similar outbreaks of methylmercury poisoning occurred in Iraq, Pakistan, and Guatemala. These and similar events were factors leading to the Occupational Health and Safety Act (OSHA) of 1970.

As our technology continues to advance, the potential for exposure to neurotoxins increases, as do opportunities for litigation. Attempts to link breast implants to neurologic disease and to link electrical transmission lines to leukemias and lymphomas are prime examples of the kinds of mass torts that are now clogging the courts. Both have been shown to be without merit. It is natural to sympathize with plaintiffs claiming to have suffered physical and emotional harm. However, frivolous suits delay justice for those who have valid claims, and the plaintiffs may be putting themselves in danger by delaying proper treatment for real illnesses.

A successful defense against litigation involving injury to the nervous system, be it neurotoxic exposure, or head, back, or neck injury, requires that the forensic neurology expert be thoroughly familiar with the relevant issues. The basic tenet of this book is the concept that conclusions should be based on the best available scientific data applicable to the medical/legal issues involved. There is no place for personal feelings, advocate positions, or anything less than rigorous discipline, careful data gathering, sound reasoning and scientific analysis.

§ 1-2. What Are Neurotoxins?

Neurotoxins are substances that cause temporary or permanent damage to the nervous system. The damage can be inflicted on the central, peripheral, or autonomic nervous systems. (See Table 1.1.)

Table 1.1
The Nervous System

Functions of the Nervous System

The functions of the nervous system include:

- The reception of stimuli, conversion of stimuli to nerve impulses, and the conduction of nerve impulses; and

- The activation and control of muscles and vital functions such as breathing and heartbeat.*

*The term *somatic nervous system* is used to describe the parts of the nervous system involved in controlling voluntary muscles, such as those of the arms and legs; the *visceral nervous system* controls internal organs — such as the heart, lungs, and intestines — not normally under the control of the somatic nervous system.

Basic Unit of the Nervous System

- The basic unit of the nervous system is the nerve cell or *neuron*. Neurons are conductive cells that transmit an electrical impulse under certain conditions.
- The neuron consists of a central part, called the cell body, which contains the cell nucleus.
- The neuron has one or more extensions from the cell body, *axons* and *dendrites.*
- Most neurons have one axon, which is an elongated unbranched process of the cell itself, the cytoplasm of which is continuous with that of the cell body or perikaryon. The axon conducts nerve impulses away from the cell body. Its volume tends to be much greater than that of the cell body. Dendrites, on the other hand, are short radiating processes that conduct information to the cell body of the nerve cell (neuron).

Components of the Nervous System

The major components of the nervous system are:

- Central nervous system

    —Brain

        —Cerebrum

        —Cerebellum

        —Brainstem

- Peripheral nervous system
  - —12 pairs of cranial nerves
  - —31 pairs of spinal nerves
- Autonomic nervous system
  - —parasympathetic division
  - —sympathetic division

Hundreds, perhaps thousands, of compounds are known to be associated with neurotoxic injury. They can be classified in many ways; classification by chemical structure or by effect on the nervous system are two possibilities. A classification of neurotoxins is shown in Table 1.2.

Table 1.2
A Classification of Neurotoxins

Volatile Solvents

Benzene
N-hexane
Methanol
Methyl ethyl ketone
Toluene
1,1,1 Trichloroethane
Trichloroethylene
Xylene

Heavy Metals

Arsenic
Cadmium
Lead
Mercury
Nickel

Organophosphate Insecticides

Diazinon
Dichlorvos
Malathion
Parathion

Chlorinated Hydrocarbon Insecticides

Aldrin
Chlordane; industrial chlordane and it metabolites
Dichlorodiphenyltrichloroethane (DDT)
Dieldrin
Heptachlor
Lindane

Other

Carbon monoxide
Carbon disulfide
Sarin
Plant and fungi toxins
Animal toxins (from snakes, spiders, jellyfish, etc.)

Our understanding of neurotoxins and their effects comes primarily from accidental or deliberate exposures and animal studies rather than from controlled experiments on humans. Accidental exposures can be caused by individual accidents in industrial settings, by large-scale industrial accidents affecting many individuals, or by even larger accidents, as in environmental catastrophes affecting great numbers of people. The disaster in Bhopal, India, was one such accident. But large-scale neurotoxic disasters are not confined to industrial settings or to exotic locations such as Bhopal. Tens of thousands of Americans — mostly children —are potentially exposed to lead poisoning, which slowly but insidiously damage their nervous systems, impairing their intellects, affecting organ systems, and impacting on the quality of life.

Intentional exposure to neurotoxins can occur in a variety of ways. These include homicide and suicide attempts, intentional exposure to prescribed medications resulting in unexpected toxicity such as iatrogenic neurotoxicity, and intentional exposure through drug abuse, resulting in unintentional toxicity.

In order for a neurotoxic injury to take place, the factors of toxicity, exposure, and dose must be present. Toxicity is the intrinsic capability of a substance to cause harm at some dose. Exposure is the opportunity for contact with the substance. Dose is the amount of the substance that is transferred out of the environment and that enters the body.

New information regarding the toxicity of naturally occurring substances has revealed that one of the most important messenger molecules when dealing with neurotoxicity is nitric oxide (NO). NO plays a role in relaxation of the gastrointestinal system and bladder function, as well as many other bodily functions. It is involved in communication among cells, but is a nonadrenergic and noncholonergic neurotransmitter. As a messenger molecule, NO may be the ultimate neurotoxin, as it is responsible for cell death. It may also be involved in glutamate neurotoxicity. The enzyme associated with NO is nitric oxide synthase (NOS), however, there may be more than one form of NOS. While $_{c}$NOS may be neuroprotective, $_{n}$NOS may be neurotoxic in an ischemic model of brain function.

In some cases, it is not clear if exposure to a neurotoxin has actually taken place. The so-called Gulf War Syndrome is an example. A syndrome is a clusering of symptoms and signs which constitutes potentially one diagnosis (Adams, 1997). After the war, hundreds of veterans began to complain of a vague and general set of symptoms. The symptoms included fatigue, headaches, stomach problems, aching joints, rashes, and memory loss. Some veterans developed tumors which they claimed may have been associated with exposure to chemical weapons. The Defense Department has devoted a great deal of time and money in an attempt to find some scientific basis for Gulf War Syndrome, without success. While the Defense Department maintains that Gulf War Syndrome does not exist, it was embarrassed at the revelation that some U.S. servicemen may have been exposed to low levels of nerve gas when an Iraqi storage building was destroyed. The Gulf War Syndrome issues are still unfolding, and the final chapter on this syndrome has not been written.

It is human nature to sympathize with veterans who risked their lives in the service of our country. However, the Gulf War Syndrome issue, as any other, must be resolved on the basis of rigorous scientific discipline.

§ 1-3. Neurotoxicity Defined.

According to the Office of Technology Assessment and the Environmental Protection Agency, neurotoxicity (or neurotoxic effect) is defined as:

> *An adverse change in the structure and function of the nervous system following exposure to a chemical agent.* (Office of Technology Assessment, 1990)

There is considerable disagreement over the meaning of the word "adverse," and over the meanings of the terms "neurotoxic effect" and "adverse change." Some authorities state that "neurotoxic effect" refers to an irreversible pathologic change in the nervous system. Others maintain that the term describes both reversible and irreversible effects. The trend of opinion, however, has been to consider "neurotoxic effects" as those marked by pathologic, irreversible changes in the nervous system. "Adverse effects" are any effects on the nervous system, including those that are transient and irreversible.

§ 1-4. Acute and Chronic Neurotoxicity.

Acute and chronic are recognized generally as the two major categories of neurotoxicity. Because of the relationship of acute and chronic neurotoxicity to the issue of temporary (reversible) versus permanent (irreversible) effects, the difference between these categories is important. (See Table 1.3.) Pathologic injury to the central nervous system is generally irreversible, while injuries to the peripheral nervous system are frequently reversible with an anticipated full recovery of all functions.

Acute neurotoxicity is associated with physiologic changes in the nervous system, generally referred to as adverse effects, which are usually rapidly reversible *if* there are no accompanying pathologic changes or degeneration of neuronal elements. Chronic neurotoxicity is usually associated with pathologic changes of the neuronal elements, generally referred to as neurotoxic effects, which are generally irreversible or, at best, incompletely reversible.

Table 1.3
Acute and Chronic Toxicity*

Acute	Chronic
Associated with physiologic change	Associated with pathologic changes of neuronal elements
Usually no pathologic change; rapidly reversible	Completely irreversible or incompletely reversible
Referred to as an adverse effect typically associated with a single large exposure	Referred to as a neurotoxic effect typically associated with repeated moderate or large exposure

*These characteristics are generalizations; many exceptions are known.

Table 1.4
Intermediate Syndrome

Intermediate
Associated with organophosphate exposure
Associated with NTE (Neuropathic target esterase enzyme), a class of membrane-bound hydrolases, molecular weight 155-178,000 daltons, found in bran and spinal cord
Causes delayed neurotoxicity called OPIDN (organophosphate-induced delayed neuropathy). This appears 8-21 days following exposure

There are multiple varied and different manifestations. Minimal manifestations may include headache, dizziness, visual changes, confusion, memory loss, numbness, tingling, and "pins and needles" sensations (paresthesias). More severe manifestations may be seizure activity, paralysis, loss of consciousness, coma, and death. The capacity of a toxicant to poison or functionally impair is important to understand. Neurotoxicity is any toxic effect on the central, peripheral, or autonomic system function, including, but not exclusively, structural, chemical, or physiological effects. Behavioral changes, as in toxic encephalopathy, must be included as well.

§ 1-5. Relating a Substance to a Toxic Effect.

The classic Henle-Koch Postulates for determining if there is a causal relationship between a microorganism and an infectious disease can be applied to determine if a substance is causally related to a neurotoxic effect. The Henle-Koch Postulates state that the suspected microorganism must be isolated from the patient with the disease and subsequently grown in a pure culture. Then the cultured organism must be inoculated into a healthy but susceptible animal. If the susceptible animal develops the disease and if the microorganism is subsequently isolated from that animal, the microorganism is verified as the causal agent.

In applying the postulates to neurotoxicology, the neurotoxin needs to be a necessary condition for the occurrence of the neurotoxic effects. Also required is experimental evidence of a causal relationship between the patient's symptoms and the suspected neurotoxin.

§ 1-5(a). Evaluating Neurotoxicity.

When evaluating the possibility of neurotoxic effects, the following must be considered:

1. Strength of association;
2. Consistency of association;
3. Specificity of relationship;
4. Temporality (when did it happen?);
5. Lag time (the time between exposure and onset of symptoms);
6. Documentation of body burden or dose relationship;
7. Biologic plausibility;
8. Coherence of evidence; and
9. Dose-response relationship.

1. *Strength of Association.*

There must be sufficient strength of association. That is, the judgment of an association between the syndrome and the neurotoxin must be based on hard scientific evidence, and not on prejudice or feelings of sympathy for the allegedly afflicted person. An association between the patient's symptoms and the specific neurotoxin in question must have been established in the medical/scientific literature and in clinical practice. Common symptoms such as headache, dizziness, and blurred vision are not specific enough to establish a relationship.

2. *Consistency of Association.*

The condition and the symptoms must be consistent with what is known about the neurotoxin. If it is possible to replicate the effect(s) allegedly caused by the neurotoxin, the case for an association is strengthened. Studies must show a repeated, consistent association between exposure to a particular neurotoxin and the patient's symptoms and complaints.

3. *Specificity of Relationship.*

If possible, specific signs and symptoms must be associated with the toxin in question. Carbon monoxide poisoning, for example, is associated with headaches and dizziness. These symptoms, however, are common complaints and are not specific to exposure to any one toxin. Carbon monoxide is known, however, to dull mental ability and occasionally to induce a "cherry red" skin flush some time after the exposure. Thus, if the headache and dizziness coincide with dulled mental ability and skin flush, the case for potential carbon monoxide poisoning is made stronger.

4. *Temporality.*

Temporality is also required. That is, the exposure to the suspected neurotoxin must precede the alleged effect(s). If symptoms occurred before the patient's known exposure to the neurotoxin, the relationship between the patient's illness and the neurotoxin cannot be fully established. Often the list of symptoms includes common complaints which practically everyone has experienced, such as dizziness, pain, numbness and tingling.

5. *Time Lag.*

It is well accepted in neurotoxicology that an individual develops symptoms to a particular neurotoxin within a short period after exposure. The longer the lag time between exposure and effects, the less likely it is that the neurotoxin is the causal factor. However, there are specific neurotoxins that do not exert their adverse effects immediately or even in a few days. These neurotoxins are associated with a delayed neurotoxicity. A certain form of neurotoxicity called intermediate syndrome (OPIDN) from organophosphate insecticides may be delayed. (See Table 1.4.) Several weeks may elapse between the exposure and the effects.

6. *Documentation of Body Burden or Dose Relationship.*

In order for toxicity to exist, the toxin must be transferred from the environment into the organism. Furthermore, the dose — the amount of toxin that has entered the organism — must be sufficient to induce a toxic response. The amount of toxin in the body must be documented by appropriate testing.

7. *Biologic Plausibility.*

When evaluating toxicity, the following must be considered:

a. The suspected chemical agent must be capable of producing the toxic effects in question.

b. The chemical must be capable of producing the toxic effects at the dose level the patient received.

It is possible to be exposed to a neurotoxin and not receive a dose capable of producing a reaction. The extent of the exposure must exceed the threshold level for toxicity to occur.

8. *Coherence of Evidence.*

This refers to the soundness of cause and effect interpretations of the data studied. These conclusions should not conflict with what is known and accepted as the natural history and biology of the disease in question.

9. *Dose-Response Relationship.*

There is a positive relationship between the amount of the neurotoxin to which an individual is exposed ("dose") and the toxic effect(s) ("response"). Because individuals differ with regard to biochemical, cellular tissue, and organ characteristics, a certain degree of variability of response can be expected. Nevertheless, dose-response implies that the extent of the response to an agent is directly related to the dose of the agent. In other words, the effect of the toxin on the patient is related to the degree of exposure to and absorption of the toxin. If the dose is insufficient there will be no response. However, once a sufficient dose has been reached, the extent of the response will be proportional to the dose. The amount of toxin at which a response will occur is referred to as the "threshold." This term implies a change from a baseline steady state resulting from exposure to the chemical agent. The effect may or not be a toxic response. Threshold is also referred to as "no observed effect level" (NOEL), or "no observed adverse effect level" (NOAEL). NOEL refers to the dose at or below which no biological effect is induced. NOAEL indicates the dose at or below which no adverse effect occurs.

These nine criteria have been proposed by Sir Austin Bradford Hill in 1965 to help decide whether a reported association is causal or spurious.

§ 1-6. Toxic Effects.

A toxic effect can be defined as a response that is maintained for a sufficient length of time or intensity to result in an adverse health consequence. An adverse health consequence is a condition that can shorten life or can impair one's ability to carry out normal activities or to reproduce. Any substance may have a toxic effect. Oxygen, for example, although vital for sustaining the life of living organisms, can have a toxic effect at a sufficient dose. Without dose, however, there can be no toxicity, and without sufficient dose there can be no toxicity. Thus, if a dose associated with an exposure is not specified, the possibility of toxicity cannot be evaluated.

§ 1-7. Twenty-First Century Diseases.

In recent years, a new set of diseases has entered the medical and litigation arena. Bearing names such as sick building syndrome, multiple chemical sensitivity, and chronic fatigue syndrome, these ailments are difficult to diagnose and have few, if any, signs and symptoms that are pathognomonic. (See Table 1.5.) Often referred to collectively as "twenty-first century diseases," some are believed to be associated, at least in part, with neurotoxic exposure, and some investigators think they all are. To date, however, there is no proof of such an association. Indeed, some medical authorities do not recognize these diseases as discrete medical entities.

Table 1.5
Diseases of the Twenty-First Century

Sick Building Syndrome
Multiple Chemical Sensitivity
Fibromyalgia
Reflex Sympathetic Dystrophy
Chronic Fatigue Syndrome
Repetitive Nerve Trauma Induced Neuropathy (e.g., carpal tunnel syndrome)
Multiple "Product Liability" Diseases (e.g., breast implant-, fen-phen-, ultram-induced disease)
Video Display Terminal Disease
Electro-Magnetic Radiation Disease (high-wire exposure)

§ 1-7(a). Sick Building Syndrome.

Sick building syndrome (SBS), also referred to as "tight building syndrome," is believed to be associated with the energy-efficient features of modern architecture — such as tight insulation and windows that cannot be opened or no windows at all — that limit the indoor supply of fresh air (Riesenberg, 1986). The World Health Organization defines SBS as "an excess of work-related irritations of the skin and mucous membranes and other symptoms, including headache, fatigue, and difficulty concentrating by workers in modern office buildings." (WHO, 1983). Typically, sick building syndrome occurs in what can be thought of as an epidemic: many people working in a building begin to complain of a variety of symptoms, including fatigue, headaches, itching, dry skin, and difficulty breathing; some complain of unpleasant odor and changes in perception of taste.

Several indoor air pollutants have been proposed as possible causes of SBS. These include stored fuels, carbon monoxide, radon, paneling, foam padding, carpets, carpet adhesives, pressed wood furniture, paint and paint supplies, asbestos, tobacco smoke, pesticides, aerosols, glues and adhesives. Bacteria, mold, and even positive ions have also been suggested as causes of SBS.

The major problem with SBS and other twenty-first century diseases is that the symptoms are often general complaints that everyone has experienced. Suspicion of SBS is increased, however, if the symptoms abate on weekends, holidays and vacations. Mass outbreaks of illness among people working in the same building have indeed occurred (Burge, 1987; Taylor, 1984; Middaugh, 1992; Stenberg, 1994). In some instances, the symptoms have been related to specific contaminants (Riesenberg, 1986).

By the mid-1980s, attempts had been made at classifying different types of SBS. In one classification, six categories of SBS were identified:

- Hypersensitivity pneumonitis: Associated with microorganisms that breed in ventilation ducts, air filters, and similar sites, this is probably the least common form of SBS.
- Building-related infections: The best-known example is Legionnaire's Disease, caused by *Legionella pneumophilia.* This and similar organisms have been found in air conditioners.

- Skin and mucous membrane irritation: This has been associated with airborne fiberglass and mineral wools. These fibers can also cause eye irritation.
- Allergens such as dust mites and mold spores: As suggested by the word allergy, not everyone is affected. Asthma-like symptoms are the usual manifestations in susceptible individuals.
- Mass hysteria: After a few people report symptoms, large numbers of people in the same building begin to feel sick. Investigations into causes of the illness reveal nothing.
- Annoyance-irritation syndrome: This is characterized by vague complaints that may often be nothing more than an unconscious expression of job dissatisfaction.

  Secondary gain: Malingering, symptom magnification, factitious illness, or simply "faking" for the sake of litigation.

There is still considerable controversy over the relationship between indoor air supply and SBS. A study of 4,373 office workers in England yielded evidence suggesting that symptoms of SBS were twice as likely to occur in buildings with indoor air control systems, such as air conditioning, than in buildings with natural ventilation (Burge, 1987). In a study in Canada, however, it was found that increases in the supply of outdoor air did not reduce reporting of symptoms considered typical of SBS (Menzies, 1993). Nevertheless, the American Society of Heating, Refrigeration, and Air-Conditioning Engineers has recommended increasing the minimal supply of outdoor air from 10 to 20 cubic feet per minute per person (ASHRAE, 1989). It is quite probable that controversy and complex litigation will continue into the twenty-first century.

§ 1-7(b). Multiple Chemical Sensitivity.

Multiple Chemical Sensitivity (MCS) has emerged as a possible disease entity over the past twenty years (Cullen, 1987; Hileman,

1991). As is the case with other syndromes characterized as twenty-first century diseases, there is controversy over the existence of MCS (Salvaggio, 1988), and the reported symptoms are vague and general. Dizziness, lethargy, reduced attention time, concentration problems, and skin rash are among the more frequently reported symptoms. People considered to be at risk include male industrial workers, female occupants of tight buildings, and residents of contaminated communities. More females than males have reported MCS. The patients tend to be thirty to fifty years old, white, middle to upper class, and professional.

The National Academy of Sciences recommended research on MCS, and a set of diagnostic criteria emerged (Hileman, 1991):

- Patients must have symptoms related to chemical exposure at concentrations tolerated by the general population;
- Symptoms must wax and wane with exposure; and
- Symptoms may be expressed in more than one organ system.

Additional diagnostic criteria have been proposed by some investigators, including the recurrence and abatement of symptoms in response to predictable stimuli, the eliciting of symptoms by chemicals of diverse structural class and mode of action, the occurrence of adverse reactions at exposures that are demonstrable but well below those known to cause adverse human responses, and the failure of any single generally available test of organ symptom function to explain the symptoms (Cullen, 1987; Salvaggio, 1988).

Although there is still uncertainty over the definition of MCS and doubt over its validity as a specific disease entity, several federal and state agencies recognize MCS as a disease qualifying for disability entitlement (Ashford, 1991; Bascom, 1988).

The number of litigations involving alleged MCS will probably increase in the twenty-first century. A thorough and complete history and a general and comprehensive neurologic exam are vital parts of the patient evaluation. The history should include a comprehensive environmental survey of the patient, starting well before the first report of symptoms. The physical examination should include tests to rule out other possible causes of the patient's symptoms in all involved organ systems. Laboratory evaluations should include regular blood work and urine analysis, as well as assessment of the immune system and testing for the presence of autoantibodies. Diagnostic testing should include appropriate neurometric studies such as electroencephalography (EEG) and semi-quantitative sensory evaluations (thermal, vibratory) for small fiber sensory neuropathy evaluations. Electromyography and nerve conduction studies can be done. Evoked potentials and other appropriate neurodiagnostic studies should also be considered. Magnetic resonance imaging (MRI), positron emission tomography (PET), and single photon emission computerized tomography (SPECT) can also be done where indicated. Neuropsychometric studies (neuropsychological testing) are also frequently done. Fat biopsies and skin biopsies may be helpful in certain chemical exposure situations.

§ 1-7(c). Fibromyalgia.

Fibromyalgia is a painful muscular condition that is believed to originate in the connective tissue associated with muscles and joints. It is characterized by aching, stiffness, fatigue, poor sleep, and the presence of multiple, reproducible tender points. These tender points include the occiput (back of the head), low cervical (lower neck), trapezius (upper back), gluteal (buttocks), and knee (Bonica, 1990; Wolfe, 1990). Also reported are fatigue, neurologic symptoms, allergic symptoms, affective disorder, cardiac symptoms, pulmonary symptoms, and gastrointestinal symptoms.

It has been estimated that 2 to 4% of patients presenting to general practitioners report symptoms of fibromyalgia (Felson, 1989; Wolfe, 1995). About 80 to 95% of patients reporting symptoms are women between 30 and 80 years of age (Powers, 1993; Waylonis, 1992).

The etiology of fibromyalgia is not known. Various etiologies have been proposed including viral, immunologic, endocrine, neurologic, genetic, toxic exposure, and combinations of these. A proposed connection to the toxic exposure hypothesis is that chronic exposure to environmental and dietary immunoreactants disrupts the homeostasis of the psychoneuroimmune control system. The disruption of homeostasis leads to symptoms of fibromyalgia, including pain, fatigue, and mood and sleep disorders. Agents causing frequent hypersensitivity reactions in patients with symptoms of fibromyalgia include MSG, *Candida albicans*, caffeine, chocolate, food colorings, xylene, cadmium, lead and sodium benzoate (Jaffe, 1996).

Treatment programs include moderate exercise, education, behavior modification, and medications. Among the medications that have been tried are tricyclic antidepressants — including amitriptyline and cyclobenzaprine, NSAIDS, and serotonin reuptake inhibitors — and vitamin and mineral supplements (Jaffe, 1996).

§ 1-7(d). Reflex Sympathetic Dystrophy.

Reflex sympathetic dystrophy (RSD) is an arthritic disease that may begin gradually or may manifest in a few hours. It occurs in acute, dystrophic, and atrophic stages. In the acute stage, there is burning pain that is exacerbated by physical contact or emotional upset, edema, hypothermia or hyperthermia. In the dystrophic stage, the swollen tissue becomes hard and cool, and takes on a bluish tinge. The patient may lose hair and sweat profusely, and the nails may become ridged, brittle and cracked. In the atrophic stage, the pain spreads, the skin may become thin and shiny, and the fingertips may become wasted. In addition, there may be vasomotor instability and bone demineralization. Motion of the shoulder may become painful and restricted. A subclinical form of the disease has also been identified (Gilliland, 1994).

The pathogenesis of RSD is unknown. However, a precipitating event can be identified in about two-thirds of cases. Precipitating events include trauma, myocardial infarction, peripheral nerve damage, and ingestion of medications including antituberculosis drugs, barbiturates, and cyclosporin (Gilliland, 1994).

Clinical evaluation includes laboratory testing and physical examination. Diagnosis may require x-rays, scintigraphy (triple phase bone scan examination), and thermography. Scintigraphy may show abnormal blood flow to bones (Gilliland, 1994).

If treated in the early stages, RDS may be reversed. However, successful treatment becomes less likely as the disease progresses. Therapy includes corticosteroids, physical therapy, regional nerve blocks, and various surgical procedures (Gilliland, 1994).

§ 1-7(e). Chronic Fatigue Syndrome.

Chronic Fatigue Syndrome (CFS) is another disease that has generated controversy. There is controversy concerning its existence as a disease entity, its etiology and pathogenesis, and the possibility that CFS and fibromyalgia may be the same disease. There is even controversy over whether to call it CFS. Other proposed names include post-viral fatigue syndrome, chronic mononucleosis, chronic Epstein-Barr virus, and myalgic encephalomyelitis.

Chronic fatigue syndrome appears to be a genuine but poorly understood illness. It is a syndromic diagnosis defined by a set of symptoms out of proportion to pathology. In 1988, the Centers for Disease Control and Prevention (CDC) published a case definition for chronic fatigue syndrome. To meet the case definition, a patient must fulfill two major criteria, and either eight of eleven symptom criteria or two objective and six symptom criteria.

The first major criterion is fatigue which is severe and debilitating and present for six months or more. The second major criterion is the absence of an identifiable medical or psychiatric etiology for fatigue.

The minor criteria include generalized headache, fever, sore throat, painful lymph nodes, arthralgia, myalgia, muscle weakness, sleep disturbance, prolonged fatigue after exercise, and neuropsychological symptoms.

The objective criteria include low-grade fever, nonexudative pharyngitis and palpable or tender cervical or axillary lymph nodes.

In 1992, the National Institutes of Health (NIH) published recommended modification of the definition. In this new modification, some patients with specific psychiatric diagnoses and certain post-infectious fatigue syndromes are excluded, while certain other patients are included. It is now recognized that chronic fatigue syndrome, fibromyalgia, and certain psychiatric disorders seem to overlap.

Again, the symptoms are vague, variable, and general. Frequent symptoms include low-grade fever, sore throat, swollen lymph nodes, muscle and joint pain, headache, sleep disturbance, anxiety, depression, and cognitive dysfunction.

The etiology of CFS is unknown, but many hypotheses have been proposed. Quite often, CFS begins after an acute flu-like or gastrointestinal illness. In some cases, symptoms start without a precipitating event. Symptoms may be aggravated by stress or exertion. Proposed etiologies include infection (usually by Epstein-Barr virus, but human herpes virus and enteroviruses are also candidates), immune dysfunction, metabolic disorders, abnormal vitamin and mineral metabolism, neuroendocrine dysfunction, psychological disturbances, and toxic exposure. The last possibility, toxic exposure, is most likely to initiate litigation. However, symptoms attributed to toxic exposure could also be interpreted as MCS or SBS.

§ 1-7(f). Reactions Relating to Dental Care.

There have been an increasing number of reports of unusual reactions and potentially deleterious sequelae after the use of chemicals commonly used in dentistry. Sodium hypochlorite, which is used as an agent to clean away unwanted tissue in preparation for root canal surgery, has been associated with unusual neurological manifestations. A 52-year old woman had a fatal intra-cerebral hemorrhage after visiting her dentist for treatment of an abscess adjacent to a right maxillary tooth. This calamity occurred after a series of treatments. The etiology of the intra-cerebral hemorrhage was based on biochemical evidence favoring a certain chain of events: sudden unexpected trigemina nerve stimulation caused by hypochlorite, followed by pain; immediate elevation of blood pressure; and intra-cerebral hemorrhage from unprotected artierioles in the left cerebral hemisphere. Acute rises in blood pressure and tachycardia accompany pain in humans and animals, and may follow mechanical or electrical stimulation of the trigeminal nerve (Barbas, 1987; Hunter, 1980; Youmans, 1982; Sweet, 1985; Haines, 1978).

§ 1-7(g). Diethylene Glycol Poisoning.

An epidemic of severe systemic toxicity and death, as well as neurotoxicity, from diethylene glycol poisoning as a result of contaminated acetaminophen (Tylenol) syrup occurred in Haiti between November 1995 and May 1996. This outbreak was an unusual occurrence, but not unique; and it could happen again. Special problems exist in developing countries where the techniques to apply U.S. health and safety standards may not be available (O'Brien, 1998; Woolf, 1998).

The later part of the twentieth century has seen numerous developments in medication and treatments, which continue today. They promise to change the course of disease and relieve symptoms. There is a brave new world in the field of pharmacology. However, problems, complications and adverse drug reactions (ADRs) occur on a daily basis. For all medications, treatments and interventions, the essential issue is whether the benefits of treatment outweigh the risks (Lazarou, 1998).

§ 1-7(h). Electric and Magnetic Field Exposure.

There has been litigation involving cases of extremely low frequency (ELF) fields produced by electric power lines and other sources. It has been claimed that the ELF fields promote changes in mood, sleep disturbances, cancer, leukemia, and other diseases (Foster, 1993). In April 1998, the Science Review Symposium plans to release human health effects resulting from exposure to electric and magnetic fields (EMFs). The National Institute of Environmental

Health Sciences (NIEHS) and the Department of Energy will produce a report at their June 1998 meeting, which will summarize what is known about these effects. That report will be used by NIEHS for its own report to Congress on EMF exposure and adverse human health effects (OHS, 1998).

§ 1-7(i). Video Display Terminals.

A few lawsuits have presented claims for illness arising from the use of video display terminals (Roel, 1990). In 1980, two women in Chicago who worked together at computer terminals developed cancer. One of the women died. The surviving woman sued Raytheon, the manufacturer of the terminal at which she worked. Unsuccessful worker's compensation claims have been filed against AT&T by women who developed skin rashes attributed to the use of video display terminals (Foster, 1993).

§ 1-8. Potentially Toxic Products.

Occasionally, consumer products that are developed to meet marketplace demands ultimately raise questions regarding safety. Several popular and widely used products have gained public attention due to their suspected neurotoxicity. These include Phen-Fen (the diet drug) and silicone breast implants.

§ 1-8(a). Phen-Fen.

Recently, phentermine (Phen) and phenfluramine (Fen) have been combined in a new administration as Phen-Fen. They are amphetamine derivatives prescribed as appetite suppressants for weight reduction (Atkinson, 1994). Phen's appetite suppression action occurs via central dopamine release. Fen asserts its appetite suppressant effects by causing 5 hydroxytryptophan (5HT) release from central 5HT terminals (Hoebel, 1989).

Long-term and adverse effects from consuming this combination are unknown, although recently certain cardiac valvular abnormalities have been identified using echocardiogram. In animal studies, these drugs have been neurotoxic in rats, guinea pigs and monkeys. Alterations in 5HT, which is a precursor to 5 hydroxytryptamine (seratonin), have been associated with sleep disturbance, nervousness, depression and memory loss (Roth, 1994).

Other medications/drugs may prove to be neurotoxic or to cause symptoms of neurotoxicity. Careful assessment and evaluation are necessary to alleviate symptoms and prevent long-term effects.

§ 1-8(b). Silicone Breast Implants.

In recent years, significant concern has been raised regarding silicone breast implants. Dating back to 1967, unique case reports and several animal studies have indicated that silicone may cause immunological and systemic pathology in animals and humans (Angell, 1994). Specifically, it has been argued both at the bedside and in the courtroom that silicone breast implants harm women. There was a major pubic outcry via the media, which resulted in a ban of silicone breast implants for cosmetic purposes in 1992.

Starting with the early Japanese experience in the 1960s, silicone implants have been allegedly associated with chronic rheumatic disease (Sanchez-Guerrero, 1994) and connective tissue disease (Gabriel, 1994). Scleradoma, rheumatoid arthritis, systemic lupus, erythematosus and polymyositis have been associated with silicone breast implants. A group of patients have been diagnosed as having human adjuvant disease, due to particular symptoms and positive laboratory findings. Some individuals have even claimed specific neurological disease associated with silicone breast implants.

The author has had significant experience in researching this issue and has examined over 100 patients with silicone breast implants. Leakage of silicone through the intact envelope may occur (Kumagai, 1984). The silicone may be transferred via the lymphatic system, and has been found in lymph nodes in the axilla. This was associated with phagocytosis by histiocytes at the site of introduction. While the discomfort of some patients is undeniable, and, in some cases, numerous corrective surgeries have been required due to leakage, rupture and "bleed," a causal relationship between silicone breast implants and neurological disease remains uncertain (Bernad, 1995; Ferguson, 1998; Winther, 1998; Nyren, 1998).

§ 1-8(c). Human Products.

In association with giving patients various products derived from immunoglobulin-G and various blood products (as in transfusions, tissue/organ transplantation, human growth hormones from cadavers), neurotoxicologic consequences have led to various debilitating illnesses and even death. Human growth hormone was given to newborn infants and young children from the 1960s to the 1980s. It is thought that this practice is associated with a rare form of neurologic disorder called Creutzfeldt-Jakob disease (CJD). This is a progressive disease of the cortex, basal ganglia, and spinal cord, and is seen in middle-aged and elderly individuals. It is now recognized that this condition is caused by a transmissible spongiform encephalopaphy agent. The natural disease is relatively rare, with an incidence rate of about one case per million people annually. This incidence is the same throughout the world, except for the higher incidence reported among Libyan Jews. Approximately 10-15% of cases occur in a familial pattern. The agent responsible for the transmission is known as a prion (proteinaceous infectious agent). Inadvertent human-to-human transmission has been reported following corneal transplantation, the use of inadequately sterilized stereotactic brain electrodes, the use of human duramatter graft, the use of human growth hormone from cadavers, and eating of beef tainted with so-called "mad cow" disease.

One of the most interesting conditions resulting from the use of human products followed the use of human growth hormone in infants and the subsequent development of CJD 15-20 years later. This led to the withdrawal of all human growth hormone treatment. A synthetic form of human growth hormone developed by the pharmaceutical industry is now used routinely. Similarly, there are new forms of treatment using intravenous immunogloblin (IVIg). This has been shown to be beneficial in the treatment of several immune regulation disorders, such as relapsing-remitting multiple sclerosis, Guillain-Barre syndrome, various types of peripheral neuropathies and Myasthenia Gravis, poly-myositis, chronic demyelinating inflammatory polyneuritis. Occasionally, a shortage of IVIg is announced. One of the reasons for the shortage among the manufacturers has been the recall of IVIg fueled by fears of the spread of CJD. In 1997, the FDA ordered over a dozen recalls of IVIg products after learning of donors with CJD or those at risk of developing it. The recalls took place even though, according to industry spokesmen, no scientific proof that CJD can be transmitted through blood or blood products has been documented. Because of past experience, manufacturers willingly comply with the FDA's conservative policy, "just in case" (Bernad, 1987; Bernad, 1989).

§ 1-9. Monitoring Toxic Exposure.

While exposure to neurotoxins can happen to anyone, most exposures are occupational. In addition to federal regulations from agencies such as the Occupational Safety and Health Administration (OSHA), there are industrial associations that establish safety standards as guidelines for industry to follow in maintaining a safe environment in the work place.

OSHA was established in 1970 as an agency within the Department of Labor. The act creating it also created the National Institute of Occupational Safety and Health (NIOSH). NIOSH conducts research on occupational safety, and OSHA uses the research to establish standards. NIOSH publishes the registry of Toxic Effects of Chemical Substances and offers technical services, such as on-site inspections.

The American Conference of Governmental Industrial Hygienists (ACGIH) issues the most widely followed standards: Threshold Limit Values (TLVs) and Biological Exposure Indices (BEIs). These are considered to be recommendations that should be followed. However, ACGIH disclaims liability in association with the use of TLVs. TLVs and other indices are constantly being changed. Every year, the TLV

Committee of ACGIH issues a "Notice of Intended Changes." The notice provides opportunity for comment and for the addition of new substances.

§ 1-9(a). Categories of TLVs.

Threshold Limit Value — Time Weighted Average (TLV-TWA): The TWA is the concentration of toxin for a normal 8-hour workday and a 40-hour work week, to which nearly all workers may be repeatedly exposed, day after day, without adverse effect (ACGIH, 1987).

Threshold Limit Value — Short-Term Exposure Limit (TLV-STEL): The STEL is the concentration of toxin to which workers can be exposed continuously for a short period of time without suffering from irritation, chronic or irreversible tissue damage, or narcosis of sufficient degree to increase the likelihood of accidental injury, interference with self-rescue, or substantially reduced work efficiency, provided that the TLV-TWA is not exceeded. The TLV-STEL is not intended to be a separate, independent exposure limit. It supplements the TWA limit when there are known acute effects from a substance with toxic effects that are usually chronic. It is recommended only in situations where toxic effects have been reported in high short-term exposures in humans or animals (ACGIH, 1987).

A STEL is defined as a 15-minute exposure that should not be exceeded during the workday, even if the 8-hour TWA is within the TLV. Exposures at STEL should be limited to 15 minutes, and should be limited to no more than 4 a day, with at least a 60-minute interval between each exposure (ACGIH, 1987).

Threshold Limit Value — Ceiling (TLV-C): This is the concentration of toxin that should not be exceeded during any part of the working exposure. The usual industrial method in assessing a TLV-C is to sample over a 15-minute period, except for substances that may cause immediate irritation (ACGIH, 1987).

§ 1-9(b). BEIs.

Biological Exposure Indices (BEIs): Biological monitoring involves assessing levels of toxins in the body of the worker. The levels are assessed by means of a variety of tests, including tests of blood, urine, breath, hair, and bone. The BEI represents the levels most likely to be observed in specimens collected from a healthy worker who has been exposed to chemicals to the same extent as a worker with inhalation exposure to the TLV (ACGIH, 1987).

Two standards are set by OSHA: Recommended Exposure Limits (RELs) and Permissible Exposure Limits (PELs). RELs are published by NIOSH, and are based on extensive reviews of appropriate scientific and medical literature. They are intended to serve as the basis for legally binding standards of OSHA. Since they come from an agency whose mandate is to protect the health of workers, they are generally the most conservative occupational health standards. PELs are issued by OSHA and are legally binding. Because PELs are issued by an agency that must take into account economic feasibility, they are usually the least conservative occupational health standards (Ford, 1994).

References.

ACGIH, *Threshold Limit Values and Biological Exposure Indices for 1986-87.* Cincinnati, American Conference of Governmental Industrial Hygienists, 1987.

Adams, R.D., Victor, M., Ropper, A.H., Principles of Neurology, 6th Ed. New York: McGraw-Hill, 1997.

Angell, M. *Do Breast Implants Cause Systemic Disease?* N. Eng. J. Med. Editorial. 1994; 330:1748-1749.

Ashford, N.A., Miller, C.S., Chemical Exposures: Low Levels and High Stakes, New York: Van Nostrand Rheinhold; 1991.

ASHRAE, *Standard 62-1989: Ventilation For Acceptable Indoor Air Quality*, Atlanta, American Society of Heating, Refrigeration, and Air-Conditioning Engineers, 1989.

Atkinson, H.L., Hubbard, V.S., *Report on the NIH Workshop on the Pharmacologic Treatment of Obesity*. Am. J. Clin. Nutr. 1994; 60:153-156.

Barbas, N., Caplan, L., Baquis, G., Adelman, L., Moskowitz, M., *Dental Chair Intra-Cerribral Hemmorage*. Neurology. 1987; 37:511-512.

Bascom, R., *Chemical Hypersensitivity Syndrome Study*. State of Maryland, Department of the Environment, 1988.

Bernad, P.G., *Ask Your Doctor – Many Patients Endure Several Misdiagnoses before They Are Diagnosed with Myasthenia Gravis. Why is Myasthenia Gravis So Difficult to Diagnose?* Myasthenia Gravis Foundation. August 28, 1995; 17.

Bernad, P.G., et al., *Creutzfeldt-Jakob Disease, Human Growth Hormone, and Its Replacement with Synthetic Growth Hormone*. In: Edlivich, S.A. (ed), Pharmacoepidemiology, Vol. I. Chelsea, MI: Lewis Publishers. 1989. Presented at the proceedings of the 3rd International Conference on Pharmacoepidemiology, Univ. of Minneapolis, MN. November 1987.

Bernad, P.G., *Guidelines: Relevance of Infectious Diseases for Electroencephalogram and Other Neurophysiology Laboratories*. Clinical Electroencephalography. 1989; 23.

Bonica, J.J., *Other Painful Musculoskeletal Disorders*. In: The Management of Pain, 1990: 389.

Burge, S., Hedge, A., Wilson, S., et al., *Sick Building Syndrome: A Study of 4373 Office Workers*. Ann. Occup. Hyg. 1987; 31:493-504.

Cullen, M.F., *The Worker with Multiple Chemical Sensitivities: An Overview*. In: M.F. Cullen (ed.), Occupational Medicine: State of the Art Reviews: Workers with Multiple Chemical Sensitivities. Philadelphia: Hanley and Belfus, 1987.

Felson, D.T., *Epidemiologic Research in Fibromyalgia*. J. Rheumatol. 1989;16 (Supp. 19): 7-11.

Ferguson, J.H., *Breast Implant Redux: This Time with Data*. Neurology 1998; 50(4):849-852.

Ford, D.P., Schwartz, B.S., Rothman, N., *Assessment of Exposure and Dose in Neurotoxicology: Clinical and Epidemiologic Applications.* In: M.I. Bleecker, J.A. Hansen (eds.), Occupational Neurology and Clinical Neurotoxicology. Baltimore: William and Wilkins, 1994: 23-42.

Foster, K.R., Bernstein, D.E., Huber, P.W. (eds), Phantom Risk: Scientific Inference and the Law. Cambridge, MA: MIT Press, 1993.

Gabriel, S.E., O'Fallon, W.M., et al. *Risk of Connective Tissue Diseases and Other Disorders after Breast Implantation.* N. Eng. J. Med. 1994; 330: 1697-1702.

Gilliland, B.C., *Relapsing Polychondritis and Miscellaneous Arthritides.* In: K.J. Isselbacher, E. Braunwald, J.D. Wilson (eds.), Harrison's Principles of Internal Medicine, 13th Ed. New York: McGraw-Hill, 1994: 1703-1710.

Goldenberg, G.L., Simms, R.W., Geiger, A., Komaroff, A.L., *High Frequency of Firbromyalgia in Patients of Chronic Fatigue Seen in a Primary Care Practice.* Arthritis Rheum. 1990; 33:381-387.

Haines, S., Marom, J., Janetta, P., *Supra-Tentorial Intra-Cerebral Hemmorage Following Posterior Fossa Surgery.* J. Neurosurg. 1978; 49:881-886.

Hileman, B. *Multiple Chemical Sensitivity.* Chem. Engineering News 1991; July 22, pp.26-42.

Hill, A.B., *The Environment and Disease: Association or Causation?* 58 Proceedings of the Royal Society of Medicine, 1965: 295-300.

Hoebel, B.G., et al. *Microdialysis Studies of Brain Norepinephrine Seratonin and Dopamine Release during Ingestive Behavior: Theoretical and Clinical Implications.* Ann. NY Acad. Sci. 1989; 575:171-191.

Holmes, G.P., Kaplan, J.E., Gantz, N.M., et al., *CFS: A Working Case Definition.* Ann. of Int. Med., 1988; 108: 387-389.

Hunter, A.R., *Anesthesia for Neurosurgery.* In: Gray, T.C., Utting, J.E., Nunn, J.F. (eds), General Anesthesia, 4th Ed. London: Butterworth. 1980; 1231-1232.

Jaffe, R.J., *A Case Study: Fibromyalgia and Chronic Fatigue Syndrome.* Presented at the 1996 Meeting of the American Association for the Advancement of Science, February 8, 1996.

Klonoff, D.C., *Chronic Fatigue Syndrome.* Clin. Infec. Dis. 1992; 15:812-823.

Lazarou, J., Pomeranz, B.H., Corey, P.N., *Incidence of Adverse Drug Reactions in Hospitalized Patients: A Meta-Analysis of Prospective Studies*. JAMA. April 15, 1998; 279(15):1200-1205.

Menzies, R., Tamblyn, R., Ferrand, J-P., *The Effect of Varying Levels of Outdoor-Air Supply on the Symptoms of Sick Building Syndrome.* N. Engl. J. Med. 1993; 328:821-827.

Middaugh, D.A., Pinney, S.M., Linz, D.H., *Sick Building Syndrome.* J. Occup. Med. 1992; 34:1197-1203.

Nyren, O., McLighlin, J.K., Nyin, L., Josefsson, S., Engqvist, M., et al., *Breast Implants and Risk of Neurologic Disease: A Population Based Cohort.* Neurology 1998; 50(4):956-960.

O'Brien, K.L., Selanikio, J.D., et al., *Epidemic of Pediatric Deaths from Acute Renal Failure Caused by Diethylene Glycol Poisoning.* JAMA. April 15, 1998; 279(15):1175-1180.

Occupational Health & Safety (*newsletter update*). April, 1998; 8.

Powers, R., *Fibromyalgia*: *An Age-Old Malady Begging for Respect.* J. Gen. Int. Med. 1993; 8:93-105.

Riesenberg, D.E., *"Sick Building" Syndrome Plagues Workers, Dwellers*. JAMA 1986; 255:3063.

Roel, R.E., *Low Level Radiation becomes High Level Concern.* Newsday. March 25, 1990; 70.

Roth, B.L. *Multiple Seratonin Receptors: Clinical and Experimental Aspects*. Ann Clin. Psychiatry. 1994; 6:67-78.

Salvaggio, J.E., *Special Diagnostic and Immunologic Considerations.* In: C. Zenz, O.B. Dickerson, H.P. Horvath (eds.), Occupational Medicine, 3d Edition. St. Louis: Mosby, 1988: 159-163.

Sanchez-Guerrero, J., Schur, P.H., Sergent, J.S., Liang, M.H. *Silicone Breast Implants and Rheumatic Disease*. Arthritis & Rheumatism. 1994; 37: 158-168.

Schluederberg, A., Straus, S.E., Grufferman, F. (eds.), *Considerations in the Design of Studies of CFS.* Rev. Infect. Disease, 1991; 13:S1-S140.

Stenberg, B., Eriksson, N., Hoog, J., et al., *The Sick Building Syndrome (SBS) in Office Workers.* Int. J. Epidemiol. 1994; 23:1190-1197.

Sweet, W.H., Poletti, C.E., Roberts, J.T., *Dangerous Rises in Blood Pressure upon Heating of Trigeminal Rootlets: Increased Bleeding Times in Patients with Trigeminal Neuralgia.* Neurosurg. 1985; 17:843-848.

Takeuchi, T., Eto., N, Eto, K., *Neuropathology of Childhood Cases of Methylmercury Poisoning (Minamata Disease) with Prolonged Symptoms, with Particular Reference to the Decortication Syndrome.* Neurotoxicology 1977; 1-20.

Taylor, P.R., Dell'Acqua, B.J., Baptiste, M.S., *Illness in an Office Building with Limited Fresh Air Access.* J. Environ, Health 1984; 47:24-27.

Waylonis, G.W., Heck, W., *Fibromyalgia Syndrome: New Associations.* Am. J. Phys. Med. Rehab. 1992; 71:343-348.

Wellton, C.L., Salit, I., Moldofsky, H., Sleep, *EBV Infection, Musculoskeletal Pain and Depressive Symptoms in CFS.* J. Rheumatol. 1992; 19:939-943.

Winther, J.F., Bach, S.W., Friis, S., Blot, W.J., Mellenkjaer, L., et al., *Neurologic Disease Among Women with Breast Implants.* Neurology 1998; 50(4):951-955.

Wolfe, F., *Fibromyalgia.* Rheumatol. Dis. Clin. N. Am. 1990; 16:681.

Wolfe, F., Ross, K., Anderson, J., et al., *The Prevalence and Characteristics of Fibromyalgia in the General Population.* Arthritis Rheum. 1995; 38:19-28.

Woolf, A.D., *The Haitian Diethylene Glycol Poisoning Tragedy: A Dark Woods Revisited.* JAMA. April 15, 1998; 279(15):1215-1216.

World Health Organization. *Indoor Air Pollutants: Exposure and Health Effects.* Copenhagen: World Health Organization, 1983.

Youmans, J.R., Neurological Surgery, Vol. II, 2d Ed. Philadelphia: W.B. Saunders. 1982; 1129-1131.

Chapter 2

MEDICAL HISTORY

I shall be telling this with a sigh
Somewhere ages and ages hence;
Two roads diverged in a wood, and I—
I took the one less traveled by,
And that has made all the difference.

—Robert Frost, Stanza 4 of *The Road Not Taken* (1916).

§ 2-1. Medical History.

The symptoms and signs of illness from exposure to neurotoxic agents are similar to those of many other neurologic disorders. A complete history is therefore essential in the diagnosis of neurologic illness, particularly when legal issues are involved, to determine if a patient's symptoms stem from an illness preceding the alleged toxic exposure.

In obtaining a neurologic history, care must be taken to establish rapport with the patient in order that a reliable history be obtained. The cooperation of the patient is critical in determining the nature, extent, and content of the symptoms in the sensory aspect of the clinical presentation. After all, it is only the patient who is able to fully describe his sensory symptomatologies. The patient will tell the examining neurotoxicologist what he smells, feels, hears, or thinks. Special care must be taken to prevent suggestion to the patient regarding his medical symptomatologies. The doctor can frequently confuse the history by suggestion or in some other way. There may be errors or inconsistencies in a recorded history that is based on poor technique on the part of the examining neurotoxicologist.

In the field of neurotoxicology, it has been the experience of this practitioner that patients will come in with a "diagnosis" and essentially distort the critical element of history taking. It is far better to ask a patient to describe his symptoms in his own words (preferably single and simple words), and to be as accurate as possible. Knowledgeable family members, friends, and neutral observers such as coworkers and supervisors should also be allowed to give some history so as to verify the patient's subjective complaints. The patient may bring his own notes and recollections to the examination.

The nature of the illness and the way it evolved, as well as its course, are also critical. It is important to remember that some neurotoxicants affect the higher cortical functioning of the brain and may derange the thinking perception and awareness of the patient. The patient's memory and attention may be altered, and his thinking may be inadequate. In these cases, history must be obtained from others. In episodic illnesses such as seizures, the patient's memory may be totally altered, and other observers will have to give their impressions of the events in question.

The history should be taken as soon as possible after the exposure to the neurotoxin has occurred. It should include medical, personal, and occupational information. Data on symptomatology should also be included, particularly observable abnormalities such as tremor, vertigo, seizure history, and weakness. Documentation of the main complaint and the onset of the present illness are also important (Bernad, 1990).

A comprehensive questionnaire should be given to patients. The questionnaire should solicit information on occupational duties, personal health habits, potential exposures, hobbies, and lifestyle. See Table 2.1 for a representative questionnaire. This questionnaire is used by the author's institution to evaluate chemical exposure patients, particularly those with exposure to pesticides (Bernad, 1990).

Past medical history should be investigated for underlying systemic diseases and for prior neurologic injuries such as head trauma. Socioeconomic factors should also be included. Low income, for example, may necessitate a diet that is deficient in certain nutrients. Occupational history provides information on the timing of potential exposures and whether similar symptoms have occurred in coworkers with the same potential exposure. The occupational history should include all job titles and descriptions of the types of work performed in all jobs held by the patient. Since some hobbies involve the use of substances that can be neurotoxic, such as glues and paints, information on these pastimes should also be included in the history.

Information on all prescribed and over-the-counter medications in use at present and in the past should be included in the history. Neurotoxic reactions, including toxic dementias, have been associated with and caused by a wide variety of legally prescribed medications. Medications with direct actions on the nervous system — including antipsychotics, hypnotics, sedatives, anticonvulsants, anticholinergics and various analgesics — can induce encephalopathy. Higher cortical functions can be impaired, altered, or diminished by benzodiazepines often prescribed as antidepressants. Long-term use of anticonvulsants can result in subtle central nervous system effects. Chemotherapeutic agents such as vincristine and cisplatin may also have adverse neurologic effects (Bernad, 1990).

Other sources of neurotoxins include carbon monoxide, recreational drugs, and a wide variety of pollutants such as insecticides. Occult exposure to carbon monoxide can result in headache and nausea and more profound effects on the central nervous system. Alcohol and recreational drugs such as marijuana, cocaine, heroin, amphetamines, and solvents (glue sniffing) can also have profound neurotoxic effects. Some agricultural workers are at risk of exposure to insecticides.

Consumers, too, may be at risk of exposure to insecticides as a result of consuming produce bearing insecticide residues. Consumers could also be at risk from some categories of household cleaners and insecticides. Queries about cleaning products and insecticides used in the home should therefore be included in the questionnaire.

Table 2.1
Clinical Neurotoxic Exposure Data

Date: ________________ Record #: ________________

PATIENT INFORMATION:

A. Patient name____
B. Home telephone ________________ Work telephone ________________
C. Address: Street ____
City ________________________ State ________ ZIP _______
D. Weight: ______________ Height: ____________ Birth Date: __________
E. Smoker? _________ If yes, how, many packs/day?____________________
F. Drink alcohol? _________ If yes, how, many drinks/week? _____________
G. Other medications?____
H. Patient's primary physician's name:_______________________________
I. Telephone __________________ City __________________ State _______

EXPOSURE LOCATION:

1. Exposure location (State) ________________________ Age of building _____
2. Type of building (check one):

_____ Single family dwelling
_____ Townhouse/Rowhouse
_____ Apartment
_____ House trailer
_____ Office
_____ Commercial
_____ Other ____

PESTICIDE APPLICATION:

3. Date of LAST pesticide application: ______________________________
4. Number of prior applications ______ Dates: ___________________________
5. Pesticide type:

_____ Chlordane/Heptachlor
_____ Aldrin/Dieldrin
_____ Other Cyclodienes
_____ Other

6. If Chlordane, which of the following:

_____ Gold Crest C-100
_____ Gold Crest Termide
_____ Orkin Chlorhepton
_____ Dursban TC

APPLICATON METHOD:

7. Please check all of the following that apply:

Areas Injected:

_____ Foundation (inside)
_____ Foundation (outside)
_____ Sub-slab
_____ Rod and trench

Areas Sprayed:

_____ Outside
_____ Living area
_____ Crawl space
_____ Ground
_____ Foundation
_____ Joists/floor

8. Misapplication: _____ admitted
_____ verified
_____ suspected
_____ none

9. Evaluated by: _____ EPA, _____ Dept. of Agri., _____ OSHA, _____ Bureau Tox. Subst., _____ Other

PATIENT SYMPTOMS:

10. Date exposure to pesticide began: ______________________________
11. Length of time exposed (weeks, months, years) ______________________
12. Are you still exposed to this pesticide? __________________________
13. Circle all of the following symptoms you have experienced since exposure began:

General symptoms:

weight gain
fevers or chills
muscle/body aches
weight loss
rash/itching
other _______________

Gastrointestinal:

noticed odor
nausea
diarrhea
stomach pain
dark urine
loss of appetite
vomiting
unusual taste
yellow jaundice
other _______________

Neurological:

headache
trouble sleeping
nervous/agitated
no concentration
feel depressed
shakes/tremors
pins & needles
uncoordinated
dizzy
tired/no energy
irritable/grouchy
memory/forgetful
confusion
seizures/fits
numbness
weak/no strength
walking different
other ___________________

Respiratory:

dry/sore throat
short of breath
wheezing
pneumonia
other ___________________
coughing
painful breathing
bronchitis

Eyes:

blurring
painful eyes
other ___________________
double vision
swell around eyes

Endocrine:

changes in menstrual periods
pregnancy since exposure began
impotence
other ___________________

Immunology:

changes in frequency of infections
other ___________________

ENVIRONMENTAL MEASUREMENTS:

14. Were pesticides measured in the area you were exposed?
______ Yes ______ No

15. If you answered yes to question 14, please record measurements below:

Sources of measurement: air (μg/m^3). water (μg /L), wipe (μg /ft^2), soil (ppm), carpet (μg /ft^2), clothing (ppm), lumber (ppm).

Source	Date	Chlordane	Heptachlor	Dursban	Other:

____
____
____
____
____

16. Please check which agency took the above listed measurements.

   ______ EPA ______ OSHA ______ Dept. of Agriculture
   ______ Other: ____

17. To your knowledge, have you ever been exposed to lead, mercury, or arsenic? If yes, explain the circumstances.

18. Have you ever taken chemotherapeutic agents, such as chloramphenicol, vincristine, cisplatin, and/or Adriamycin?

19. To your knowledge, have you ever been exposed to acrylamide, sulfites, pesticides, or termiticides?

20. Have you or any of your relatives had diabetes mellitus?

21. Do you consume alcohol or other recreational drugs? If yes, please list.

22. Is there a history of liver or kidney disease in your family?

23. Please list your hobbies.

24. Do you use chemicals (insect killers, concentrated cleaning solutions, etc.) around the home? If yes, please list.

25. Are there features in you neighborhood that you feel may be a threat to health (example: factory pollution, dumps)? If yes, please describe.

PATIENT SYMPTOMS:

26. Check any of the following difficulties you have:

______ Cramps/twitching/weakness
______ Difficulty opening jars
______ Tingling/pins and needles
______ Tremors, incoordination
______ Unsteady hands or walk
______ Burning in hands or feet
______ Difficulties in urination
______ Impotence
______ Menstrual period changes
______ Weight loss
______ Loss of appetite
______ Cracked/itchy skin
______ Itchy eyes/nose/throat
______ Frequent bloody nose
______ Shortness of breath
______ Ringing/noise in ears
______ Cough a lot
______ Heart disease

______ Headaches
______ Tired/lack of energy
______ Difficulty sleeping
______ Irritability/grouchiness
______ Nervous/agitated
______ Difficulty concentrating
______ Depression
______ Shakes/tremors
______ Birth defects/miscarriages (both sexes answer)
______ Nausea/vomiting
______ Yellow jaundice
______ Changes in urine color
______ Joint pain
______ Constipation
______ Memory problems
______ Seizures/fits
______ Changes in walking
______ Dizziness

OCCUPATIONAL HISTORY:

27. Current employment status (check one):

______ employed full-time
______ temporarily laid-off
______ retired
______ employed part-time
______ unemployed
______ disabled

28. Please list your employment history beginning with your current or most recent job.

Job Title (type of work)	Employer & City	Date Start	Date End	Hrs/Week

29. Check any of the following items you have been exposed to through hobbies or any of your jobs. Please list exposure dates and include exposures from other nearby workstations.

	Item	Exposure Dates
______	Dusty workplace	______
______	Asbestos (see below*)	______
______	Rock dusts (incl. sandblasting, foundry molds, concrete, mine/ore dust)	______
______	Coke oven fumes/tars/pitch/soot	______
______	Vegetable dust (incl. sawdust, cotton dust, flours)	______
______	Metal dusts (example: grinding)	______

_____ Molten metals or metal fumes _____
_____ Welding/acetylene torch _____
_____ Machine or cutting pils _____
_____ Solvent/degreasers/cleaning fluid _____
_____ Paint/varnishes/coating _____
_____ Chemical dyes _____
_____ Plastic/rubber/polymer chemicals _____
_____ Chemical manufacture _____
_____ Gasoline/other fuels _____
_____ Corrosives (acids, alkalis) _____
_____ Insect, rodent, or weed killers _____
_____ Other chemical liquids or vapors _____
_____ Gases (used, product, or byproducts) _____
_____ Smoke (from burning materials) _____
_____ Engine exhaust or carbon monoxide _____
_____ Loud noise _____
_____ Vibration (example: air hammer) _____
_____ Extremes of heat or cold _____
_____ Long-term standing _____
_____ Heavy lifting _____
_____ Repetitive motions all day _____
_____ Video Display Terminal (VDT) _____
_____ Job stress ("pressure") _____
_____ Infections or infectious material _____
_____ X-rays/direct radiation _____
_____ Radioactive materials _____
_____ Infrared/ultraviolet/laser _____
_____ Other ______________________ _____

*Asbestos mining, milling, textiles, brake linings or repair, insulation (especially pipes), ship building, cement manufacture.

30. Have you worked with any materials that you believe or were told were harmful? If yes, please list.

31. Do any materials at work frequently, get on your skin or in the air you breathe? If yes, please list.

32. Have you ever been exposed to unusually large amounts of hazardous materials at work (examples: accidents, spills, fires)? If yes, describe.

33. Has an industrial hygienist ever measured exposure to hazards at your job?

34. Do you smoke cigarettes, cigar, or pipe? If yes, do you smoke while at work?

35. At your current or most recent job, do you eat or drink in the same room you work in?

36. At your current or most recent job, are your work clothes cleaned at work?

37. At your current or most recent job, are showers suggested by your employer before returning home?

38. Do you drink more than 2 beers/alcoholic beverages a day?

39. Check any of the following protective equipment items you have been advised to use:

	Item	Equipment used: as advised	sometimes	never
_____	Goggles	_____	_____	_____
_____	Hearing protection	_____	_____	_____
_____	Respirator/face mask	_____	_____	_____
_____	Ventilation hood/fan/suction	_____	_____	_____
_____	Gloves	_____	_____	_____
_____	Protective apron/suit	_____	_____	_____
_____	Barrier cream (skin)	_____	_____	_____
_____	Other	_____	_____	_____

40. Do you have any health problems that you think are caused by or made worse by your job? If yes, please describe.

41. If you answered yes to the previous question, do these symptoms occur:

	Yes	No
a. Increasingly as the work day or week goes on?	_____	_____
b. Worse at the beginning of the work week?	_____	_____
c. Worse for some hours after work?	_____	_____

42. Do you have symptoms (for example, cough or dizziness) that appear *mainly at* or *after* work? If yes, please describe.

43. Do other workers in your workplace complain of job-related health problems? If yes, please explain.

44. Do you receive any regular physical examinations or testing (hearing tests, blood tests, x-rays) on the job?

45. Have you ever had injury or illness related to work? If yes, please describe (also state which job).

46. Have you ever applied for worker's compensation? If yes, please explain.

47. FOR WOMEN:

	Yes	No
a. Are you between 15 and 45 years old?	_____	_____
b. Are you planning a child in the future?	_____	_____
c. Are you pregnant now?	_____	_____

Abbreviations: EPA, Environmental Protection Agency; Dept. of Agri., Department of Agriculture; OSHA, Occupational Safety Hazards Administration; Bureau Tox. Subst., Bureau of Toxic Substances.

Courtesy of Neurentox International, Inc., Washington, DC.

References.

Adams, R.D., Victor, M., Ropper, A.H., Principles of Neurology, 6th Ed. New York: McGraw-Hill, 1997.

Bernad, P.G., Saunders, G., *Clinical and Laboratory Evaluation of Patients Exposed to Neurotoxicants*. Clin. Lab. Med. 1990; 10:387-402.

Chapter 3

PHYSICAL AND NEUROLOGIC EXAMINATIONS

I feel more confident and more satisfied when I reflect that I have two professions and not one. Medicine is my lawful wife and literature is my mistress. When I get tired of one, I spend the night with the other. Though it's disorderly, it's not so dull, and besides, neither really loses anything through my infidelity.

—Anton Pavlovich Chekhov, from a letter to A.S. Suvorin, September 11, 1888.

§ 3-1. Introduction.

Toxic chemicals such as pesticides and organic solvents can induce a variety of neurologic illnesses. These diseases are neither infectious, genetic, nor degenerative diseases. However, the symptoms and signs of illness due to toxic exposure are, in many instances, similar to those of other diseases. Careful and complete general and neurologic examinations, as well as a comprehensive patient history, are therefore essential in evaluating neurotoxic exposure. The physician must develop a complete differential diagnosis accounting for all probabilities associated with all potential causal agents.

§ 3-2. Physical Examination.

A complete physical examination should include measurements of weight, height. and the vital signs of blood pressure and pulse. The head, neck, eyes, ears, nose and throat should be included in the examination. Particular attention should be paid to the skin, lymph nodes, and spleen.

§ 3-3. Neurologic Examination.

The nervous system has three main branches: the central nervous system (CNS), peripheral nervous system (PNS), and autonomic nervous system (ANS). The central nervous system consists of the brain, brainstem and spinal cord. The brain has three main divisions, the cerebrum, cerebellum and brainstem. The cerebrum (also called encephalon), the largest part of the brain, is composed of two cerebral hemispheres. The cerebral cortex is the outer layer of cells or gray matter. The cerebellum, situated under the cerebrum, coordinates voluntary muscular movement. The brainstem contains centers that control involuntary functions such as breathing, heartbeat, digestion, and excretion.

The peripheral nervous system consists of the twelve pairs cranial nerves and their branches, and thirty-one pairs of spinal nerves. The cranial nerves originate from the brainstem, and the spinal nerves originate from the spinal cord.

The autonomic nervous system controls involuntary functions.

§ 3-3(a). Cranial Nerve Examination.

The cranial nerves are those that originate within the brain and brainstem. There are twelve pairs of cranial nerves, and they exit the skull to innervate the head and neck regions. The peripheral nerves are those that exit from the spinal cord. One cranial nerve, the vagus, has fibers that extend beyond the head and neck to supply autonomic innervation to the heart, lungs, esophagus, and stomach. Nerves are subject to injury from trauma, infections, toxic agents, and vascular and metabolic disorders. Trauma is most often the cause of localized injury to a single nerve. Toxic exposure and metabolic disorders usually affect more than one nerve.

Cranial Nerve I (Olfactory Nerve): The olfactory nerve carries the sense of smell. It originates at the base of the brain over the eyes, and extends downward over the orbits into the top of the nasal region. Patients with olfactory nerve disorders complain of loss or alteration of the sense of smell. They also usually complain of loss or alteration of taste because human perception of flavor is a combination of smell and taste. Toxic exposure can cause such alterations to the sense of smell. However, alterations to the sense of smell can also result from many other causes, ranging from the common cold to central nervous system damage from injury or disease.

The olfactory nerve can be tested by having the patient smell different odors such as those of perfumes, colognes, after-shave lotions, coffee, flowers and other aromatic substances.

Cranial Nerve II (Optic Nerve): The optic nerves, which carry impulses of vision, originate in the retina of each eye. Optic nerve fibers extend back through the orbit into the skull. Fibers from both eyes converge at the optic chiasm, where some decussate or cross to the side of the brain opposite the eye of origin, while others stay on the same side. Damage to the optic nerve can result in loss of vision, impairment of the pupillary light reflexes, and abnormalities in the size of the pupil. Optic nerve function can be assessed by examining visual acuity, pupillary response to light, and field of vision. Looking into the eye can reveal swelling of the optic disk, which is indicative of an increase in intracranial pressure.

The optic nerve is subject to damage from many causes. Toxic substances known to injure the optic nerve include ethyl alcohol, methyl alcohol, tobacco, quinine, thallium, mercury, lead and pentavalent aresenicals. Exposure to toxic substances can induce lesions of the optic nerve generally referred to as optic neuritis. Manifestations include loss of visual acuity with or without changes in the peripheral fields of vision. An early manifestation of neruotoxicity may be the finding of color desaturation or loss of color acuity. Optic neuritis also occurs in association with degenerative and inflammatory disorders such as mutiple sclerosis or other demyelinating diseases.

Cranial Nerve III (Oculomotor Nerve): This nerve innervates four of the six muscles that move the eyes. It also controls pupil size and the position of the eyelid. Oculomotor nerve function is tested by observing eyelid position, pupillary reactivity, and the ability of the eye to move in, out, up, and down. Lead poisoning is associated with adverse effects on the function of this nerve and two others — the trochlear and abducens — that control movement of the eye.

Cranial Nerve IV (Trochlear Nerve): This nerve controls a single eye muscle, the superior oblique, which turns the eyeball downward and inward. This nerve is difficult to examine because of the weakness of the muscle it innervates. However, patients with disorders of the trochlear nerve often complain of double vision in a vertical plane.

Cranial Nerve V (Trigeminal Nerve): As the name implies, this nerve has three major branches: the ophthalmic, or uppermost, branch, innervates the forehead and scalp back to the ear; the maxillary, or middle branch, innervates the cheek and the gums of the upper teeth; and the mandibular, or lower branch, innervates the chin extending up the jaw to the ear.

This nerve has both sensoiy and motor functions. It controls the movement of the muscles of chewing, sensory input from the face, and the corneal and sneezing reflex. Damage to the nerve can be associated with paralysis of the chewing muscles or loss of ability to perceive soft tactile, thermal, and painful sensations in the face, depending upon which branch is damaged. Sensation in the areas innervated by the trigeminal nerve can be assessed using a pin for pain, a wisp of cotton for soft tactile sensation, and a cool object to test thermal sensation. The corneal reflex can be elicited by lightly brushing the cornea. It is usually diminished in patients who have a lesion of the ophthalmic branch. Patients with a lesion in the mandibular branch may demonstrate a deviation of the jaw toward the side of the lesion.

Cranial Nerve VI (Abducens Nerve): This nerve controls the muscle that moves the eye laterally. It is tested by having the patient look in several directions while the examiner observes for weaknesses or asymmetry in eye movement. Abducens nerve lesions can produce a horizontal double vision that worsens when the patient looks in the direction of the weak muscle.

Cranial Nerve VII (Facial Nerve): The facial nerve innervates the muscles of facial expression, including those that make a smile, furrow the forehead, close the eye, and wrinkle the nose. Lesions of the facial nerve result in a painless weakness of the entire face called Bell palsy. This condition can be the result of trauma to the area anterior to the ear, skull fractures, tumors or infections. It has also occurred following surgery on nearby structures such as the removal of tumors of the acoustic nerve or parotid gland. In some cases, the etiology of Bell palsy is unknown. The facial nerve is tested by having the patient forcibly close the eyes, furrow the brow, wrinkle the nose and smile on command.

Cranial Nerve VIII (Acoustic Nerve): The acoustic nerve has two divisions: the cochlear and the vestibular. The cochlear portion carries impulses originating in specialized nerve cells in the inner ear that respond to sound. The impulses are carried to the auditory brain centers and are perceived as sound. The vestibular portion of the acoustic nerve carries impulses from the labyrinth, or balance center, which is also located in the inner ear. Lesions of the acoustic nerve can cause deafness, tinnitus (ringing in the ears), and vertigo (dizziness). Lesions can result from a variety of sources including, trauma, toxic exposure, tumors, and some medications, particularly some antineoplastic agents used as chemotherapy for the treatment of cancer (Elveskoski, 1996; Schweitzer, 1993; Kretschmar, 1990).

Hearing can be tested in a number of ways, ranging from the simple expedient of seeing how far from the ear the patient can detect the ticking of a watch to sophisticated electronic and computerized audiometry. A tuning fork is a simple but effective method. Most sounds are conducted through the air to the eardrum. However, the bone around the hearing structures also conducts sound. The tuning fork can test both air and bone conductance. Air conductance is tested by striking the tuning fork and holding it away from the ear at various distances. Bone conductance is tested by touching the base of the tuning fork to the mastoid bone behind the ear. The Rinne test compares bone and air conductance: a normal ear can hear the tuning fork twice as long by air conductance as by bone conductance. In the Weber test, the tuning fork is placed on the vertex of the skull. The normal result of this test is that the sound is heard equally by both ears. If the cochlear nerve is damaged, sound will be heard better on the normal side. These simple office procedures can be used to determine whether more sophisticated audiology should be carried out by an audiologist.

Cranial Nerve IX (Glossopharyngeal Nerve): The glossopharyngeal nerve carries the sensory impulses of taste from the posterior third of the tongue, and, with the vagus nerve, controls palatal function. It cannot be tested alone, but is examined along with the vagus nerve by observing palatal motion and assessing the gag reflex.

Cranial Nerve X (Vagus Nerve): The vagus nerve is the longest cranial nerve and it has the most extensive distribution. Its fibers pass through the neck and into the thorax and abdomen. It has fibers comprising the autonomic nervous system, which controls involuntary functions such as respiration, heartbeat, digestion and excretion. It has sensory fibers that innervate the skin of the posterior surface of the external ear and the external auditory meatus, the tube leading from the ear opening to the eardrum. It also has fibers that control voluntary muscles of the larynx, pharynx, and palate. Injuries to the vagus nerve are rare. Damage to one vagus nerve could result in paralysis of the vocal cords. Injury to both vagus nerves could result in respiratory arrest. Injuries are often manifested as hoarseness.

Cranial Nerve XI (Accessory Nerve): This nerve has two divisions: the cranial and the spinal. The cranial part originates from the medulla behind the vagus and spinal nerves at the upper five or six segments of the spinal cord. This part of the accessory nerve joins the vagus to innervate the larynx and pharynx. The spinal portion of the accessory nerve controls movement of the sternocleidomastoid (neck) and trapezius (upper back) muscles. This nerve is evaluated by observing for weakness in the trapezius or inability to elevate the arm above the horizontal plane.

Cranial Nerve XII (Hypoglossal Nerve): This nerve innervates both sides of the tongue, controlling motor or movement function. Lesions of the nerve can cause weakness on one side of the tongue, causing it to deviate. Damage to the right side causes the tongue to deviate to the left, and damage to the left side causes the tongue to deviate to the right. A good way to test this nerve is to have the patient push the tongue to the side against the cheek and the examiner's fingers.

§ 3-3(b). Spinal Nerves.

The spinal nerves are those that arise from the spinal cord, the large fiber tract system that extends from the brainstem through the foramen magnum, a large opening at the base of the skull. The spinal nerves branch to form peripheral nerves. The perhipheral nerves provide nerve impulses to control voluntary muscles, such as those of the arms and legs, and to conduct sensory impulses to the spinal cord and brain.

§ 3-3(c). Motor and Sensory Examination.

Motor nerves supply nerve fibers for the movement of voluntary muscles. These nerves are assessed by testing the muscles they innervate. Sensory function is evaluated by applying various stimuli, such as sharp or dull pinpricks, to the skin.

§ 3-3(d). Mental Status Examination.

Though often not performed adequately, the mental status examination is extremely important. In the mental status examination, the neurologist attempts to establish if the patient has the ability to remember in detail, to express himself or herself, and to comprehend probing questions. Frequently, physicians describe a patient as either awake, stuporous, or comatose. However, it is often preferable to describe exactly what the patient is doing and what the examiner observes. For example, the patient may be sleeping rather than comatose. Or the patient may be muttering incoherently. Orientation, ability to calculate, language function skills, and general appearance are also important in evaluating mental status. Higher cortical function testing remains an important part of the overall neurotoxic examination. Memory, insight, judgment, overall affect, attitude during evaluation and various language skills all need to be assessed.

§ 3-3(e). Tests of Motor Function.

When evaluating motor function the examiner needs to assess the speed and strength of movements as well as evaluating coordination. The muscles are evaluated in terms of their bulk, size and tone. Evaluating the arms, which should be exposed while outstretched in the prone and supine position, is also important. Strength testing in the upper and lower extremities is also recommended. Look for evidence of atrophy, loss of muscle and fasciculations. Abnormal tone and movements are also noted.

§ 3-3(f). Testing of Gait and Stance.

Testing of gait, stance, and the ability to ambulate is also important in the toxicological evaluation. An abnormality in gait or stance may be the only neurologic manifestation and may represent cerebellar or frontal lobe disorder. An abnormality of posture or movements such as walking may provide the first clue of an extrapyramidal disorder. Pendem gait is evaluated. Posturing of the patient, both in terms of the body or arms or legs, is noted. As part of the evaluation, the patient is asked to get up on his toes as well as on his heels and to hop in place.

§ 3-3(g). Cerebellar Testing.

This evaluates equilibrium and is tested with the patient's eyes closed. Cerebellar testing may represent a sensory problem as well, as in Romberg testing.

§ 3-3(h). Testing of Reflex Function.

Each of the reflexes is tested in turn. These include the biceps, triceps, and supinator reflexes in the upper extremities. In the lower extremities, the patellar, and Achilles reflexes are tested. When testing for the deep tendon reflexes, the involved muscles must be relaxed. Using the Jendrassik maneuver is helpful in eliciting underactive reflexes or when the patient is very anxious and is resisting reflex evaluation. This maneuver is done by voluntary contraction of muscles other than those being evaluated. A special reflex that needs to be tested in all evaluations is the Babinski sign. This is a reflex obtained by stimulating the sole of the foot along its outer borders, causing a dorsi flexion of the toe, the foot, and occasionally the knee and hip.

§ 3-3(i). Testing of Sensory Function.

This is the most difficult part of any neurologic examination. Patients frequently are unable or unwilling to give accurate responses. This test should be done fairly quickly. Some patients are more introspective and tend to be obsessive-compulsive about their reporting of stimulus. Sensory testing is the least objective part of the neurologic examination. Quantitative testing or semi-quantitative testing is needed to support the qualitative nature of the sensory evaluation.

§ 3-4. Infants and Small Children.

It is important to recognize that infants and small children also have neurotoxicological exposures. The neurologic examination should be tailored towards the infant or child, depending on the development of the individual.

§ 3-5. Fundamental Approach to the Exam.

The author learned the fundamental principles of medicine and neurology from R.D. Adams, C.M. Fisher, and E.P. Richardson, Jr. An approach based on fundamental principles is the soundest approach to the physical and neurologic examinations. The following five principles derive from *Principles of Neurology,* 6th Edition, by R.D. Adams, M. Victor, and A.H. Ropper:

1. Symptoms and signs are obtained by means of the history and physical exam.
2. Symptoms and signs are interpreted in terms of physiology and anatomy.
3. Correlations of symptoms and signs localize the disease process anatomically or topographically.
4. From this anatomic diagnosis and other medical data, including the mode of onset, evolution, and course of the illness, the involvement of other organ systems, the relevant past and family histories, and the important laboratory findings, one is able to identify a pathologic diagnosis. And when the mechanism and causation of the disease are determined, then the etiologic diagnosis is made.
5. The neurotoxicologist needs to asses the degree of disability and determine whether it is temporary or permanent. This functional diagnosis is important in managing the patient's illness, and in judging the potential for any improvement.

In the medicolegal context, this approach is extremely valuable and important in terms of the opinion of a neurotoxicologic expert. Not infrequently, a court may ask for an opinion from the expert. It is only with careful and judicious circumspection, review, and analysis of data that a medical or medicolegal opinion should be given.

References.

Adams, R.D., Victor, M., Ropper, A.H., Principles of Neurology, 6th Ed. New York: McGraw-Hill, 1997.

Elveskoski, I., Saarine, U.M., Wiklund, T., et al., *Ototoxicity in Children with Malignant Brain Tumors Treated with the "8 in 1" Chemotherapy Protocol.* Med. Pediatr. Oncol. 1996; 27:26-31.

Kretschmar, C.S., Warren, M.P., Lavally, B.L., et al., *Ototoxicity of Preradiation Cisplatin for Children with Central Nervous System Tumors.* J. Clin. Oncol. 1990; 8:1191-1198.

Mayo Clinic and Mayo Foundation, Clinical Examinations in Neurology, 6th Ed. St. Louis: Mosby Yearbook, 1991.

Schweitzer, V.G., *Ototoxicity of Chemotherapeutic Agents.* Otolaryngol. Clin. N. Am. 1993; 26:759-789.

Chapter 4

LABORATORY ANALYSIS

The Art of Detachment, the Virtue of Method, and the Qualities of Thoroughness may make you students, in the true sense of the word, successful practitioners or even great investigators, but your characters may still lack that which can alone give permanence to powers — the Grace of Humility.

—Sir William Osler, *Aequanimitas* (1904).

§ 4-1. In General.

Laboratory analyses are an essential part of any complete evaluation of a patient who may have acute or chronic heavy metal toxicity. Since all heavy metals bind to sulfhydryl groups located throughout the body, they tend to produce multi-system failure, including the following organ systems: gastrointestinal, renal, cardiovascular, and nervous. Chronic low-level toxicity has more subtle effects involving the nervous and renal systems, skin, bones, connective tissues, anemias, and neoplasms in various tissues (Bernad, 1990). Frequently used laboratory procedures include tests of biologic specimens, biopsies and spinal taps. While existing analytic laboratory methods can detect the presence of toxins, their usefulness in this application is limited. Analyses of biologic specimens such as urine, blood, and stool are not always conclusive because toxins are almost always present at baseline levels. Also, the biologic clearance mechanisms of detoxification, metabolism and excretion may obscure exposure levels (Bernad, 1990).

§ 4-2. Sampling and Storage.

Proper sampling, storage, and shipping of biologic specimens for analysis are extremely important, from both the health evaluation and forensic/legal aspects. False positives or negatives can result from faulty techniques, and opposing attorneys are quick to exploit any suggestion of improper handling of samples. The importance of avoiding contamination is obvious. If the laboratory to which the sample is being sent has specified procedures for sample collection, storage, and shipment, it is best to follow them. It is also important to use the same laboratory for a series of tests from the same patient or group of patients. Procedures, equipment and standards differ from one lab to another, and these differences can affect results. Because of the possibility of infection, great care must be exercised when handling samples of tissue and body fluids. The HIV virus has been transmitted by careless handling of samples. In response to this concern, OSHA blood pathogen rules are now mandated for clinical labs.

In addition to the following methods of analysis, sweat patches may be used to determine dermal exposure. Saliva may also yield useful information when collected and analyzed.

§ 4-2(a). The Time Factor.

The timing of sample collection is critical. In cases of acute toxic exposure, samples of urine, whole blood, or serum should be collected as soon as possible, preferably within 72 hours of the exposure incident. Many toxins are metabolized and excreted within that time frame, and chances of identifying suspected toxins are therefore greatly reduced if samples are collected more than 72 hours after exposure. The timing of collection is less critical when chronic exposure is being investigated (Hill, 1988).

§ 4-2(b). Urine.

Urine samples can be placed into general categories on the basis of collection time:

- 24-hour specimen, which includes all voidings over a 24-hour period;
- Pooled or combined specimen, which is a combination of voidings over a period of several hours;
- Single-spot specimen; and
- First morning specimen.

Since a 24-hour specimen is most representative of the average body burden of a toxin, it has the most potential for providing useful information. However, it is not the method of choice for collecting specimens at the workplace. In order to avoid contamination, the 24-hour sample must be collected under strictly controlled conditions that can usually be met only in a hospital. The pooled specimen is also representative, but avoiding contamination is quite difficult. The single-spot specimen is the easiest to collect, but it is generally not very representative of total body burden. Single-spot specimens are often collected at the end of a work shift or in a doctor's office. A first morning specimen is usually more concentrated than other specimens, and is often the method of choice for identifying unknown exposures. This specimen is usually collected at home in a container that the patient received the day before. A disadvantage is that one must depend on the patient to avoid contamination (Hill, 1988). It is also important to determine the half-life of the substance being measured so that it can be determined if the patient was on the ascending or descending part of the absorption or metabolite curve. Timed urines, e.g., for organophosphate metabolites, could be coordinated with cholinesterase panel levels for the 0-6 hour, 6-24 hour, and 24-48 hour post-admittance time following an organophosphate poisoning. A complete patient history that determines chronic exposure, in addition to acute exposure incidents, is also helpful in coordinating sampling times.

§ 4-2(c). Blood.

Blood tests can be classified into four basic categories: hematology, chemistry, microbiology, and toxicology. Hematology is concerned with the components and characteristics of blood itself. Frequently used techniques included complete blood count (CBC), which provides information on the number of red blood cells (erythrocytes) and white blood cells (leukocytes), and hematocrit, the determination of hemoglobin levels. Elevated white cell count, for example, can be an indication of infection, while low hematocrit can be a sign of anemia.

A great many analytical methods are available for testing blood chemistry. There are tests for determining levels of foreign substances such as toxins and other exogenous materials. Vital diagnostic information can be obtained by determining levels of endogenous chemicals such as electrolytes, which are salts of important minerals, including potassium, sodium, copper, calcium, fluorine, and others. Also included in blood chemistry are hormones, enzymes, and metabolites, all of which could, in some circumstances, provide information indicating the presence of toxins. Levels of antibodies and other immune system components can be indicative of infection or immune system malfunction. Information regarding the blood level of the exposure chemical may be helpful in cases of acute poisoning.

Microbiologic blood work is designed to test for the presence of microorganisms in the blood. These microorganisms may include bacteria, viruses, rickettsiae, or protozoa and other parasites. In many instances, the blood is drawn directly into tubes containing growth media for bacteria. Testing for protozoa, such as those that cause malaria, usually involves direct examination of the blood facilitated by smearing and staining techniques that help to identify the organisms.

Blood samples are usually collected by venipuncture. Modern methods involve the use of vacuum tubes into which the blood flows following the insertion of the needle. The contents of the tube vary according to the blood component that is to be tested. Whole blood consists of the blood cells, the so-called "solid components," and plasma, the liquid part of the blood. Serum is plasma from which the clotting factors have been removed. If whole blood is needed, a vacuum tube containing an anticoagulant is used for the collection of the sample. The rubber stoppers of the tubes are color-coded to indicate which anticoagulant is being used.

Serum is used frequently in tests to identify neurotoxins. Blood intended for serum extraction is collected into tubes containing no additives. The blood is allowed to clot for 30 minutes at room temperature, after which the tube is centrifuged to separate the blood cells to the bottom of the tube. The serum at the top is then transferred to a clean tube, using a disposable pipette. When the suspected neurotoxin is an organic solvent (e.g., toluene, styrene), it is very important that the blood not be allowed to come into contact with the rubber or plastic stopper. Such contact may contaminate the blood with organic substances contained in the stoppers. The tubes themselves could also be contaminated with trace amounts of metals. Tubes certified to be free of metal contamination are available for use when metals are the suspected toxins (Hill, 1988).

§ 4-2(d). Stool.

Stool specimens can be used for a variety of tests, ranging from microscopic examination for eggs of parasites to analyses of chemicals present in the specimen. While the kidneys are the major organs of excretion, the liver also plays an important excretory role. Many chemicals are metabolized in the liver, and the metabolic products are taken up into a liquid called bile. The bile is collected in the gall bladder, which is connected to the small intestine via a tube called the bile duct. At irregular intervals, the gall bladder contracts to force bile into the small intestine, where it is incorporated into the stool and eliminated.

The bile/stool elimination route serves to keep some metabolites out of the bloodstream, and avoids distribution to other parts of the body. The liver is the site of important detoxification processes, and direct excretion into the bile keeps the detoxification products out of the body.

§ 4-2(e). Biopsy.

Biopsy involves taking a piece of tissue for laboratory analysis. Many techniques and procedures have been developed to obtain specimens from almost all parts of the body, both external and internal. An endoscope, for example, can be inserted into the mouth and directed into the esophagus to take biopsy specimens from any site in the digestive tract, from the esophagus to the small intestine. Similarly, the endoscope can be directed into the trachea and downward into the bronchi and lungs. The endoscope can also be directed into the anus and large intestine to obtain specimens from those body sites. Endoscopes are equipped with lighting and optical systems that enable visualization of the operative sites.

The most frequently used biopsy technique is the needle biopsy. A needle is inserted into the tissue and the specimen is aspirated into a syringe. Biopsies of muscle and external body fat, for example, are usually obtained with a needle biopsy. Needles can also be inserted through the skin into organs such as the liver.

Fat biopsies are often effective for detecting organic solvents, such as trichloroacetic acid and trichloroethanol, because of the highly lipophilic nature of these substances. The specimen is usually obtained by needle biopsy from the buttocks. In some instances, a small surgical procedure is needed (Hirsh, 1960; Daum, 1978). Again, the specimen should not be allowed to come into contact with rubber, most plastics or any other substance that may contaminate it. Teflon will not contaminate the specimen, so many containers for fat specimens are made of this material.

§ 4-2(f). Hair.

Metals such as mercury, lead and arsenic tend to deposit in hair. Hair analysis, therefore, can help to determine if there has been chronic exposure to these or other metals. Hair samples can also reveal the use of some drugs, such as cocaine. Hair is usually collected from the back of the head at the nape of the neck, as close to the scalp as possible. A problem with hair analysis is the deposition of the toxin in question on the surface of the hair. For that reason, the hair collection should be done at the workplace or other site suspected to be the source of exposure. Some hair products, such as shampoos, hair sprays, and colorings, may affect analyses for trace metals. The patient should be questioned about use of these products, and about the brand names used (Hill, 1988).

§ 4-2(g). Breath Sampling.

Breath sampling has been proposed as a means of monitoring the exposure of workers in factories, for example, to a toxic substance. Breath sampling is restricted to volatile substances, those that exist as gases and vapors. However, this restriction is not as limiting as it might seem. Many substances are used as liquids, but vaporize to enter the body through inhalation. Also, some substances that enter the body in the nonvolatile state may be metabolized to volatile substances (Wells, 1974).

Gases appropriate for breath monitoring include hydrogen disulfide, carbon monoxide, and freon. Also appropriate for breath monitoring are liquid substances that vaporize, including metallic mercury, ethers, alcohols, and various solvents such as toluene and xylene. Reactive gases that might damage mucous membranes if inhaled, such as ammonia and hydrochloric acid, are not suitable for breath monitoring (Hill, 1988).

Breath monitoring can be used to determine whether a person has actually been exposed to a particular compound and, with the proper analytic technique, the total body burden or overall dose the person has received. Breath monitoring can also be used to check the effects of some toxic substances. Such a technique has sometimes been used in medicine as a diagnostic parameter. The acetone-like breath of diabetics is a well-known example. Other examples include monitoring of the compounds in relation to liver disorders (Manolis, 1983), and of amines that may indicate kidney disorders. These applications are beginning to be used in occupational medicine (Frank, 1983).

The usual procedure in breath monitoring is for the subject to exhale into a container, which can be a plastic or rubber bag, a glass tube, or a solid adsorbent such as activated charcoal or silica gel. Tedlar bags are now recommended for sample collection, since they can be directly analyzed with little interference in the lab and can be directly hooked to "purge and trap" equipment. Several types of instruments are available for analyzing the sample. Some are direct-reading portable devices that include the analyzing component. Others are limited to the collection container only, and the sample is transferred to a laboratory for analysis (Hill, 1988).

§ 4-3. Analytical Methods.

A wide variety of methods are available for use in chemical analysis, and new types are always in development. Most current analytic methods can be classified into five categories: spectroscopic, radiochemical, electrochemical (See Tables 4.1 and 4.2), chromatography and nuclear.

Spectroscopic techniques are most commonly used in chemical analysis today. Spectroscopy makes use of the interaction between electromagnetic radiation (EMR) and matter. Electromagnetic radiation is emitted from sources such as the sun and from devices such as light bulbs, radio transmitters and x-ray machines. Different kinds of EMR are characterized by their wavelengths. The full range of EMR from the shortest to the longest wavelengths is called the electromagnetic spectrum. Some familiar EMRs, listed in order from longest to shortest wavelength, include radio waves, microwaves, infrared radiation, visible light, ultraviolet light, and x-rays. When matter interacts with EMR, some radiation is absorbed and some is emitted. The result is a pattern, or spectrum, characteristic of the substance involved. Some of the instruments used in spectroscopy are referred to as spectrophotometers, spectrometers, mass spectrometers, and spectroscopes.

§ 4-3(a). Types of Spectrometry.

Atomic Absorption and Atomic Emission Spectroscopy: The sample is heated to very high temperature and decomposes into atoms that absorb or emit visible or ultraviolet EMR in energy patterns characteristic of the elements in the sample. These techniques are particularly useful for detecting low concentrations of metallic elements.

Absorption Spectrophotometry: In this technique, the relative transparency of a solution is measured before and after adding a chemical that changes the solution's color. The result is a decrease in transparency that is analyzed to determine the concentration of the substance under consideration. This is a widely used technique for the analysis of both inorganic and organic substances.

Fluorescence Spectroscopy: In this method, molecules are induced to emit light. The light is emitted at energies that are characteristic of the molecular structure of the substance being identified. The intensity of the light varies with the concentration of the substance. This method is quite sensitive and is used when accurate quantitative results are needed.

Infrared Absorption Spectrophotometry: This technique measures the absorption of different frequencies of infrared radiation by the samples being analyzed. It is often used for alcohols and other organic molecules.

Mass Spectroscopy: The sample to be analyzed is placed in a vacuum, where it is vaporized and ionized with energy input. This treatment serves to fragment the molecules of the sample. Electric and magnetic fields in a mass analyzer then sort out the molecules by their weights. Spectral patterns, or mass spectrums, are produced. A mass spectrum is a unique "fingerprint" of a molecule of a particular substance.

X-ray Fluorescence Spectroscopy: This technique is used for the analysis of metallic elements. The sample is bombarded by a high-energy x-ray source, and the sample, in turn, gives off x-rays with energies characteristic of the element(s) present.

§ 4-3(b). Radiochemical Techniques.

In these techniques, radioactivity emitted from the sample as alpha and beta particles and gamma rays is analyzed. One method used to induce the release of radiation is *neutron activation*, in which the sample is bombarded with neutrons. The radioactivity is emitted in patterns characteristic of the substance being analyzed. This procedure is often used to identify metals in a sample. Neutron activation analysis (NAA) is also useful for fingerprinting the source of environmental contaminants that may have caused exposure. NAA is very sensitive for metal analysis in biological specimens. It is non-destructive, so the sample can be used for other analysis, as well.

§ 4-3(c). Electrochemical Techniques.

This technique is based on the movement of electrically charged ions in a solution. When an electric potential is applied to a positive electrode and a negative electrode in a solution containing ions, the positively charged ions (cations) move toward the negative electrode (cathode), and the negatively charged ions (anions) move toward the positive electrode (anode). The result is an electric current flowing between the electrodes. The strength of the current depends on the electrical potential between the electrodes and on the concentration of the ions in the solution. Thus, the technique can be used to quantitatively measure the concentration of an ion in solution.

Specific Ion Electrode: Electrodes specially constructed to accept only specific ions are used in this technique, which determines the concentration of sodium or calcium ions in a solution, as well as the pH of the solution. The major application is clinical analysis.

§ 4-3(d). Chromatography.

Before analysis can be done, in many instances, it is necessary to separate the substance to be analyzed from the sample. Chromatography is the procedure most often used to effect this separation. Chromatography is based on the principle of selective adsorption, a type of adhesion. Because of differing degrees of adhesion, different substances in a solution will move through an adsorption medium at different rates of speed. Paper chromatography is the simplest form. If a spot of the solution is placed on a strip of paper of suitable composition, the various components of the solution will appear at different points along the paper. Many variations are in use today, and in almost all, results are obtained from data analyzed by a computer. In some instances, the identity of the substance can be determined by means of chromatography alone.

Column chromatography is the most frequently used method. A glass tube is filled with the adsorbent, and the solution is introduced. The result is a series of bands of material at different levels of the tube. A wide range of adsorbents is available for different applications. Among the variations is high-performance liquid chromatography, which involves the use of a pump to move the adsorbed liquids on very small, uniform particles, and which provides high sensitivity. In thin-layer chromatography, the adsorbent is placed on a film of glass or plastic.

Another method is gas-liquid chromatography. In this technique, gases or substances that can be vaporized by heat and separated from mixtures are forced by an inert gas through a coiled tube packed with suitable adsorbents. In ion-exchange chromatography, gases can be converted to ions by various methods including passing them through a hydrogen flame, bombarding them with x-rays or radioactive material, or using adsorbents that exchange ions with substances in the sample. In gel-permeation chromatography, molecules are separated according to their size.

Table 4.1
Methods Used in Selected Analyses of Toxins

Substance	Sample	Method
Aluminum	Serum	AAS
Arsenic	Urine	AAS
Cadmium	Blood	AAS
Chlorinated Hydrocarbons	Serum	GC
DDT	Serum	GC
Mercury	Urine	SP
Manganese (Organic)	Urine	AES
Methyl ethyl ketone	Blood	GC
Methylmercury	Urine, Blood	AAS
Selenium	Urine, Blood	AAS
Styrene	Breath	GC

Substance	Sample	Method
Tetrachloroethylene	Breath	GC
Toluene	Breath	GC

Abbreviations: AAS — atomic absorption spectrophotometry; AES — atomic emission spectroscopy; GC — gas chromatography; SP — spectrophotometry (Robbins, 1983)

Table 4.2
Analysis of Toxic Substance Metabolites

Substance	Metabolite	Sample	Method
Ethanol	Propanediol and butanediols	Serum	GC
Styrene	Mandelic Acid	Urine	GC
Toluene	Hippuric Acid	Urine	HPLC

Abbreviations: GC — gas chromatography; HPLC — high pressure liquid chromatography (Hill, 1988).

§ 4-3(e). Nuclear Techniques.

Nuclear techniques for measuring the levels of chemical elements in the body have been in use since the 1960s. A major advantage of these methods is that they are noninvasive. Results are quite accurate and they have advanced our knowledge of many clinical disorders. A disadvantage is the need for exposure of the patient to radiation. Maximum radiation limits have been established. Some elements cannot be measured with these techniques because the exposure time is too high. However, in all cases of permissible nuclear procedures, the radiation dose is less than that involved in x-ray examination of the same body region.

The basic procedure involves directing a collimated beam of neutrons, photons, or x-rays to the organ or tissue under investigation.

Various types of radiation are then given off by the excited atoms in the tissue being examined. This radiation in picked up by a detector, amplified, converted to digital signals, processed by pulse-height analysis, and analyzed by computers. Elements that have been measured with this technique include lead, mercury, aluminum and silicon. Regions and organs that are frequently examined include the liver, kidneys, brain, lungs, teeth, fingers and hand, and the whole body (Ellis, 1988).

Whole body counting of the amount of naturally occurring potassium was one of the earliest nuclear techniques (Ellis, 1988). Today, the most widely used nuclear techniques are x-ray fluorescence (XRF) and neutron activation analysis (NAA). A variation of NAA is called prompt gamma neutron activation analysis (PNAA).

§ 4-4. Testing for Specific Neurotoxins.

Careful and thorough clinical evaluation of all patients with suspected neurotoxic exposure is necessary for proper diagnosis and treatment. A complete assessment includes a medical and occupational history, physical examination, neuropsychological evaluation and laboratory tests (Bernad, 1990).

§ 4-4(a). Lead.

Lead and its compounds are among the most toxic substances in the world. While lead is ubiquitous in nature, occurring in soil, food, air, water and dust, there is no known physiologic use for this metal in humans. In addition to the lead found in nature, industrial processes and automobiles have greatly increased the concentration of lead in the atmosphere. Children are more susceptible to lead toxicity than are adults. A major source of lead in children is the ingestion of lead-based paint chips peeling from the walls of older, poorly maintained buildings. Exposed children may suffer from a variety of ailments, including low scores in psychological tests (Graef, 1979). With the banning of the use of paints containing lead pigment for internal use, and with the use of lead-free fuels in automobiles, mean blood lead levels in both children and adults have dropped over the past 30 years (Gochfeld, 1995). However, lead poisoning is still a problem in our society, particularly in children, and the use of appropriate analytical tests is vital.

Lead interferes with several enzymes required for the synthesis of hemoglobin, the compound in blood cells that binds to and transports oxygen. Anemia and decreased reticulocyte counts result. At high concentrations of lead, brain damage and symptoms of acute encephalopathy may occur.

Lead levels can be determined by screening serum, urine, hair, and the deciduous teeth of children. Blood concentration of lead is an indication of relatively recent exposure, as is lead concentration in a 24-hour urine sample. In cases involving long-term exposure and chronic effects, analyses of teeth are useful. Determining levels in deciduous teeth is particularly useful in determining past exposure in children.

Testing blood and urine for biochemicals that are products of the physiologic activities of lead can also provide useful measures. Calcium disodium edetate (EDTA, or versene), a compound used to treat acute lead encephalopathy, can be used to mobilize body stores of lead, which can then be measured in a 24-hour urine sample. Results can give some idea of past exposure. One of the enzymes deactivated by lead is delta aminolevulinic acid dehydratase (ALAD). This deactivation occurs at fairly low levels of lead intoxication, and the degree of deactivation can be correlated with the blood lead concentration (EPA, 1977). The inhibition results in an accumulation of delta aminolevulinic acid in the urine when the blood lead concentration of ALAD is about 40 μ/dL. An earlier indication is provided by free erythrocyte protoporphyrin (FEP). Elevated urine FEP levels may be present when blood levels of ALAD are as low as 15 μ/dL (CDC, 1985; Piomelli, 1984). A lead blood level of 30 μ/dL and higher, and an FEP level of 60 μ/dL are considered to be indicative of acute lead intoxication even in the absence of symptoms (Bernad, 1990). Lead can be effectively detoxified by chelation, which forms stable ring compounds via the coordination of electrons between the lead and an organic compound. Chemet (DMSA) is the preferred chelator, unless the patient has very high levels of lead poisoning or is significantly symptomatic. In such cases, dimercaprol (BAL) may be more helpful (NYC Poison Control Center, 1989).

§ 4-4(b). Mercury.

Chronic mercury poisoning may originate from the element in either organic or inorganic form. Inorganic elemental mercury (quicksilver) is more volatile than organic mercury compounds found in commercial products, such as paint and amalgam dental fillings (Bernad, 1990). There is no test that provides an early warning of subclinical effects of mercury poisoning. Symptoms of poisoning with methylmercury, the most toxic mercury compound, do not become evident until quite some time after ingestion. A mercury blood level of 10 μ/dL or below is generally considered to be normal.

Mercury can be detected in blood, urine, and hair. Hair analysis can provide useful information on the body burden of mercury. Each segment of a hair sample reflects the blood methylmercury concentration at the hair follicle at some point in the patient's life. The hair concentration of methylmercury is about 250 times greater than that of the blood at a given time (WHO, 1976). Hair is not a particularly good indicator for mercury vapor because of the problem of external deposition. Urinalysis is one of the more frequently used monitoring tests in occupational settings. Some investigators have found a good correlation between urine and blood concentrations, but the results may be less reliable when the exposure involves mercury vapor (Smith, 1970).

§ 4-4(c). Arsenic.

One widely used method of testing for arsenic involves changing the arsenic in a urine sample to arsine, which is then measured by spectrophotometry. The urine sample is digested in nitric, sulfuric, and perchloric acids. This digestion converts the pentavalent arsenic to trivalent arsenic, resulting in generation of arsine. The amount of arsine produced is measured by colorimetric techniques and compared to a graph of known standards indicating the amount of arsenic. A variation of this method involves the use of atomic absorption spectrophotometry.

§ 4-4(d). Cadmium.

The basic procedure for determining the level of cadmium in blood involves using nitric acid to remove the protein from a blood sample. The sample is then spun down with a centrifuge. The liquid remaining in the upper part of the centrifuge tube (supernatant) is subjected to atomic absorption analysis in a device called a graphite furnace (Nackowski, 1988).

§ 4-4(e). Thallium.

Thallium is primarily utilized by the semiconductor industry, but other commercial uses include the manufacturing of pigment, paint, optical lenses, cement, and semi-precious stones for jewelry. Almost all thallium toxicity occurs from exposure to inorganic compound forms (thallium salts). Although dermal and nasal mucosal absorption have been reported, thallium is most readily absorbed from the gastrointestinal tract. It has a short half-life of two days and is largely eliminated in feces. Thallium is taken up into cells like potassium and binds to sulfhydryl groups, especially enzymes of oxidative phosphorylation. Early symptoms include nausea, vomiting and diarrhea, which give way to coma, psychosis and/or seizures. Late-stage symptoms include Mei's lines and skin abnormalities. Urine is an unreliable indicator of thallium poisoning, but hair, x-rays of the abdomen, and blood screening for thallium levels above 30 mcg/dL are all helpful (NYC Poison Control Center, 1998).

References.

Bakir, F., Damluji, S.F., Amin-Zaki, L., et al., *Methylmercury Poisoning in Iraq.* Science 1973; 181:230.

Bernad, P.G., Saunders, G., *Clinical and Laboratory Evaluation of Patients Exposed to Neurotoxins.* Clin. Lab. Med. 1990; 10:387-402.

Center for Disease Control (CDC), *Preventing Lead Poisoning in Young Children.* Atlanta, GA: U.S. Department of Health and Human Resources, 1985; CDC 99:2230.

Daum, S., et al., *A Simple Technique of Fat Biopsy of PBB-Exposed Individuals.* Environ. Health Perspectives 1978; 23:183-185.

Ellis, K.J., *In Vivo Monitoring Techniques.* In: T.J. Kneip, J.V. Crable (eds.), Methods for Biological Monitoring. Washington, D.C.: American Public Health Association, 1988: 65-80.

Environmental Protection Agency, *Air Quality Criteria for Lead.* Washington, D.C.: U.S. Environmental Protection Agency, EPA 600/8-77-107, 1977.

Frank, H., Duerk, H., *Determination of Alkanes in Breath to Monitor Lipid Peroxidation in the Presence of Volatile Toxicants and Metabolites.* Arch. Toxicol. 1983; 53:213-223.

Gochfeld, M., *Chemical Agents.* In: Brooks, et al., Environmental Medicine. St. Louis: Mosby-Year Books, 1995; 53:608.

Graef, J.W., *Clinical Aspects of Lead Poisoning.* In: P.G. Vinken, C.W. Bruyn (eds.), Handbook of Clinical Neurology. Amsterdam: North Holland Publishing Co., 1979: 1-11.

Hill, R.H. Jr., Guikkemin, Droz, PO, *Sample Collection.* In: T.J. Kneip, J.V. Crable (eds.), Methods for Biological Monitoring. Washington, D.C.: American Public Health Association, 1988: 37-63.

Hill, R.H. Jr., M*easurement of Levels of Hazardous Agents.* In: T.J. Kneip, J.V. Crable (eds.), Methods for Biological Monitoring. Washington, D.C.: American Public Health Association, 1988: v-xii.

Hirsh, J., et al., *Studies of Adipose Tissue in Man.* Am. J. Clin. Nutr. 1960; 8:499.

Manolis, A., *The Diagnostic Potential of Breath Analysis.* Clin. Chem. 1983; 29:5-15.

Nackowski, S.B., *Cadmium in Blood.* In: T.J. Kneip, J.V. Crable (eds.), Methods for Biological Monitoring. Washington, D.C.: American Public Health Association, 1988: 161-164.

New York Poison Control Center, et al., *An Intensive Review Course in Clinical Toxicology.* Course Materials 1998; 249-254.

Piomelli, S., Davidow, B., *The FEP (free erythrocyte porphyrin) Concentration: a Promising Screening Test for Lead Poisoning.* Pediatr. Res. 1972; 6:366.

Piomelli, S., Rosen, J.F., Chisolm, J.J., et al., J. Pediatr. 1984. 105:523-532.

Robbins, D.A., *Measurements of Levels of Hazardous Agents.* In: T.J. Kneip, J.V. Crable (eds.), Methods for Biological Monitoring. Washington, D.C.: American Public Health Association, 1988: i-xii.

Smith, R.G., *The Effects of Exposure to Mercury in the Manufacture of Chlorine.* Am. Ind. Hyg. Assoc. Lett. 1970; 31:687.

Wells, J., Kowes, E., *Detection of Carbon Disulphide (A Disulfiram Metabolite) in Expired Air by Gas Chromatography.* J. Chromatogr. 1974; 92:442-444.

World Health Organization (WHO), *Conference on Intoxication Due to Alkyl-Mercury Treated Seed.* Bull. World. Hlth. Org. 1976; 53(Supp.).

Chapter 5

PSYCHOMETRICS; NEUROPSYCHOLOGICAL ASSESSMENT

First, do no harm.

—Hippocrates (c. 460-377 BCE), *Epidemis*, Book I, chapter 11.

§ 5-1. In General.

Damage to the central nervous system from disease, trauma, or exposure to toxic substances often induces cognitive, motor sensory, or behavioral impairments that can be detected with appropriate neuropsychological tests. In many instances, the results of these tests suggest specific pathologies that can be confirmed with other diagnostic evaluations such as x-ray, computerized tomography (CT) or magnetic resonance imaging (MRI). Neuropsychological testing has been shown to be particularly useful for the diagnosis of dementia.

The term "dementia" is frequently used to describe the effects of brain damage in which acquired cognitive impairments produces dysfunction in thinking, communicating, or in occupational settings and in social functioning. "Psychoorganic syndrome" or "organic brain syndrome" are other terms so used. A difficulty with dementia and other such descriptive terms is the lack of a clear definition. The fourth edition of the *Diagnostic and Standard Manual of Mental Disord*ers (DSM-IV) lists diagnostic criteria for different kinds of dementia based on etiology. According to DSM-IV, all are characterized by "the development of multiple cognitive defects (including memory impairment) that are due to the direct physiological effects of a general medical condition, to the persisting effects of a substance, or to multiple etiologies" (APA, 1994). Another widely accepted definition was put forth by Lishman in 1978: "An acquired global impairment of intellect, memory and personality, but without impairment of consciousness.... The syndrome consists of a constellation of symptoms, which suggests chronic and widespread brain dysfunction." Dementia is generally considered to be a manifestation of diffuse cerebral damage.

Neuropsychology deals with the cognitive, emotional, and behavioral expressions of brain function and dysfunction. Neuropsychological testing assesses changes in intellect, personality, or behavioral relationships using standardized tests. Neuropsychological testing often complements the clinical neurological examination, which tends to be most useful for evaluating some motor and sensory processes, but may be less useful in evaluating higher cortical functioning. The evaluation of higher cortical functioning, however, is the basis of neuropsychological testing. It is also useful for limited evaluations of motor-sensory processes (Lynch, 1983).

Early in its history, neuropsychological testing was used in hospital and clinical settings and in research laboratories to evaluate patients with known brain disorders, such as epilepsy, stroke, trauma, tumor, toxic exposure, and other disorders. Initial research correlated the results of psychological testing with clinical findings obtained from radiologic and surgical diagnoses in order to gain better understanding of brain functioning. Neuropsychological testing was found to have predictive value which allowed comparisons to be made in patients with the same kind of lesions. It also provided a noninvasive means for follow-up of patients. Patients who are to undergo surgical removal of a brain lesion such as a tumor or epileptic foci would be studied before and after the procedure. The results of the neuropsychological tests would be studied, compared, and analyzed with regard to the known neuroanatomy and neuropathology.

In recent years, neuropsychological testing has moved from the hospital to the psychologist's office where it is used to "diagnose" abnormalities in patients who have had normal neurophysiologic and other medical diagnostic test results. Neuropsychological testing is now used widely as a primary diagnostic method, particularly for patients who have had normal or negative results from other neurologic and neurodiagnostic tests. There has thus been a complete overturn of the original goals. The point of view of the neuropsychologist has become that of the diagnostician, rather than that of the researcher working to confirm the existence of lesions diagnosed by other methods.

While psychological tests can provide useful information, they do have limitations. Batteries of tests are sensitive, but tend to lack specificity as to what the results actually mean. Tests must be done properly, in appropriate surroundings and circumstances. The neuropsychologist needs to consider the effects of a patient's medications, level of alertness, and motivation. Patients should be free of all medications (if medically not contraindicated), fully alert, and highly motivated to do the tests. Interpretation of the results must be done by qualified practitioners.

The interpretation of what the results actually mean can become a point of controversy. The basic assumption in psychological testing has always been that patients were motivated to do as well as they could on the test; they wanted to be helped and were willing to participate in research not only to help themselves, but also to contribute to the expansion of scientific knowledge that could help others as well. Today, however, many people undergoing neuropsychological testing are involved in litigation. They may have a personal stake in displaying their injuries as they understand them or as they believe and want them to be. They may believe that poor test results will help convince attorneys, judges, and juries that their injuries are real. It is important, however, to underscore that malingering, dissimulation, symptom magnification and faking on testing are seen in only a small minority of patients.

Brain damage from any cause, be it trauma, toxic exposure, metabolic disease, or tumor, can be manifested as deficits of intellect, emotion, cognition, and behavior. Neuropsychological tests focus on the identification and measurement of these psychological deficits. Any psychological function can be affected by brain damage, and each may be affected in varying degrees depending on the circumstances.

Neuropsychological tests have been used to assess the long-term and short-term effects of neurotoxins such as organic solvents on behavior. Reaction time, vigilance, and other measures of psychomotor function were found to be adversely affected. Exposed workers have also shown increased fatigue and mood changes (Cherry, 1983). Painters with more than ten years' exposure were found to do poorly on memory tests (Baker, 1988). A study of printers with long-term exposure to toluene demonstrated high incidences of fatigue and memory deficits (Larsen, 1988). The organic solvent styrene, widely used in the plastics industry, has also been associated with impaired performances on neuropsychological tests.

§ 5-2. History.

In the 1870s, in the course of treating soldiers wounded in the Franco-Prussian War, Paul Broca discovered that an area of the anterior left cerebral cortex is important to the production of speech. Some ten years later, Carl Wernicke described an area in the posterior left hemisphere that is important for comprehension of speech (Becker, 1986). These pivotal discoveries led to further research and to the realization that many localized areas of the brain are involved in discrete behavioral functions. Because of these discoveries, early rehabilitation programs based on neuropsychological research were developed. In the late 1930s and early 1940s, K. Goldstein began neuropsychological rehabilitation of brain-damaged World War I soldiers. In the 1950s, Wepman worked with aphasic soldiers who had sustained brain-damaging wounds in World War II. At this time, Halstead established the first neuropsychology laboratory at the University of Chicago. Reitan, a student of Halstead, built on Halstead's concepts of objective and quantitative measures of correlating behavioral deficits with evidence of neurologic pathology. Reitan applied Halstead's laboratory methods to clinical practice and devised a battery of assessment tests that, with modifications, is still used today.

§ 5-3. The Role of Psychological Testing.

Neuropsychological tests are used to describe and predict behavior, and to modify or control it. They measure the nature and extent of behavioral impairment, and the results are used as diagnostic aids and to document the course of the disorder and the effects of treatment. The tests are useful in differentiating between psychiatric and neurologic disorders and may also help to validate a patients' complaints. Patients exposed to neurotoxic substances often experience behavioral changes. Psychological test results can help the patient to understand and to deal with the anxiety and confusion surrounding the behavioral changes.

Neuropsychological assessments are often used in legal proceedings in which monetary compensation is sought for claims of injury and loss of function. In these cases, results of neuropsychological and other tests are used to determine the extent of physical and behavioral impairment, the potential for rehabilitation, and the need for future care (Lezak, 1981).

More than 200 psychological tests and assessment techniques are currently available. The selection of test must be based on an individual's needs and limitations. Some tests, such as the Wechsler Adult Intelligence Scale (WAIS-III), are quite popular and constitute the foundation of the most widely used test batteries. Others are more specific and fit specialized needs. The examination procedures — usually consisting of assessment interviews, scaled tests, and questionnaires — provide relatively precise and sensitive indices of behavior. (See Tables 5.1, 5.2, 5.3, 5.4)

Table 5.1
Selected Intellectual Ability Tests

Wechsler Adult Intelligence Scale (WAIS-III)
Wechsler Intelligence Scale for Children (WISC-R)
Wechsler Intelligence Scale for Children — Revised (WISC-R)
Wechsler Preschool and Primary Scale of Intelligence — Revised
The Stanford-Binet Intelligence Scale
The Peabody Individual Achievement Test (PIAT-R)
The Wide Range Achievement Test (WRAT)
The Wide Range Achievement Test — Revised (WRAT-III)
The Pictorial Test of Intelligence (PTI)
The Leiter International Performance Scale
Army General Classification Test (AGCT)

Army Classification Battery (ACB)
Differential Aptitude Tests (DAT)
General Aptitude Test Battery (GATB)
Peabody Picture Vocabulary Test (PPVT-R)
The Full Range Picture Vocabulary Test (FRPV)
The Quick Test
Raven's Progressive Matrices (RPM)
Detroit Tests of Learning Aptitude-2 (DTLA-2)
Paced Auditory Serial Addition Test

Table 5.2
Memory Tests

Wechsler Memory Scale — (WMS-III)
Memory Assessment Scale
Rey Auditory Verbal Learning Test

Table 5.3
Verbal Function Tests

The Porch Test of Communicative Ability (PTCA)
The Minnesota Test for Differential Diagnosis of Aphasia
Neurosensory Center Comprehensive Examination for Aphasia
The Language Modalities Test for Aphasia
Aphasia Screening Test by Halstead and Wepman
The Revised Token Test

Word Naming (Stanford-Binet)
Controlled Word Association Test
Controlled Word Fluency
Speed of Writing
Gates-McGinty Reading Diagnostic Tests
Gray Oral Reading Tests — III

Table 5.4
Sensory Function Tests

Visual

The Hooper Visual Organization Test (VOT)
The Minnesota Paper Form Board Test
Visual-Aural Digit Span Test (VADS)
Perceptual Maze Test
Field of Search
Counting Spots
Visual Tracking Tests
Talland's Line Tracing Task

Auditory

The Seashore Rhythm Test
Speech Sounds Perception Test

---

§ 5-4. Neuropsychological Referrals.

A neurotoxicologist may refer patients for psychological testing on the basis of clinical findings, or patients receiving therapy from a psychologist may be referred to a neurotoxicologist on the basis of psychological test findings.

The neuropsychologist should be a professional trained in neuroanatomy, physiology, and clinical neurology, in addition to the basis of psychological curriculum. Standards for the training and qualification of neuropsychologists have been adopted by the American Board of Clinical Neuropsychology, under the aegis of the American Board of Professional Psychology and the sponsorship of the American Psychological Association. Basic for acceptance as a diplomate is a requirement of five years' postdoctoral experience in neuropsychology, the submission of extensive work samples, and the satisfactory completion of oral and written examinations.

§ 5-5. Advantages of Neuropsychological Testing.

The major advantage of neuropsychological testing over most other neurodiagnostic procedures is that the patient does not experience pain and discomfort, and there is no risk of morbidity or mortality during testing. Neuropsychological testing has other advantages as well: it is less expensive than the technologically advanced neurologic tests used today, and the neuropsychological tests are interesting to most patients. While neuropsychological tests do not replace neurologic evaluation, they do provide descriptive and prognostic information that other techniques cannot, such as the effects of brain dysfunction on the patient's intellectual, social, or vocational adjustment (Becker, 1986).

§ 5-6. Assessing Behavior.

Behavior can be divided into three categories: intellect, emotionality, and control. Intellect deals with how information is processed, emotionality with motivation and feelings, and control involves how specific behavior is expressed. Behavior is the interaction of each of these behavior categories. If toxic exposure disturbs an area of the brain that is involved with intellect, for example, the behavior expressed will encompass intellect, emotionality, and control.

§ 5-6(a). Intellectual Functioning.

Intellectual functioning is perhaps the most important element in a psychological assessment. Intellectual impairment is often seen in cases of both acute and chronic exposure to neurotoxins. Intellectual impairment in children associated with exposure to lead is one of the most extensively studied neuropsychologic disorders. However, specific brain lesions may not reflect an adverse effect on intellectual function. There is no evidence that a general intellectual function is served by any one part of the brain.

Intellectual functioning can be divided further into several functions: receptive, cognitive, memory, learning, and expressive functions. All these functions are interdependent, and the behavior measured by testing them is directly referable to specific intellectual functions. Testing of intellectual function is an evaluation of the patient's ability to perform many different intellectual tasks at about the same level of proficiency recognized before the brain injury.

Receptive Functions: Receptive functions involve the ability to acquire, process, classify and integrate information. The major receptive function is sensation, which includes visual, tactile, auditory, and olfactory perception. Chronic exposure to solvents has been associated with impaired visual function (Härkönen, 1978; Mergler, 1987; Mergler, 1991; Mergler, Bowler, 1991), and vestibular problems (Morrow, 1988).

Cognitive Functions: The primary cognitive function is essentially the ability to think, to mentally organize and reorganize information. Thinking involves computation, reasoning, judgment, formation of concepts, abstraction, generalization, organization and planning. Reasoning, abstraction, judgment, analysis and synthesis are categorized as higher intellectual functions. These functions are generally more susceptible to diffuse brain injury, while most specific receptive, expressive or memory functions remain essentially intact (Lezak, 1981). Thinking is a function of the entire brain; no localized area is responsible for control of cognitive functions. Specific cognitive defects have been found in association with acute exposure to solvents, particularly toluene abuse (glue and paint sniffing) (Tsushima, 1977). Chronic exposure has been associated with a variety of cognitive defects assessed with neuropsychological testing. Among these were deficits in forward and reversed digit span. These are measures of short term memory. Other deficits are in different aspects of memory and slowness in responding to stimuli (Anger, 1990; Anger, 1992; Morrow, 1992; Bowler, 1991; Bowler, 1992).

Memory and Learning Functions: The memory and learning functions are the ability to store and to recall information. Memory deficits can be short-term or long-term. They can be mild, moderate or severe. Mild to moderately impaired memory can have a disorienting effect. Memory deficits have been observed in association with toxic exposure.

Expressive Functions: Expressive functions comprise the ability to communicate information or to take actions based on information. Examples of expressive communication include speaking, drawing, writing, gestures, and facial expressions. Apraxia is the medical term for deficits in expressive function.

§ 5-6(b). Emotionality.

Emotional and personality changes have been associated with acute and chronic toxic exposure. The changes may include dulling or emotional flaccidity, inhibition or diminution of anxiety with associated emotional blandness, mild depressed moods, and hypersensitivity in social interactions. These changes may be expressed as depression, anxiety, irritability, restlessness, low frustration tolerance, and apathy. Exposure to solvents has been associated with depression, anxiety, and social withdrawal. These reactions have been known to persist for as long as two years after exposure (Bowler, 1989; Bowler, 1991; Linz, 1986).

Personality changes can develop as a direct result of toxic exposure. They may also arise through a patient's frustration at not being able to carry out certain tasks as well as he or she could before the exposure.

§ 5-6(c). Control.

Control is the ability to stop or alter the rate of an action, to inhibit or display excitement, and to modify or regulate activities. Brain damage can almost always be associated with some aspect of control, and some behavioral control abnormalities suggest damage in specific areas of the brain. Symptoms of impaired control include a heightened tendency to excitability, impulsive acts, erratic carelessness, rigidity and difficulty in ongoing behavior, shifting attention, and decreased tolerance for alcohol (Lezak, 1995).

§ 5-6(d). Measuring Intellectual and Emotional and Control Abilities.

Measuring intellectual abilities is easier than measuring emotional or control functions. Numerous reliable and well-standardized tests are available for identifying, defining, grading, measuring, and comparing intellectual abilities. Results of tests for assessing personality are generally descriptive rather than specific, calculated measurements. Control deficits are usually assessed in terms of their effects on specific intellectual functions or personality characteristics, rather than by direct measurement of the deficits themselves.

Psychological measurement can be difficult. There is no standard baseline that can be applied to an individual. Instead, comparative norms that can be applied to populations are used. Patient histories and family interviews provide additional sources of comparative information. The finding of defensible and meaningful standards of comparison is the responsibility of the examiner. If a series of neuropsychological assessments are needed, individual comparison standards can be used to measure change.

§ 5-7. Basic Assumptions in Interpretation of Neuropsychological Testing Results.

Several basic assumptions are extensively applied in neuropsychological testing. First, it is assumed that a normal individual's intellectual performance level remains constant across a battery of intellectual test measurements. Thus, if a patient has higher than average reading ability, that individual's language ability will also be higher than average. Significant differences in a patient's skills from those which existed before the testing are evidence of brain injury in the absence of other developmental, cultural, or emotional contributions.

A second assumption is that intellectual performance is governed by an individual's biological capacity. If a person is not endowed with a high level of intellect, they will not achieve beyond their biological limitations no matter how hard they try.

Third, no one functions at maximum endowed potential. Environmental and cultural factors do have an effect on intellectual abilities. Thus the ability to perform a task is indicative of the performance level for that task only.

Finally, it is assumed that the patient's levels of functioning before the exposure can be estimated from historical facts and behavioral observations. Thus, there is a need for in-depth interviews of patients and their relatives, as well as a review of prior medical records, behavior, and performance.

These assumptions form the foundation for the interpretation of neuropsychological tests. In essence, the examiner collects historical information, develops a standard of comparison based on norms, administers a thorough battery of tests to measure current levels, compares those with the standard, notes discrepancies, analyzes the discrepancies for statistical significance, and interprets and reports the findings.

Many tests must be used to provide a comprehensive picture of the patient's behavior. In the interpretation of the tests, the neuropsychologist looks for patterns of deficits which can be compared to patterns known to be associated with a class of neurotoxin. It is usually not possible to identify a specific neurotoxin from the results of neuropsychological tests alone.

Neuropsychological testing following exposure to neurotoxic substances has objectives that differ somewhat from those of testing following trauma, degenerative diseases, or metabolic disorders. It most instances, it is known, for example, that a head injury has indeed occurred, and the testing is done to determine the effects of the injury. In many instances of reported toxic exposure, however, the testing is done to secure evidence that the exposure actually occurred, and, if there was indeed exposure, to determine whether the level of exposure was sufficient to be considered a possible cause of deficits in testing performance.

§ 5-8. The Neuropsychological Examination.

A comprehensive neuropsychological examination should cover the major areas of cognitive function: intelligence, attention, memory, concentration, language, problem-solving, abstract thinking, achievement in basic reading, spelling and calculating skills, sensation and perception, motor abilities, vigilance, mental stamina, and personality (Becker, 1986).

Each patient is different and each will require a personalized series of tests. A flexible and imaginative approach, therefore, is required in the preparation of the neuropsychological examination. Patients with sensory or motor handicaps, for example, will require special tests for evaluation in these areas; a blind person will need to be evaluated with verbally administered test methods.

Neuropsychological examinations are time-consuming. They may take from eight to twelve hours to complete, and more than one session may be necessary. Patience is required of both the examiner and the patient if accurate results are to be obtained. Care must be taken to prevent patient fatigue, which could cause poor results.

There are problems with neuropsychological testing. More than 200 tests are in frequent use today and there are no national standards for many of them. Many tests in use today are outdated. Cultural and environmental biases must be taken into account to obtain reliable results. Test-taking skills differ from one individual to another, and there may also be differences in the qualifications of neuropsychologists. Most are well trained, but many who administer tests have no background in neuroanatomy, neuropsychology, neurochemistry, or neuropathology.

Although changes in brain morphology, neurochemistry, structure and organization after neurotoxic damage (as in most mild to moderate closed head injuries) cannot be visualized with neurodiagnostic testing such as x-ray, CAT, and MRI, neuropsychological testing can be quite useful in the overall diagnosis, evaluation, and treatment of the injury (Bernad, 1994).

§ 5-9. Tests for Intellectual Ability.

The Wechsler Adult Intelligence Scale — Revised (WAIS-III) is one of the more frequently used neuropsychological tests of intelligence. The scale is a composite of many tests in recognition of the fact that intellect is made up of many skill components. The battery is composed of eleven test subsets: verbal, comprehension, arithmetic, similarities, digit span, vocabulary, digit symbol, picture completion, block design, picture arrangement and object assembly.

Numerical scores are used to grade each WAIS-III subject, the sum of which produces an IQ score. The IQ scores are averaged estimates of intellectual performance representing many different kinds of functions. So, the overall estimates of general, verbal and nonverbal skills may not pinpoint specific neuropsychological disorders.

The WAIS-III test is usually administered along with paper and pencil tests of basic communication, arithmetic and special skills, and individually administered tests involving mental tracking, recent memory, and learning. A limitation of the Wechsler scales is that scores may not show specific memory deficits or frontal lobe dysfunction.

Deficits in orientation and attention often accompany some form of neurotoxic damage. With an emphasis on academic skills that primarily test verbal conceptual functions, it is particularly useful for patients with left hemisphere damage (Heaton, 1987). No complex motor responses are required of the patient, making the test useful for patients with physical handicaps.

The Paced Auditory Serial Addition Test (PASAT) measures the ability of the patient to add pairs of randomized digits. For example, if the examiner presents the digits 3-1-7-4-8, the correct response would be 4-8-11-12. The digits are presented at different rates of speed by means of a taped presentation. Results are assessed in terms of the percentage of correct responses. Patients who have suffered a concussion perform below the established norm for this test (Stuss, 1989). Performance returns to normal for most patients from 30 to 60 days postconcussion. Some patients, however, never regain their previous level of performance (Leininger, 1990). The PASAT has been reported to be quite sensitive to deficits in information processing ability (Gronwall, 1981). A problem with the test is that many patients find it to be stressful, feel pressured to "pass," and have a feeling of failure even when they are doing well. Warning the patient about these possible pitfalls before administering the test can be helpful. Suspected neurotoxic insult may be evaluated with PASAT.

The Stroop Test has been in use since the end of the nineteenth century and is still quite popular. It is primarily a test of concentration. The test involves identifying the colors of patches and the colors of printed names of colors. It is known that it takes longer to read printed names of colors when the ink color is not the same as the color designated by the name. According to one investigator, the test requires the selective processing of "only one visual feature while continuously blocking out the processing of others" (Shum, 1990). The difference between the word and the color is a distracter when combined with the different color that has a less habituated response (Lezak, 1995).

§ 5-10. Standardized Test Batteries.

Several popular and well-known standardized test batteries are used frequently as the basis of the neuropsychological examination. The three most commonly used batteries are the Halstead-Reitan Battery (see Table 5.5), Luria's Neuropsychological Investigation, and the Luria-Nebraska Neuropsychological Battery. The Michigan Neuropsychology Test Battery is also popular. These test batteries are designed so that they may be modified to meet individual evaluation requirements and to suit the particular circumstances of the patient.

Table 5.5
Halstead-Reitan Battery (Adults 15 and Older)

Test Name	Brief Description	What the Test Measures
Halstead's Tests		
Category Test	208 slides divided into 7 subsets are presented on a rear-projection screen. Patient must discern a consistent organizing principle or concept for subtest in trial-and-error fashion, with immediate feedback provided by a bell (correct) or buzzer (incorrect). Score is given as the number of errors.	Attention, concentration, visual problem solving, ability to generate and test hypotheses, abstract reasoning, ability to attend to and make constructive use of feedback, ability to generalize from familiar to new-but-similar situations.
Tactual Performance Test	A modified Sequin-Goddard form board is employed. Patient is blindfolded; empty board and loose blocks are placed before patient. Patient must replace as many blocks as possible with a time limit	Motor problem solving, stamina, transfer of training from one trial to the next, tactile-motor-spatial integration, spatial and tactile memories, incidental learning.

Test Name	Brief Description	What the Test Measures
	(10-15 min.) Dominant, nondominant, and both-handed trials are obtained consecutively. After board and blocks are hidden, blindfold is removed and patient must draw a picture of the board, correctly depicting as many of the shapes as possible in their proper relative locations. Score is given as total time, blocks correctly recalled (memory), and blocks correctly located (localization).	
Rhythm Test	Presented on audio tape, the test items consist of 30 pairs of monotonic rhythmic patterns. Patient must indicate "same" or "different" for each pair (15 are same; 15 are different). Score is again given as either a scaled score (1-10) or as number of errors.	Attention, concentration, nonverbal auditory discrimination, nonverbal memory.
Seashore Perception Test	Presented on audio tape are 60 nonsense words in sets of 10; patient must underline on an answer sheet the correct choice among four alternatives for each item. Score given as number of errors.	Attention and concentration, verbal auditory discrimination, visual discrimination, high-frequency sound perception.
Finger Tapping Test	Using a mechanical counter affixed to a 9 × 9.5 inch board, patient taps as rapidly as possible with index finder for 10 seconds. Preferred and nonpreferred hands are used	Motor speed (although there is a small visual proprioceptive component). The ability to establish and sustain a regular rhythm of tapping is required, and

Test Name	Brief Description	What the Test Measures
	alternately until five trials are obtained which vary by less than five taps from one another. Score is given as the mean number of taps for five trials with the preferred hand. (Although not contributing to the Impairment Index, the nonpreferred hand's performance is recorded for comparison).	therefore basal ganglia or cerebellar dysfunction may impair performance.
Additional Measures:		
Grip Strength	Using a hand dynamometer calibrated in kilograms, the relative strength of each hand grip is measured (two trials per hand). Score is given as the mean number of kilograms, across two trials, with each hand.	Strength of the upper extremities.
Trail Making Tests	Using a pen or pencil, patient must rapidly draw a line sequentially connecting 25 circles scattered on an 8½ × 11-inch sheet of paper. On Part A, the circles contain both numbers (1-13) and letters (A-L). On Part B, the patient connects the circles in a number-letter-number-letter sequence. Score is given as the number of seconds required to complete each part. Errors (incorrect sequences) are also recorded.	Visual-motor speed, scanning and searching, ability to deal with numeric and linquistic symbols, ability to execute a sequential sensory-motor activity, ability to maintain and alternate smoothly between parallel mental sets.

Test Name	Brief Description	What the Test Measures
Aphasia Screening Test	32 items, dealing with aspects of language, constructional skill, articulation, and right-left orientation are presented either verbally or by means of a booklet of small stimuli cards. Scoring of a plus-minus or pass-fail variety. No total score is used, although some researchers have attached weight to the items.	Communicative abilities (naming, reading, writing, spelling), auditory comprehension, calculating, drawing ability, recognition of body parts, clarity of speech, ability to imagine and carry out a motor set.
Sensory Perceptual Examination	Basic tactile, auditory, and visual signal detection are evaluated. Bilateral simultaneous stimulation is also carried out in each modality. Finger localization, number writing perception, and tactile object recognition are evaluated. Visual fields are approximated by confrontation.	Cortical sensory functions. The presence of sensory "neglect" (suppression or inattention) is measured, along with the ability to locate one's fingers, graphesthesia, stereognosis, and integrity of visual fields.

Permission to reprint granted by F.A. Davis Co., Philadelphia, PA.

The Halstead-Reitan Battery (HRB) (Reitan, 1993) is possibly the most widely used battery for neuropsychological assessment. The earliest version was a battery of seven tests intended to differentiate between patients with lesions on the frontal lobes of the brain and those with other lesions or no lesions. Administration time varies from six to eight hours, depending on how much of the test is used. The part of the battery developed by Halstead includes: 1. Category Test; 2. Tactual Performance test; 3. Rhythm Test; 4. Speech Sounds Perception Test; and 5. Finger Oscillation Test (also called Finger Tapping Test). Seven scores are obtained from these five tests. The Tactual Performance Test yields:

- Remembering the shapes of blocks;
- Remembering the location of blocks;
- Total time to accurately place blocks in corresponding spaces.

A single score is obtained from each of the remaining tests. An Impairment Index is derived from the number of test scores in the range established as indicating an impairment (Lezak, 1995).

Tests recommended for inclusion in the battery by Reitan include Grip Strength, Trail-Making Test, Aphasia Screening Test, and Sensory Perceptual Examination, and the MMPI-II.

The Halstead-Reitan Battery has been studied extensively, and has had its share of critics. The original norms of the battery were based on a small sample, consisting of only twenty-eight individuals, only eight of whom were women (Boll, 1981; Halstead, 1947). Ten were servicemen with psychiatric problems, including three who were scheduled for lobotomies because of behavior dangerous to themselves and others. Another criticism is that the norms were based on a young population. Scores have been noted to fall off with age (Heaton, 1986; Cullum, 1989). However, age-graded norms have been developed. These are available in *Comprehensive Norms for an Expanded Halstead-Reitan Battery* (Heaton, 1991). These norms control for both age and gender.

The Halstead-Reitan Battery is not suitable for patients with sensory or motor handicaps. Although it has limitations, it is a study which yields ever increasing means for assessing neuropsychological functioning.

Luria's Neuropsychological Investigation has ten subsets: preliminary conversation, motor functions, acousticomotor organization, higher cutaneous and kinesthetic functions, higher visual functions, impressive speech, expressive speech, writing and reading, arithmetic skill, and memory and intellectual processes.

The Luria-Nebraska Neuropsychological Battery consists of 269 items organized into fourteen scales: motor functions, rhythm or acousticomotor organization, tactile or higher cutaneous and kinesthetic functions, visual functions, receptive (impressive) speech, expressive speech, writing, reading skills, arithmetic skills, memory, intellectual processes, pathognomonic, right hemisphere, and left hemisphere.

A battery may include more items than are required for a particular patient, and at other times there may be an insufficient number of items to meet the requirements of a particular case. Screening tests can be used for patients who do not require a full battery of tests. However, complete documentation is usually required in cases involving litigation. Also full assessments are more useful in follow-up comparisons. A frequently used screening test is the Bender Visual Motor Gestalt Test. In this test, the patient copies a number of simple designs to detect the presence of organic brain damage.

§ 5-10(a). Advantages and Limitations of Standardized Neuropsychological Test Batteries.

Standardized neuropsychological test batteries have a number of advantages and limitations:

Advantages:

1. Research findings extend the examiner's experience and understanding of the procedure's value and limitations;
2. There is an extended individual experience, particularly with feedback from interviewing, records, clinical experience, etc.; and
3. Local norms are developed because of larger numbers.

Limitations:

1. The tests are not designed for an outpatient population with primarily diffuse brain damage;
2. The tests do not assess adaptive functioning, and ignore personality, mood disorders, or the sense of self of the brain-damaged patient;
3. There is a lack of national norms;

4. The latest version or revision of standard procedures is not always used;
5. The tests are limited in the range of their exploration;
6. The tests rely on out-of-date or inappropriate theories; and
7. Individuals with particular demographic characteristics may require special documentation.

§ 5-11. Test Batteries for Assessing Effects of Neurotoxicity.

In recent years, several test batteries designed for assessing the neuropsychological effects of exposure to neurotoxins have been developed. The need for batteries of this kind has grown with increased regulation of occupational safety, concerns about environmental toxicity, and the related increased potential for litigation. Most are compilations of other tests, and they rely on the standardization data for those tests. These test batteries are similar in content in that they include at least one test of general mental ability, and most have at least one test of memory, abstract reasoning, attention, visuospatial skills, motor speed and coordination.

Agency for Toxic Substances and Disease Registry Battery (ATSDR) (Hutchinson, 1992): This battery is divided into four domains: cognitive, motor, sensory, and affect. It is designed to be used in the field, as well as in a doctor's office or laboratory, and is considered to be particularly appropriate for assessing the effects of airborne toxins. The cognitive domain consists of the Auditory Verbal Learning Test, Simple Reaction Time, Raven's Progressive Matrices, and computerized versions of the Serial Digit Learning Format, the Symbol-Digit Modalities Test, and Vocabulary. The motor domain includes the Hand Dynamometer, the Grooved Pegboard, and a computerized test for tapping speed. The sensory domain consists of tests of visual acuity, contrast sensitivity, and the Lanthony d15 Color Vision test, as well as tests for vibrotactile threshold. Affect is assessed with a computerized Mood Scale.

California Neuropsychological Screening Battery (Bowler, 1986): This battery includes fourteen tests of cognitive function and a Neurotoxic Anxiety Scale, which is a collection of anxiety items from the Minnesota Multiphasic Personality Inventory. These items deal with emotional distress and other symptoms frequently reported by persons exposed to neurotoxins. The evaluation is based on comparisons with matched control groups, using published test norms.

Individual Neuropsychological Testing for Neurotoxicity (Singer, 1990): This battery is designed for flexibility of use. It consists of the Wechsler Adult Intelligence Scale — (WAIS-III) and eight tests of specific cognitive functions, such as memory and attention. The use of Dot Counting and Memorization of fifteen items is recommended for detecting malingering. For a brief examination, using Digit Symbol and Vocabulary from the WAIS-III battery is suggested. Using both the Digit Symbol and Trail Making Tests is recommended for Group Administration. Two brief tests for the evaluation of emotional status are also included.

Neurobehavioral Test Battery (Baker, 1983): This battery was developed by administering a large number of tests to foundry workers who had been exposed to lead. Relationships were identified between the test results and visuomotor performance, mood, verbal intelligence/organizational ability, and memory. The tests which had the highest loadings for these factors and which took the least time to complete were kept in the battery of nine cognitive tests plus the Profile of Mood States. Qualified personnel can administer this battery in forty minutes.

Pittsburgh Occupational Exposure Test (POET) (Ryan, 1987): The Pittsburgh Occupational Exposure Test is a battery of tests intended to assess the effects of likely workplace exposures on worker's neuropsychological function. Normative data has been established for factory workers based on the results of these tests. While acute exposure can and does occur in the workplace, most exposure is chronic at so-called subclinical levels of exposure. Large epidemiological studies generally do not show statistically significant differences between controls and groups of workers with subclinical exposure. However, it is more than likely that individual workers in that cohort will have been adversely affected by the exposure. There is a need for a brief yet comprehensive battery of tests known to be sensitive to toxic exposure to provide accurate assessment of neurobehavioral deficits in exposed workers. POET is intended to meet this need.

The POET battery contains the following tests:

- Wechsler Intelligence Subtests;
- Verbal Associative Learning;
- Symbol-Digit Learning;
- Incidental Memory;
- Recurring words;
- Boston Embedded Figures;
- Mental Rotation;
- Trail Making; and
- Grooved Pegboard.

As is the case with many test batteries, the scores are affected by age and education. In the trials that were carried out to establish norms, the sample was divided into four age groups (Ryan, 1987). No association between test results and alcohol consumption was found.

§ 5-12. Differentiation Between Organic and Functional (Psychological) Impairments.

Patients who are referred to a neuropsychologist for analysis after trauma or toxic exposure may be suffering from concurrent emotional and personality impairments. The sometimes vague complaints associated with exposure to neurotoxins are often similar to those of neurosis, creating a diagnostic challenge. Confounding variables include depression, degenerative lesions, congenital lesions, head trauma, medications, and other neurologic diseases, such as multiple sclerosis. Lezak offered the following suggestions on how neuropsychological testing can be of help in differentiation:

> Functional impairment is suggested by signs of inappropriate, usually bland or indifferent reaction to the complaints, symbolic meaningfulness of the symptoms, secondary gains, perpetuation of a dependent or irresponsible lifestyle, a close association between stress and the appearance of the patient's problem, and an unlikely or inconsistently manifested pattern of psychological impairment, regardless of the patient's neurological status. (Lezak, 1995).

§ 5-12(a). Malingering.

Malingering is antisocial, adaptive behavior where the individual, under voluntary control, produces symptoms in an attempt to obtain compensation or avoid responsibility. The individual may malinger or feign deficits for many reasons, including financial obligations, avoidance of work, avoidance of military duty, or for social empathy. Persons may also feign deficits to gain special care from the family, additional attention from a physician, or a release from job responsibilities.

Malingering can be detected during neuropsychological testing via inconsistencies that do not make sense in terms of the patient's overall levels of functioning and history. Thorough neuropsychological examinations combined with neuropsychological testing a malingerer can be distinguished from truly impaired individuals. In-patient observation or videotaped surveillance may be required for detection in some cases.

Malingering may be encouraged by the compensation and retirement policies of some companies, which give the impression that it makes financial sense for the individual not to get well. In toxic tort, significant financial incentives may stimulate individuals to exaggerate their symptoms. Therefore, extreme care must be taken with interpretation of neuropsychological data. The number of patients who fake or exaggerate deficits on neuropsychological testing is not known, but malingering should be a consideration, particularly when incentives for the patient to resort to it exist through compensation litigation or competency disputes in criminal trials.

It is important to differentiate malingering from true organic disorder in conditions such as factitious illness, hysteria, other secondary gain, somatization disorder, dissimulation, and symptom magnification. Occasionally, behavior after neurotoxic exposure may appear to suggest a neurologic diagnosis of dementia. Upon more careful analysis, this condition is more likely to be pseudodementia (Gade, 1994).

§ 5-12(b). Deficit Faking.

Attempts have been made to quantitatively determine if a malingerer's neuropsychological test scores could be distinguished from those of nonmalingering patients. Heaton carried out a study of volunteer malingerers and diagnosed brain-damaged individuals (Heaton, 1978). The Minnesota Multiphasic Personality Inventory (MMPI-II) and other neuropsychological tests were used as assessment tools. MMPI-II scales and formulas have been developed for detecting conscious malingering and other test-taking attitudes that may affect MMPI-II profile validity or serve as moderator variables in profile interpretation.

Ten neuropsychologists attempted to determine whether the test scores were produced by a malingerer or a non-malingering brain-damaged patient. The success of the judges ranged from chance-level to prediction rates of about 20% better than chance. The results suggested that malingerers can show significant abnormalities on testing, but that the patterns of their strengths and deficits differ from those produced by genuinely injured patients However, patients who are coached in the faking of deficits may be more difficult to detect. The research data are instructive and suggest the need for further evaluation and investigation of organic and nonorganic lesions in neurotoxicologic brain and nerve damage.

References.

American Psychiatric Association. Diagnostic and Statistical Manual of Mental Disorders, 4th rev. ed. Washington, D.C.: 1994.

Anger, W.K., *Assessment of Neurotoxicity in Humans.* In: H. Tilson, C. Mitchell (eds.), Neurotoxicology. New York: Raven Press, 1992.

Anger, W.K., *Worksite Behavioral Research: Results, Sensitive Methods, Test Batteries and the Transition From Laboratory Data to Human Health.* Neurotoxicology. 1990; 1:629-720.

Baker, E.L., Feldman, R.G., White, R.F., et al., *Monitoring Neurotoxins in Industry: Development of a Neurobehavioral Test Battery.* J. Occup. Med. 1983; 25:125-130.

Baker, E.L., Letz, R.E., Eisen, B.A., et al., *Neurobehavioral Effects of Solvents in Painters.* J. Occup. Med. 1988; 30:116-123.

Becker, B., Kay, G.G., *Neuropsychological Consultation in Psychiatric Practice.* Psychiatr. Clin. N. Am. 1986; 9:255-265.

Bernad, P.G., Closed Head Injury: A Clinical Source Book. Charlottesville, VA: Michie, 1994.

Boll, T.J., *The Halstead-Reitan Neuropsychology Battery.* In: S.B. Filksov, T.J. Boll (eds.), Handbook of Clinical Neuropsychology. New York: Wiley-Interscience, 1981.

Bowler, R.M., Mergler, D., Rauch, S.S., Bowler, R.P., *Stability of Psychological Impairment: Two year Follow-up of Former Microelectronics Workers' Affective and Personality Disturbance.* Women & Health. 1992; 18:27-48.

Bowler, R.M., Mergler, D., Rauch, S.S., et al., *Affective and Personality Disturbances Among Female Former Microelectronics Workers.* J. Clin. Psychol. 1991; 47:41-52.

Bowler, R.M., Rauch, S.S., Becker, C.H., et al., *Three Patterns of MMPI Profiles Following Neurotoxin Exposure.* Am J. Forensic Pathol. 1989; 7:15-31.

Bowler, R.M., Sudia, S., Mergler, D., Harrison, R., *Comparison of Digit Symbol and Symbol Digit Modalities Tests for Assessing Neurotoxic Exposure.* Clinical Neuropsychologist. 1992a; 6(1):103-104.

Bowler, R.M., Thaler, C.D., Becker, C.E., *California Neuropsychological Screening Battery.* J. Clin. Psychol. 1986; 42:946-955.

Cherry, N., Rodgers, B., Venables, H., Walchron, H.A., Wells, G.G., *Acute Behavioral Effects of Styrene Exposure: A Further Analysis.* British Journal of Industrial Medicine. 1981; 38:346-350.

Cherry, N., Waldron, H.A. (Eds), *The Neuropsychological Effects of Solvent Exposure.* Havant, Hampshire: Colt Foundation.

Cullum, C.M., Thompson, L.L., Heaton, B.K., *The Use of the Halstead-Reitan test Battery with Older Adults.* In: F.J. Pirozzolo (ed.), Clinics in Geriatric Medicine, Vol. 5, No. 3. Philadelphia: W.B. Saunders, 1989.

Gade, A.E., Mortensen, L., Bruhn, P., *Chronic Painter's Syndrome: A Reanalysis of Psychological Test Data in a Group of Diagnosed Cases, Based on Comparisons with Matched Controls.* Acta. Neurol. Scand. 1988; 77:293-306.

Gade, A.E., Mortensen, L., Udesen, H., *The Pattern of Intellectual Impairment in Toxic Encephalopathy, or a Study of the Pattern, Degree, and Validity of Intellectual Impairment in Toxic Encephalopathy.* Presented at the International Conference on Organic Solvent Toxicity. October 15-17, 1984, Stockholm, Sweden.

Gronwall, D., Wrightson, P., *Memory and Information Processing Capacity After Closed Head Injury.* J. Neurology, Neurosurg. Psychiatry 1981; 44:889-895.

Halstead, W.C., Brain and Intelligence. Chicago: University of Chicago Press, 1947.

Härkönen, H., Lindström. K., Seppälänen, A.M., et al., *Exposure-Response Relationship Between Styrene Exposure and Central Nervous Functions.* Scand. J. Work Environ. Health 1978; 4:53-59.

Heaton, R.K., Grant, I., Matthews, C.G., *Comprehensive Norms for an Expanded Halstead-Reitan Battery: Demographic Corrections, Research Findings, and Clinical Applications.* Odessa, FL: Psychological Assessment Resources. 1991.

Heaton, R.K., Grant, I., Matthews, C.G., *Differences in Neuropsychological Test Performance Associated with Age and Sex.* In: I. Grant, K.M. Adams, Neuropsychological Assessment of Neuropsychiatric Disorders. New York: Oxford University Press, 1986.

Heaton, R.K., Schmitz, S.P., Avitable, N., et al., *Effects of Lateralized Cerebral Lesions on Oral Reading, Reading Comprehension, and Spelling*. J. Clin. Experiment. Neuropsych. 1987; 9:711-721.

Heaton, R.K., Smith, H.H., Lehman, R.A.W., et al., *Prospects for Faking Believable Deficits on Neuropsychological Testing.* J. Consult. Clin. Psych. 1978; 46:137-140.

Hutchinson, L.J., Amker, R.W., Lybarger, J.A., Chappell, W., *Neurobehavioral Test Batteries for Use in Environmental Health Field Studies.* Atlanta, Agency for Toxic Substances and Disease Registry, Public Health Service, 1992.

Leininger,B.E., Grambling, S.E., Farrell, A.D., *Neuropsychological Deficits in Symptomatic Minor Head Injury Patients After Concussion and Mild Concussion.* J. Neurology Neurosurg. Psychiatry 1990; 53:293-296.

Lezak, M.D., Neuropsychological Assessment, 3d Ed. New York: Oxford University Press, 1995.

Linz, D.H., deGarmo, P.L., Morton, W.E., et al., *Organic Solvent-Induced Encephalopathy in Industrial Patients.* J. Occup. Med. 1986; 28:119-125.

Lishman, W.A., Organic Psychiatry. The Psychologic Consequences of Cerebral Disorder. Oxford: Blackwell Scientific, 1978.

Lynch, W.J., *Neuropsychologic Assessment.* In: M. Rosenthal, E.R. Griffith,. J.D. Miller, Rehabilitation of the Head-Injured Adult. Philadelphia: F.A. Davis Co., 1983.

Mergler, D., Blain, L., *Assessing Color Vision Loss Among Solvent-Exposed Workers.* Am. J. Indust. Med. 1987; 12:195-203.

Mergler, D., Frenette, B., Legault-Belanger, S., et al., *Relationship Between Subjective Symptoms of Visual Dysfunction and Measurements of Vision in a Population of Former Microelectronics Workers.* J. Occup. Med. 1991; 3:75-82.

Mergler, D., Huel, G., Bowler, R. et al. *Visual Dysfunction Among Former Electronics Workers*. Arch. Environ. Health 1991; 46:326-334.

Morrow, L.A., Furman, M.R., Ryan, C.M., et al., *Neuropsychological Deficits Associated with Vestibular Abnormalities in Solvent Exposed Workers*. Clin Neuropsychologist 1988; 2:272-273 (abs).

Morrow, L.A., Kamis, H., Hodgson, M.J., *Psychiatric Symptomatology in Persons with Organic Solvent Exposure*. Journal of Consulting and Clinical Psychology 1993; 61:261-269.

Morrow, L.A., Robin, N., Hodgson, M.A., Kamis, H., *Assessment of Attention and Memory Efficiency in Persons with Solvent Neurotoxicity*. Neuropsychologica. 1992; 30:911-922.

Morrow, L.A., Ryan, C.M., Goldstein, G., Hodgson, M.J., *A Distinct Pattern of Personality Disturbance Following Exposure to Mixtures of Organic Solvents*. J. Occup. Med. 1989; 31:743-746.

Morrow, L.A., Ryan, C.M., Hodgson, J.J., Robin, N., *Risk Factors Associated with Persistence of Neuropsychological Deficits in Persons with Organic Solvent Exposure*. J. of Nerv. Ment. Dis. 1991; 179:540-545.

Morrow, L.A., Steinhauer, S.R., Hodgson, M.J., *Delay in P300 Latency in Patients with Organic Solvent Exposure*. Archives of Neurology 1992a; 49:315-320.

Reitan, R.M., Wolfson, D., The Halstead-Reitan Neuropsychological Test Battery: Theory and Clinical Interpretation. Tucson, AZ: Neuropsychology Press, 1993.

Ryan, C.M., Morrow, L., Parkinson, D., Branet, E., *Low-level Lead Exposure and Neurobehavioral Dysfunction Associated with Occupational Exposure to Mixtures of Organic Solvents*. Am. J. Psychiatry 1987; 36:26-39.

Ryan, C.M., Morrow, L., Parkinson, D., Branet, E., Parkinson, D.K., *Assessment of Neuropsychological Function in the Workplace: Normative Data from the Pittsburgh Occupational Exposure Test Battery*. J. Clin. Exp. Neuropsychol. 1987; 9:665-679.

Shum, D.H., McFarland, K.A., Bain, J.D., *Construct Validity of Eight Tests of Attention: Comparison of Normal and Closed Head Injured Samples.* Clin Neuropsychologist 1990; 4:151-152.

Singer, R.M., Neurotoxicity Guidebook. New York: Van Nostrand Reinhold, 1990.

Stuss, D.T., Stethem, L.L., Hungenholtz, H., Richards, M.T., *Traumatic Brain Injury.* Clin. Neuropsychologist 1989; 3:145-156.

Tsushima, W.T., Towne, W.S., *Effects of Paint Sniffing on Neuropsychological Test Performance.* J. Abnormal Psychol. 1977; 86:402-407.

Chapter 6

IMAGING AND NEUROPHYSIOLOGIC STUDIES

Technological advances can also exert deleterious non-genetic effects at first unnoticed. Environmental pollution illustrates how many of the adjustments that facilitate life in a hostile environment, commonly express themselves later in disease and human misery.

—Rene Dubos, *Man, Medicine and Environment* (1970).

§ 6-1. In General.

While patient history, physical and neurologic examination, as well as psychological testing can provide valuable information for the diagnosis and treatment of neurotoxic disease, neurometric examinations are required to specifically locate and characterize specific lesions associated with the disease. X-rays, or roentgenography imaging, was the first neurometric examination to be made available. While it has limited application in neurotoxicology, it is still useful. In recent years, many new diagnostic techniques have been developed.

Neurodiagnostic procedures can be classified into two broad categories: imaging, and neurophysiologic.

Table 6.1
Neurodiagnostic Testing

Imaging

X-ray

Computerized Tomography (CT) Scan

Angiography

Magnetic Resonance Imaging (MRI)

Ultrasound

Positron Emission Tomography (PET)

Single Photon Emission Computed Tomography (SPECT)

Neurophysiologic Testing

Electroencephalogram (EEG)

Quantitative Electroencephalogram (QEEG)

Brainstem Auditory Evoked Potential

Visual Evoked Potential (VEP)

Somatosensory Evoked Potential (SEP)

Cortical Evoked Potential (CEP)

Electromyography

Nerve Conduction Studies

Electronystagmography (ENG)

Visual Field Testing

Visual Acuity Testing

Auditory Testing

Quantitative Sensory Testing

---

§ 6-2. Imaging.

§ 6-2(a). X-Ray.

X-ray examination has been in use since the early 1900s. So-called "plain film" X-rays have little value in diagnosing neurotoxic disease, except in those instances where the disease may also have a direct effect on bone.

§ 6-2(b). Angiography.

Angiography is X-ray examination with the use of radiopaque or contrast media dyes. In cerebral angiography, for example, the dye is injected into a blood vessel in the leg or arm from which it travels in the blood to vessels in the brain. The contrast media provide negative or positive shadows that allow visualization of the brain's vascular system. Problems include reactions to the contrast media, which can result in irritation, transient pain, fever, and elevated cerebrospinal fluid cell counts. The contrast media themselves, at times, may prove neurotoxic in some individuals. Seizures and anaphylactic reactions are rare occurrences. Cerebral angiography is being replaced by CT scanning and MRI in many applications.

§ 6-2(c). Spinal Myelography.

Myelography involves injecting a radiopaque substance into the subarachnoid space via a lumbar puncture (spinal tap). It is used to visualize pathologic conditions resulting in gross structural changes in the spinal cord and related tissues. It can demonstrate the presence of a lesion in the intradural or extradural compartments of the spinal canal. Fluoroscopic observation of the flow of the dye within the spinal subarachnoid space provides the most valuable information. Problems include possible reactions to the dye. Some patients complain of sharp pain when the dye is removed. Another potential complication is headache, and even seizure activity has been documented with certain contrast material (i.e., metrizamide).

§ 6-2(d). Computerized Tomography (CT) Scanning.

Computerized tomography scanning was one of the first imaging procedures to make use of computers to enhance images. MRI also involves the use of computer image enhancement. CT scanning and MRI have become the major neurologic diagnostic procedures.

CT scanning is a radiographic imaging method. That is, it makes use of x-rays. Images are reconstructed from quantitative sets of x-ray measurements of the body from many angles. The x-ray source rotates 180 degrees around the patient, sending out pencil-thin beams at many different points. As an x-ray beam passes through the patient, an array of detectors picks up absorption rates in the varying thicknesses of tissues and bone. These are conducted to the computer, which produces "slices" of images which are as much as 100 times sharper and clearer than those obtained from conventional x-ray imaging. Contrast agents can be injected to enhance the images.

CT differentiates well between white and gray matter. It shows the main divisions between the basal ganglia and thalamus. With contrast, it shows the major arteries. CT has been superior to MRI for imaging subarachnoid hemorrhages and other intracranial blood. CT is also superior for imaging bone. It is used frequently for screening in acute evaluation of stroke, head injury and infections. With contrast, CT can detect lesions involving breakdown of the blood-brain barrier, such as brain or spinal tumors, infections and inflammations. It can also be used to rule out cerebral metastases. However, MRI enhanced with gadolinium is better for most intracranial tumors and some infections.

Advantages of CT include its speed, low cost, and availability. It is useful for patients who cannot tolerate MRI because of claustrophobia or obesity. It can be used for patients who cannot be exposed to the strong magnetic fields of MRI because they have various metallic implants, such as aneurysm clips and cardiac pacemakers, or metallic foreign bodies, particularly in the eye.

Among its disadvantages is that CT does not show the posterior fossa well because of the thickness of the bone at the base of the skull. The X-ray beams may project across the brain stem and obscure underlying lesions. CT is less effective that MRI in identifying nonhemorrhagic infarctions.

In a study of six workers exposed to styrene, CT showed cerebral atrophy in five patients. Two of these had cortical and central atrophy as well (Melgaard, 1979). CT showed cortical atrophy alone in two patients, and central atrophy only in one. These workers had a history of headache, dizziness, and a feeling of drunkenness at the end of the workday. The symptoms eventually became chronic with increased fatigue and need for sleep, lack of concentration and initiative, and emotional instability. The five whose CT scans showed cerebral atrophy also exhibited intellectual impairment on psychological examination, while the one with a normal CT scan showed no evidence of such impairment. CT has also shown cerebral atrophy in neurotoxicity associated with 1,1,1-trichloroethylene (Gresham, 1983). The patient, an 18-year-old male, was found unconscious in a vat of 1,1,1-trichloroethylene. He regained respiratory function, but did not regain consciousness, and died 39 months later. At autopsy, the brain was atrophic. The most severe atrophy was seen in the occipital gyri. Similar CT results have been obtained in individuals suffering acute poisoning with methanol and carbon monoxide. (Aquilonius, 1980; Kim, 1980).

§ 6-2(e). Magnetic Resonance Imaging (MRI).

Magnetic resonance imaging (MRI) has become a widely used diagnostic technique in recent years. It has replaced pneumoencephalography and many angiographic procedures as the diagnostic method of choice in many applications. In MRI, radio wave pulses are applied to biologic tissue, exciting some protons in the tissues into a higher energy state. After the radio pulse, the protons relax to their original energy state. This relaxation is accompanied by the emission of radio waves characteristic of the particular tissue. Differences in the emissions are picked up by a computer, which converts them into images that have a three-dimensional quality. Two tissue-specific relaxation constants, referred to as T_1 and T_2, can be measured. The differences in T_1 and T_2 relaxation values enable the production of images that distinguish bone, fat, muscle, bone marrow, and gray or white matter in the brain.

MRI images can be modified to provide for weighting of T_1 and T_2 relaxation characteristics or of proton-density characteristics. Various factors influence the weighting of these characteristics, including the imaging technique (pulse sequence), the repetition time (the interval between repetitions of the pulse sequence), and the echo time (the interval between the radio frequency excitation and the measurement of the radiowave emission or signal). Examples of imaging technique are spin-echo, gradient-echo, and inversion recovery. Spin-echo pulse sequence is one of the more useful and frequently used techniques. This technique utilizes 90. and 180. pulses and measurement of the signal after each 180. pulse. The 90. pulse induces the radiowave excitation in the tissue and the 180. rephases the signal to produce "echos," which are measured.

MRI is particularly useful in imaging intracranial and intraspinal lesions. It provides well-defined images of soft tissues, both normal and pathologic. The three-dimensional quality of the images provides information on the relationships of anatomical structures. It can also demonstrate the flow of blood and cerebrospinal fluid. A great advantage is that MRI does not expose the patient to ionizing radiation. No adverse effects have been reported.

Disadvantages include cost, time, and claustrophobia. While CT requires only seconds per "slice," MRI sequences require minutes. A complete examination can take 45 minutes to an hour or more. Most MRI units require the patient to lie motionless inside a relatively narrow tube during this time. Some obese patients just do not fit. For claustrophobic patients, the procedure can be a harrowing, if not impossible, task. Oral or intravenous sedation has been of help in these situations. More promising is the development of open MRI units, which became available in the mid-1990s. These units make MRI examinations possible for obese patients and are better tolerated by those with claustrophobia.

MRI is contraindicated in patients with some types of metallic implants, including older types of aneurysm clips, cochlear implants, cardiac pacemakers, implanted neurostimulators, and metallic foreign bodies in the eye. Individuals who have worked in industries where they were exposed to dusts of magnetic metal should also not have MRI examinations. Pregnant women are considered to be at risk, although no harmful effect of MRI on pregnant women or fetuses has been demonstrated.

MRI has revealed cerebral atrophy in some toluene abusers (Rosenberg, 1988). These patients had increased periventricular signal intensity and loss of gray-white matter demarcation. These patients exhibited cognitive impairment and cerebellar dysfunction.

§ 6-2(f). Gadolinium-Enhanced MRI.

Compounds of gadolinium, a rare heavy metal, are used as contrast media for MRI. Several types are in use. One called gadopentate dimeglumine (Gd-DPTA), crosses the blood-brain barrier. It has not been associated with a high level of adverse reactions (Katayama, 1990). It shortens the time required for image formation, and is accumulated in some types of lesions, enhancing their visibility. It has demonstrated high sensitivity in detecting malignant and inflammatory lesions, which are not detectable with CT. Gadolinium-enhanced MRI (Gd-MRI) has found metastases at a stage when surgery is still a therapeutic option (Davis, 1991). Gd-MRI has also been used successfully in detecting the following, often not found with CT:

- Schwannomas, which are small tumors along the auditory nerves; Gd-MRI has detected these even when they are inside the auditory canal;
- Gliomas, small tumors often occurring on the optic nerve and in the hypothalamus;
- Demyelinating plaques of multiple sclerosis in the brain and spinal cord; Gd-MRI can distinguish between acute and chronic lesions (Grossman, 1986); and

- Lesions associated with AIDS, meningitis, encephalitis, myelitis, and acute disseminated encephalomyelitis (Greenberg, 1995).

In some instances, differences in images before and after administration of gadolinium can provide diagnostic information. For example, noncontrast MRI can readily detect herniated discs and degenerative spondylosis before surgery. After surgery, Gd-MRI can be used to distinguish recurrent disc herniation from postsurgical scarring or fibrosis.

Gd-MRI has not been useful in cases involving headaches, low back pain, neck pain, dementia, psychosis, or head trauma. Few contrast-enhancing lesions are found in association with these disorders. Of greater potential use in these cases is directing certain special types of MRI pulse sequences to the area of the suspected lesion. A 1998 study revealed that special protocol MRI scans detected important pathologic abnormalities in 32 out of 34 cases shown to be normal by standard MRI scans (McBride, 1998).

§ 6-2(g). Magnetic Resonance Angiography.

In spin-echo images, the big arteries and veins in the neck are usually seen as a signal void because of the relatively fast flow of blood. Magnetic resonance angiography (MRA) is a technique that produces enhanced views of flowing blood. MRA uses gradient-echo technique to produce a "map" of blood vessels. That map is reconstructed as projection angiograms that can be viewed in any orientation. MRA avoids the risks of x-ray angiography while providing the advantage of views from many different angles. Diffusion-perfusion MRI and magnetic resonance spectroscopy are beginning to be used in spectroscopy and in other conditions as well (Greenberg, 1995).

§ 6-3. Advanced Imaging Techniques.

Advanced imaging techniques which provide more sensitive and specific information for evaluating the pathology and physiology of the brain are now available. Among these are positron emission tomography and single photon emission computed tomography.

§ 6-3(a). Positron Emission Tomography.

Positron emission tomography (PET) is a method of measuring the level of metabolic activity within the brain. It builds a three-dimensional image based on the distribution of a radio tracer injected into the body. PET scans of the brain produce detailed images of brain structures in a selected plane by blurring the images of structures in other planes.

In PET, radioactive water (oxygen-5-water) or glucose molecules (fluoro-2-deoxyglucose) labeled with positron-emitting radionuclides are injected into the brain via a blood vessel. The image is built from emissions induced by the interaction of the nuclides with the atomic nucleus. When the neutron-to-proton ratio in the nucleus of an atom is too low for the atom to maintain a stable state, positron decay occurs, resulting in the conversion of a proton to a neutron and a positron, which is emitted (Diksic, 1991). Unstable atoms emit electrons which are referred to as beta particles. Positrons are positively charged beta particles that exist for a short time — measured in milliseconds — before they combine with negative electrons. In an annihilation event, two high-energy photons are produced simultaneously when a positron reacts with an electron. The two photons fly away from each other and are detected by integrated crystal detectors in the PET apparatus. The simultaneous detection of the pair of electrons reveals their line of origin. A computer constructs a three-dimensional image of the brain from the detected lines of origin.

PET is used to evaluate cerebral metabolic rate, ischemia, focal epilepsy, and degenerative disorders of the central nervous system. In addition, the distribution and chemical affinities of neurotransmitters have been imaged with PET.

§ 6-3(b). Single Photon Emission Computed Tomography Scanning.

Single photon emission computed tomography (SPECT) is similar to PET scanning. Its image is of poorer quality than PET, but it is much more readily available and is practical for appropriate routine evaluations. In SPECT, a radio tracer emits gamma rays, which are detected by a scintillation camera. An image of the brain is constructed by the computer from the gamma ray detection pattern. SPECT is often used to measure cerebral blood flow, to outline specific areas of the brain, or to evaluate receptor sites (Greenberg, 1995).

§ 6-4. Neurophysiologic Studies.

Neurophysiologic studies are techniques able to identify altered brain and nervous system functioning which cannot be imaged. Among the more widely used techniques are electrophysiologic studies, which include electroencephalogrpahy, electromyography, nerve conduction studies, and evoked potential. These studies are frequently used to assess the function of the brain, spinal cord, and peripheral nervous systems (Bernad, 1987)

§ 6-4(a). Electroencephalography (EEG).

Electroencephalography (EEG), the measurement of the brain's electrical activity, has been used for more than sixty years to obtain information on brain function. EEG measures spontaneous activity recorded from the scalp. It can also measure activity that occurs as a result of stimulation. The test is noninvasive, safe, painless, and relatively inexpensive.

§ 6-4(a)(1). Basic Procedure.

To observe the electrical activity of the brain, electrodes in the form of small metal disks are attached to the scalp. A conductive gel is applied between the scalp and the electrodes. The electrode disks are attached to a lead wire which is connected to an electroencephalograph, the recording instrument. The electroencephalograph amplifies the small amount of electrical activity generated by the brain and records the amplification on a moving sheet of paper in patterns called tracings. EEG can identify specific sites at which damage to the brain has occurred.

Several electrodes, sixteen to twenty-one pairs, are applied, resulting in several tracings. Each line represents a different activity area of the brain. The EEG is a composite of many different types of brain activity, each of which is characterized by factors of frequency, amplitude, quantity, morphology, reactivity, variability, topography, and phase relationships.

The frequency bands of EEG activity are designated by Greek letters:

- Delta: up to 4 Hz (cps);
- Theta: 5 to 7 Hz;
- Alpha: 8 to 14 Hz; and
- Beta: 13 Hz or more.

The alpha rhythm is the most characteristic feature of the normal EEG of an adult during relaxed wakefulness, which occurs over the posterior regions of the head while the eyes are closed. Beta activity occurs primarily in the frontal and central regions. High-voltage beta activity is suggestive of the effects of sedative and hypnotic medications. Theta activity is usually seen during drowsiness in normal individuals. Delta activity is seen in stage 3 and stage 4 of sleep, as well as in pathologic conditions.

§ 6-4(a)(2). EEG and Toxic Exposure.

EEG can be used to obtain evidence of encephalopathies due to toxic exposure. Some toxic exposures can have profound effects on the EEG. While there is no EEG activity that is exclusive to toxic exposure, certain EEG patterns are known to occur in association with exposure to neurotoxins. The following are some of the more commonly encountered EEG abnormalities:

Diffuse slowing of background rhythms: This is the most frequently encountered EEG abnormality. This is a nonspecific finding that is often present in patients with diffuse encephalopathies of various etiologies including toxic, metabolic, degenerative and anoxic. It is also seen in association with multiple structural abnormalities.

Triphasic waves: This pattern usually consists of generalized, synchronous waves occurring in brief runs. About half of the patients with tripahsic waves have encephalopathy with toxic and metabolic etiology; the other half generally have hepatic encephalopathy.

Focal slowing: This pattern suggests a dysfunction localized in the parenchyma, the general tissue of the brain. Focal slowing is sometimes seen in patients with focal seizure disorders, i.e., those characterized by partial seizures. In some instances, focal slowing is seen in patients with seizures in the absence of lesions.

Epileptiform discharges: This pattern is considered to be the most characteristic pattern of epilepsy. It is also seen in association with some neurotoxins.

Periodic lateralizing epileptiform discharges (PLEDs): These suggest the presence of an acute destructive lesion in the cerebrum. They have been associated with acute cerebral infarctions and other mass lesions, cerebral infections, anoxia, and other conditions. Associated clinical manifestations include seizures, obtundation, and focal neurologic defects.

§ 6-4(a)(3). EEG Rhythms Associated with Specific Neurotoxins.

Toxic agents — including heavy metals, organic solvents, pesticides, drugs, some pharmaceuticals, and other natural and synthetic toxins — may induce encephalopathies that can have remarkable effects on the EEG. EEG activities associated with toxic encephalopathies include profuse nonparoxysmal and/or paroxysmal activity. While the EEG can provide evidence of toxic encephalopathy, in most instances the activity is not a specific indication of a particular toxin. However, the EEG can show the presence of encephalopathy, providing the basis for further investigation. In a few exceptional cases, because of particular affinities of a toxin for an area of the cortex, or preexisting lesions, EEG activity can be more specific.

§ 6-4(a)(3)(i). Lead.

In severe and subacute forms of toxic encephalopathy due to lead, the EEG shows considerable diffuse slowing. As the disease progresses, diffuse paroxysmal discharges are seen. Lead exposure has also been associated with a condition known as the Lennox-Gestaut syndrome, a group of childhood epileptic encephalopathies characterized by mental retardation and uncontrolled seizures. Slow spike waves are often seen in the EEG (Fejerman, 1973). In chronic lead encephalopathy, the EEG may show poor alpha development and low voltage character (Beningus, 1981; Kalaidjiev, 1983). While EEG has provided some support for early cognitive impairment from pre- and postnatal lead exposure in high concentration groups, the data are inconclusive (Burchfiel, 1980; Benignus, 1981; Otto, 1981).

§ 6-4(a)(3)(ii). Mercury.

Chronic inorganic mercury neurotoxicity is associated with increased central and autonomic nervous system excitability. In young children, involvement of the sympathetic division of the autonomic nervous system can lead to acrodynia, a multi symptom-syndrome. Symptoms of acrodynia in infants and young children include listlessness, irritability, pain, swelling and pink coloration of the fingers and toes, among others. (See Chapter 8.) Mercury interferes with the permeability of cell membranes. Atrophic cell degeneration is seen in the cortex and cerebellum. Typical late EEG findings include general slowing and epileptiform discharges. The clinical state of the patients is reflected in the EEG changes (Murai, 1982).

§ 6-4(a)(3)(iii). Manganese.

Prolonged exposure to manganese has been associated with severe Parkinsonian syndromes characterized by spasticity, epileptic seizures, and dementia. EEG data are inconclusive. Some investigators have found slowing and fast activity (Mellerio, 1977), while others have found normal activity.

§ 6-4(a)(3)(iv). Aluminum.

Aluminum can accumulate in brain tissue and induce an encephalopathy, characterized by rapid cognitive decline, and epileptic activity (Alfrey, 1972; Alfrey, 1976; Wills, 1983). These symptoms are seen frequently in patients with kidney failure on hemodialysis. There is evidence suggesting that the EEG slowing seen in dialysis patients is directly related to the accumulation of aluminum (Cutrufo, 1984; Lipman, 1988). The aluminum accumulation in dialysis patients may be related to fluid and ion shifts and changes in the sodium-potassium pump associated with the dialysis process.

§ 6-4(a)(3)(v). Other Metals.

Bismuth: Bismuth encephalopathy is associated with nonspecific neuropsychological disturbances, seizures, confusion, and ataxia. General EEG slowing is associated with the confusion, but the seizures are not associated with paroxysmal discharges (Buge, 1981).

Severe but reversible acute encephalopathy has been seen in middle-aged women taking bismuth salts for chronic constipation. Symptoms include ataxia, confusion, seizures, and dysarthria. EEG patterns seen with the syndrome include rhythmical theta action, paroxysmal bursts, and general slowing (Burns, 1974; Buge, 1974; Hazeman, 1975).

Tin: Tin neurotoxicity is generally associated with the organic ethyl and trimethyl compounds of this metal. Seizures and Intracranial hypertension with paraplegia secondary to spinal cord swelling are often seen in this encephalopathy. Severe EEG changes have been seen in association with this syndrome. These include diffuse slowing, occipital sharp wave foci, and rhythmic slow wave activity over the temporal regions (Prüll, 1970; Besser, 1987).

Thallium: This metal is used widely in rat poisons. While most of its neurotoxic effects are peripheral, some central nervous system effects have been observed involving primarily the hypothalamus and limbic structures. Sometimes referred to as "encephalopathia thallica," symptoms and signs include lethargy, headache, concentration problems, memory loss, and paranoid psychosis. EEG abnormalities are generally nonspecific (Prick, 1979).

Lithium: Compounds of lithium are used for the treatment of affective disorders. Severe EEG abnormalities — including slowing, sharp waves, and spikes — are seen frequently in patients taking these medications (Small, 1986). The toxic effects of this metal include myoclonus, confusion, tremor, and extrapyramidal movement disorder, which can be irreversible (Sansone, 1985). EEG events include excessive slowing and prominent irritative discharges, which often show a periodic pattern with short (less than 4-second) intervals (Gregory, 1979; Spatz, 1978; Smith, 1988).

§ 6-4(a)(3)(vi). Volatile Solvents.

Volatile solvents are widely used in industry. Although most industries have safety procedures for working with these materials, exposure to toxic levels still occurs. (See Chapter 7.) Exposure can be chronic or acute and can affect the central, peripheral, and autonomic nervous systems. Most severe cases of exposure involve abuse of the solvent to achieve a "high." Common findings include diffusely reduced frequencies and an excess of focal slow activity and paroxysmal activity (Seppäläinen, 1981; Seppäläinen, 1982). In one study, increased theta activity was found to be associated with memory loss in workers with acute intoxication associated with exposure to organic solvents (Chalupa, 1960).

EEGs done on some workers exposed to *n*-hexane in the Italian shoe industry showed mostly diffuse frequent slow bursts and sporadic sharp waves (Passero, 1983). In a study of industrial styrene exposure, EEG abnormalities were seen in 24% of workers. Most showed localized slow activity, diffuse theta activity, and bilateral spike and wave discharges (Härkönen, 1977). In another study, increases in fast activity in the central and frontocentral areas were seen in 27% of exposed individuals, and increments in slow activity over both hemispheres were seen in 18% (Ros.n, 1978). Immediate EEG changes have been seen in association with accidental exposure to toluene. Diffuse or focal slow activities persisted for more than six months (Biscaldi, 1981).

§ 6-4(a)(3)(vii). Insecticides.

Chlorinated hydrocarbon insecticides, the first of which was DDT, can be highly neurotoxic to both the central and peripheral nervous systems. (See Chapter 10.) Effects on EEG are inconsistent. In a study of workers in the manufacture of DDT, only 21% demonstrated EEG changes. These changes were mostly bitemporal sharp waves, sometimes associated with anterior slow activity (Mayersdorf, 1974).

Compounds known as organophosphates are also used as insecticides. (See Chapter 9.) Acute poisoning by organophosphates has resulted in death. Autopsies have shown swollen cerebral cortex, bleeding in the meninges, and lesions on the cerebellum (Preda, 1963). Chronic exposure can result in depression, memory and concentration problems, and psychotic behavior. Peripheral neuropathies can also occur. EEG changes seen in association with organophosphate toxicity include paroxysmal changes and nonspecific enhancement of slow activity (Kurt, 1976; Punkas, 1969).

§ 6-4(a)(3)(viii). Other Toxins.

Carbon Monoxide: EEG associated with carbon monoxide (CO) poisoning usually shows marked slowing, particularly in patients with prolonged loss of consciousness. Decreasing voltage may be a sign of impending fatality. Impaired consciousness may produce 1-4/second activity of high voltage. Clinical recovery may or may not be reflected in EEG changes (Van Sweden, 1993).

Methyl Alcohol (Methanol): When methanol is ingested, it is broken down into formaldehyde and formic acid. Formaldehyde is highly toxic for cells in the retina. Formic acid causes an acidosis, which is believed to be the source of CNS involvement. Encephalopathy associated with methyl alcohol intake is manifested primarily by visual loss and blindness which can be permanent because of damage to the optic nerve. Epileptic seizures, seizures, and coma may occur. The EEG shows marked slowing that correlates with the acidosis (Gilman, 1990; Jameson, 1969; Van Sweden, 1993).

Ethyl Alcohol (Ethanol); Chronic excessive intake of ethanol may be associated with a variety of neurologic disorders. Withdrawal signs following dependence may be accompanied by delirium tremens hallucinations, and seizures. Within the first 48 hours after withdrawal, EEG activity is desynchronized, and the voltages are low. EEG accompanying Wernicke-Korsakov encephalopathy, often seen in alcoholics, is variable, showing mainly diffuse slowing (Van Sweden, 1993).

§ 6-4(b). Quantitative Encephalography.

In this procedure, multiple EEG recordings are used to construct a computer-generated topographical map of the brain. This technique allows the local cortical activity to be visualized (Bernad, 1994). QEEG also has the potential to significantly improve the accuracy of the diagnosis of neurologic diseases and the monitoring of the efficacy of therapy (John, 1993). It enables a precise, quantifiable, and reproducible estimate of how much EEG data differ from what is accepted as normal (Oken, 1988). Thus quantitative assessments of the severity of brain disease and abnormal function can be made.

§ 6-4(c). Evoked Potentials.

While EEG is a measure of spontaneous brain activity, evoked potentials offer a measure of central nervous system activity in response to specific stimuli. Evoked potentials are very small electrical signals produced along sensory pathways in response to sensory stimuli. The voltage of evoked potentials is generally much lower than that of the ongoing spontaneous electrical activity of the cortex. Evoked potentials are detected through the use of signal averaging techniques.

Changes in evoked potentials caused by disease are expressed in term of either delayed responses reflecting conduction delays in sensory pathways or loss or attenuation, resulting from a blockage or dysfunction of the sensory structures generating a response, of the waveforms that are components of the response. Sensory evoked potentials can involve auditory, visual, or somatosensory (tactile) pathways. Auditory evoked potentials are also referred to as brainstem auditory potentials and can provide accurate information on the function of the peripheral nervous system, brainstem, and brain hemispheres. Furthermore, evoked potentials may be altered or obliterated by changes in arterial oxygenation, carbon dioxide content, intracranial pressure, cerebral blood flow, cerebral perfusion pressure, and hypothermia (Stone, 1988). Although evoked potentials test the functional rather than the anatomical integrity of a region, it may be possible to determine the location of brainstem lesions using short-latency signals.

Evoked potential testing has many clinical advantages, including: 1) it can be done at bedside; 2) it is noninvasive and poses no serious risk to the patient; 3) testing time is under one hour; 4) results can be quantified, stored, and subjected to on-line or off-line mathematical and statistical treatment; 5) the procedure is sensitive to central nervous system dysfunction; 6) the procedure is not seriously influenced by level of coma or by depressant medications; 7) the cost is reasonable; and 8) the information obtained from the procedure, which is not available from other procedures applied in assessing the patient, can be correlated with neurologic status (Hall, 1988).

§ 6-4(c)(1). Visual Evoked Potentials.

Visual evoked potentials (VEP) measure brain activity in response to visual stimuli such as flashing lights. The usual preferred stimulus for VEP testing is a checkerboard pattern of black and white squares. In a technique called "pattern reversal," the white squares are changed to black and the black to white to produce what is called an occipital positive signal, the P100, about 100 milliseconds after the stimulus. This technique can determine the approximate location of a lesion in the optic nerve that carry signals from the eye to the brain. The optic nerve fibers from the nasal retina (the side of each eye next to the nose) decussate, or split, at the optic chiasm. Those from the temporal area (away from the nose) do not cross. Thus, an abnormality in the P100 response to stimulation of one eye implies that the dysfunction is anterior to the optic chiasm on that side. If delayed P100s are observed following stimulation of both eyes separately, the abnormalities may be either anterior or posterior to the chiasm or at the chiasm (Emerson, 1995).

Acute optic neuritis is indicated by loss or severe attenuation of the VEP. Pattern reversal visual evoked potentials (PRVEP) are abnormal in almost all patients with a history of optic neuritis. Noncompressive optic nerve lesions such as nutritional and toxic amblyopia can also be causes of VEP, as can compressive disorders such as tumors. PREVP results have been useful in diagnosing multiple sclerosis. About 70% of multiple sclerosis patients who have no history of optic neuritis have abnormal PVREP. VEPs have been particularly useful in distinguishing malingering (Emerson, 1995).

VEP changes have been associated with exposure to *n*-hexane (Seppäläinen, 1979). In a study of workers at risk, exposure time varied from five to twelve years at levels ranging from very low (10 to 50 ppm) to moderate (500 ppm and below) to high (3000 ppm). VEP results were generally flatter in exposed workers compared to controls. Early component latencies were increased while those of later components were decreased. The changes were interpreted as indications of cerebral dysfunction.

§ 6-4(c)(2). Brainstem Auditory Evoked Potentials.

Brainstem auditory evoked potentials (BAEPs), also referred to as auditory evoked potentials, are electrical potentials generated by neural activity and associated with specific sensory, cognitive and motor processes. They reflect processes that intervene between stimulus and response, providing information about the BAEPs' time course and cerebral localization (Heinze, 1992). Metabolic and toxic encephalopathy can induce changes in BAEP.

In the BAEP procedure, a "click" stimulus is used to generate a response in the brainstem and auditory nerve. The normal response is a series of signals occurring within seven milliseconds after the stimulus. Interpretations usually based on three components: 1) wave I, which arises from the peripheral portion of the auditory nerve; 2) wave III, generated in the tegmentum of the caudal pons section of the brainstem; and 3) wave V, generated in the region of the inferior colliculus (Emerson, 1995).

There is a close relationship between BAEP changes and the pathology of the structure generating the potential. Since BAEPs are resistant to alteration by medications and metabolic disturbances, they could be useful in sorting out toxic and structural factors in comatose patients (Epstein, 1988). They are most often abnormal when structural brainstem lesions exist. BAEPs are particularly useful for the detection of tumors of the eighth cranial nerve (Emerson, 1995).

Effects of BAEP were found in a study of printing workers exposed to low levels of toluene over long periods of time (Vrca, 1996). The range of exposure among the 59 workers tested was 4 to 30 years, with a mean of 20.6 years. Significant prolongations of P1 latencies, decreased amplitudes of P1, P1, P3, P4, and P5 waves, and prolongation of P3-P5 IPLs were observed. Head injuries and the use of alcohol, coffee, or tobacco had no effect on the results. The investigators suggested that BAEPs be included in pre-employment and regular follow-up examinations of workers who would be exposed to toluene.

Toxic metals have also been shown to change evoked potentials. The neurotoxic effects of mercury vapor were shown in an evoked potential study of chloralkali workers in Taiwan. Testing included VEP, and somatosensory evoked potential (SEP), as well as BAEP. Prolonged latencies were observed in both BAEP and SEP. Higher interpeak values were seen in the VEP studies (Chang, 1995). Prolongation of BAEP latencies have been observed in rhesus monkeys exposed pre- and postnatally to lead acetate (Lilienthal, 1996).

§ 6-4(c)(3). Somatosensory Evoked Potentials.

Somatosensory evoked potentials (SEP) are often helpful in the clinical diagnosis of peripheral nerve or brachial plexus injury and of lesions of the spinal cord, brainstem, thalamus and cortex (Stone, 1988). SEPs are usually produced by stimulation of the median and posterior tibial nerves. SEPs are changed by, and are therefore useful in diagnosing, conditions that affect the somatosensory pathways. These conditions include strokes, tumors, various hereditary degenerative disorders, and vitamin E and vitamin B_{12} deficiencies (Krumholz, 1981). SEPs have also been of use in diagnosing multiple sclerosis (MS). Some 50 to 60% of MS patients demonstrate SEP abnormalities, even in the absence of clinical symptoms and signs (Emerson, 1995). SEPs of the trigeminal nerve have been used to assess workers exposed to trichloroethylene (Barret, 1987). The trigeminal nerve (fifth cranial nerve) is stimulated on the skin, and the response is detected in the facial muscle innervated by the facial nerve (seventh cranial nerve). The sensitivity and specificity of this method, however, are only 67%.

§ 6-4(c)(4). Cortical Evoked Potentials.

This technique evaluates the patient's attention and memory. It has been useful in assessing the effects of degenerative disease and head trauma. The patient is kept awake and asked to listen to sounds in the form of tones that vary every 300 milliseconds. The patient's reaction time is measured. In patients with Alzheimer's disease, for example, reaction time increases as the condition deteriorates (Bernad, 1994).

§ 6-4(c)(5). Motor Evoked Potentials.

Motor evoked potentials (MEP) are a recent development and are still regarded as experimental. In this procedure, the cortex is stimulated, either by a direct pass of a brief high-voltage electric pulse through the scalp or by using a time-varying magnetic field to induce an electric current in the brain. The action potential of appropriate muscles is recorded. It is used to assess the condition of neurologic pathways descending from the brain. This technique may be helpful in diagnosing and assessing the effect of disease processes, including toxic exposure, on the motor system.

§ 6-4(d). Electromyography and Nerve Conduction Studies (Electroneuronography).

A normal muscle at rest displays no electrical activity. When a muscle becomes active, potentials of the motor units appear. When muscles or nerves are damaged, the motor units may continue to fire, even when the muscle is at rest. This condition can be detected by electromyography (EMG).

Electromyography provides information on variations of electric potential or voltage. Electrical changes are detected by a needle electrode inserted into skeletal muscle or by electrodes placed on the skin. The activity is displayed on an oscilloscope and can also be monitored by auditory signals. EMG is only an extension of the complete neurologic exam and must be integrated with data from other neurologic tests. No specific EMG wave forms characterize a particular disease or trauma. EMG can help in the diagnosis of nerve damage after toxic exposure. EMG may detect minimal residual innervation that may not be apparent on clinical examination. Neither EMG or any other electrodiagnostic test can determine if injured nerve fibers are reversibly damaged or if they are irreversibly damaged and will degenerate.

Electroneuronography (ENG) is a measurement of sensory and motor nerve conduction velocities, information that can be useful in assessing polyneuropathy. Stimulation of a nerve initiates the propagation of the nerve impulse, the action potential, along the axon. The nerve conduction velocity is calculated by measuring the action potential at a second location within a known distance from the point of stimulation. The nature of the action potential can useful in differentiating between axonal neuropathy and a demyelinating neuropathy such as multiple sclerosis. EMG and ENG have been quite useful in investigating neuropathy associated with exposure to *n*-hexane, carbon disulfide, acrylamide, and trichloroethylene.

EMG has been used in studies of toxic exposure. In a study of workers exposed to *n*-hexane in shoe factories in Italy, EMG and nerve conduction studies were some of the diagnostic methods used to determine the prevalence of neuropathy. EMG showed varying degrees of abnormal motor unit potentials, denervation and fibrillations, which correlated with the severity of clinical findings (Passero, 1983).

§ 6-4(e). Peripheral Nerve Conduction Velocity.

Conduction velocity is the speed at which a nerve action potential moves along an axon. It is calculated in meters per second. In this procedure, stimulating electrodes are placed over a peripheral nerve. The electrodes can be placed on the skin or inserted as a needle. Nerves used frequently in motor nerve assessment include the median and radial in the arm and the tibial and peroneal in the leg. Sensory nerve conduction is more difficult to measure because sensory nerves tend to be smaller in diameter than motor nerves. Signal averaging techniques and computer programs have been used to improve the quality of information obtained in nerve conduction studies. The distribution of fibers based on their conduction velocities can be estimated with these techniques. The components of the nerve can be distinguished, and their susceptibility to neurotoxic agents can be determined (Sax, 1981).

A frequent cause of changed nerve velocity is damage to or loss of myelin, the "insulation" of nerve fibers. The speed of a nerve impulse in a demyelinated nerve fiber can be slower than in a fiber with an intact myelin covering. Other factors can also contribute. Degeneration of the axon, as well as demyelination, is involved in most neuropathies (Vinken, 1987). There is a relationship between these processes. A neurotoxic agent that attacks one will affect the other. However, changes in nerve conduction velocity are not always associated with histopathological changes in the nerve fiber (Dyck, 1984; Maxwell, 1979).

A number of neurotxins have been associated with decreases in nerve conduction velocity. Lead has been shown to slow conduction velocity, but lead-induced myelination in humans has not been clearly demonstrated (LeQuesne, 1982; Seppäläinen, 1972). Slowing of conduction velocity was shown in workers with asymptomatic sensorimotor polyneuropathy associated with exposure to elemental mercury (Albers, 1982). Among the solvents, *n*-hexane has been most frequently associated with decreased nerve conduction velocity (Mutti, 1982; Bravaccio, 1981). The normal embryology development of peripheral nerves is well understood and has been studied for many years. A number of well-respected researchers have devoted lifetimes of study to both normal and abnormal development and neuropathology of the peripheral nervous system.

§ 6-4(f). Electronystagmography.

Nystagmus is the rapid involuntary oscillation of the eyeballs. It often occurs following dizziness resulting from disease or injury to the cerebellum or to the inner ear structures known as vestibulae. Electronystagmography is used to detect the movement of the eyeballs that characterizes nystagmus. ENG is based on a voltage difference in the eye between the retina, which is negative, and the cornea, which is positive. Electrodes are placed on either side of the brain in the plane of the eye movement. Detected changes are recorded and analyzed. ENG often finds abnormalities in the vestibular system that other neurodiagnostic procedures fail to detect.

§ 6-4(g). Quantitative Sensory Evaluation.

Quantitative sensory evaluation has been useful in evaluating sensory neuropathies involving the fingers and toes, as well as the face. This technique is a semiquantitative approach to patients who have sensory symptoms such as numbness, tingling, and/or "pins and needles" sensation. This technique is performed by using thermal perception (hot and cold), vibratory sensation, and, to some extent, current perception thresholds (measuring painful sensation in distal, small sensory fibers).

References.

Albers, J.W., Cavender, G.D., Levine, S.P., Langolf, G.D., *Asymptomatic Sensorimotor Polyneuropathy in Workers Exposed.* Neurology 1982; 32:1168-

Alfrey, A.C., Mishell, J.M., Contiguglai, et al., *Syndrome of Dyspraxia and Multifocal Seizures with Chronic Hemodialysis*. Trans. Am. Soc. Artif. Intern. Organs. 1972; 18:257-261.

Alfrey, W.C., Le Gendre, G.R., Kachny, W.D., *The Dialysis Encephalopathy Syndrome. Possible Aluminum Intoxication.* New Engl. J. Med. 1976; 294:184-188.

Aquilonius, S.-M., Bergström, K., Enoksson, P., *Cerebral Computed tomography in Methanol Intoxication.* J. Comput. Assist. Tomogr. 1980; 4:425.

Barret, L., Garrel S., Danel, V., Debru, J.L., *Chronic Trichloroethylene Intoxication: a New Approach by Trigeminal-Evoked Potentials*? Arch. Environ. Health. 1987; 42:297.

Beningus, V.A., Otto, D.A., Muller, K.E., Seiple, K.J., *Effects of Age and Body Lead Burden on CNS Functions in Young Children. II. EEG Spectra.* Electroencephalogr. Clin. Neurophysiol. 1981; 52:240-248.

Bernad, P.G., *Symposium on Closed Head Injury: Clinical Aspects.* American Medical Encephalographic Association. Tucson, Arizona: March 4-8, 1987.

Bernad, P.G., *Neurodiagnostic Procedures and Examinations*. In: P.G. Bernad, Closed Head Injury: A Clinical Source Book. Charlottesville, VA: Michie, 1994: 67-109.

Besser, R., Kramer, G., Thumker, R., et al., *Acute Trimethyltin Limbic-Cerebellar Syndrome*. Neurology. 1987; 945-950.

Biscaldi, G.P., Mingardi, M., Pollini, G., et al., *Acute Toluene Poisoning. Electroneurophysiological and Vestibular Investigations.* Toxico. Eur. Res. 1981; 3:271.

Bravaccio, F., Ammendola, A., Barruffo, L., Cralomango, S., *H-Reflex Behavior in Glue (n-hexane) Neuropathy.* Clin. Toxicol. 1981; 18:1369-1375.

Buge, A., Rancurel, G., Poisson, M., et al., *Encéphalopathies Myocloniques par les sels de Bismuth.* Nouv. Presse Méd. 1974; 3:2315-2320.

Buge, A., Rancurel, G., Dechy, H., *Encephalopathies Myocloniques Bismuthiques*. Rev. Neurol. 1977; 133:401-415.

Buge, A., et al., *Epileptic Phenomina in Bismuth Toxic Encephalopathy*. J. Neurol. Neurosurg. Psychiatry 1981; 44:62.

Burchfiel, J.L., Duffy, F.H., Bartels, P.H., et al., *The Combined Descrita Rating Power of Quantitative EEG and Neuropsychologic Measures in Evaluating CNS Effects of Lead in Low Levels.* In: H.C. Needleman (ed.), Low Level lead Exposure. New York: Raven Press, 1980.

Burns, R., Thomas, W., Barron, V.J., *Reversible Encephalopathy Associated with Bismuth Subgallate Ingestion.* Br. Med. J. 1974; 1:220-223.

Chalupa, H., Synkova, J., Sevcik, M., *The Assessment of Electroencephalographic Changes and Memory Disturbances in Acute Intoxication with Industrial Poisoning.* Br. J. Ind. Med. 1960; 17:238.

Chang, Y.C., Yeh, C.Y., Wang, J.D., *Subclinical Neurotoxicity of Mercury Vapor Revealed by a Multimodality Evoked Potential Study of Chloralkali Workers.* Am. J. Ind. Med. 1995; 27:271-279.

Cutrufo, C., Caroli, S., Delle Femmine, P., *Experimental Aluminum Encephalopathy, Quantitative EEG Analysis of Aluminum Bioavailability.* J. Neurol. Neurosurg. Psychiatry. 1984; 47:202-06.

Davis, P.C., Hudgins, P.A., Peterman, S.B.L., *Diagnosis of Cerebral Metastasis: Double Dose Delayed CT Versus Contrast Enhanced MR Imaging*. AJNR. 1991; 12:293-300.

Diksic, M., Reba, R.C., Radiopharmaceuticals and Brain Pathology Studied with PET and SPECT. Boca Raton: CRC Press, 1991.

Dyck, P.J., Thomas, P.K., Lambert, E.H., Bunge, R., Peripheral Neuropathy, Vol I & II, 2d Ed. Philadelphia: W.B. Saunders Co., 1984.

Emerson, R.G., Walczak, T.S., Turner, C.A., *EEG and Evoked Potentials.* In: L.P. Rowland (ed.), Merritt's Textbook of Neurology. Baltimore: Williams and Wilkins, 1995: 67-77.

Epstein, C.M., *The Use of Brain Stem Auditory Evoked Potentials in the Evaluation of the Central Nervous System.* Neurologic Clinics. 1988; 6:771-789.

Fejerman, N., Gimenez, E.R., Vallejo, N.E., Medina, C.S., *Lennox-Gestaut Syndrome and Lead Intoxication.* Pediatrics. 1973; 52:227-234.

Gilman, A.G., et al., The Pharmacological Basis of Therapeutics, 8th Ed. New York: Pergamon Press, 1990.

Greenberg, J.O., Neuroimaging: A Comparison to Adams and Victor's Principles of Neurology. New York: McGraw-Hill, 1995.

Gregory, D.C., Jones, K.W., Cochavi, S., Bernad, P.G., *Determination of Lithium in Biological Samples with 6Li(n,x) 3H Reaction.* Bulletin of the American Physical Society 1979; 24:823.

Gresham, G.A., Treip, C.S., *Fatal Poisoning by 1,1,1-Trichloroethylene After Prolonged Survival.* Forensic Sci. Int. 1983; 23:249:

Grossman, R.I., Gonzalez-Scarano, F., Atlas, S.W., et al., *Multiple Sclerosis: Gadolinium Enhancement in MR Imaging.* Radiology 1986; 161:721-725.

Hall, J.W., *Auditory Evoked Responses in the Management of Acutely Brain-Injured Children and Adults.* Am. J. Otol. 1988; 9:36-45.

Hazeman, P., Rebello, F., Landau, J., *Encéphalopathies par le Bismuth.* Rev. EEG. Neurophysiol. 1975; 5:291-294.

Härkönen, H., *Relationship of Symptoms to Occupational Styrene Exposure and to the Findings of Electroencephalographic and Psychological Examinations.* Int. Arch. Occup. Environ. Health. 1977; 40:231.

Heinze, H-J, Munte, T.F., Gobiet, et al., *Parallel and Visual Search After Closed Head Injury: Electrophysiological Evidence for Perceptual Dysfunctions.* Neuropsychologica 1992; 30:495-514.

Jameson, H.D., Kane, R., *EEG Records During an Epidemic of Methanol Intoxication.* Electroencephalogr. Clin. Neurophysiol. 1969; 26:112 (abstract).

John, E.R., Orichep, L.S., *Principles of Neurometric Analysis of EEG and Evoked Potentials.* In: E. Niedermeyer, F. Lopes da Silva (eds.), Electroencephalography. Baltimore: Williams and Wilkins, 1993: 989-1004.

Kalaidjiev, D., *Electroencephalographic Changes in Workers Resulting from Prolonged Exposure to Lead.* Electroencephalogr. Clin. Neurophysiol. 1983; 55:25P (abstract).

Kim, K.S., Weinberg, P.E., Suh, J.H., Ho, S.U., *Acute Carbon Monoxide Poisoning: Computed Tomography of the Brain.* AJNR 1980; 1:399.

Krumholz, A., Weiss, H.D., Goldstein, P.J., Harris, K.C., *Evoked Responses in Vitamin B_{12} Deficiency.* Ann. Neurol. 1981; 9:407-409.

Kurt, D., *The EEG in Intoxications by Pesticides and Raticides.* In: A. Redmond (ed.), Handbook of Electroencephalopathy and Clinical Neurophysiology, Vol. 15C. Amsterdam: Elsevier, 1976: 105-107.

LeQuesne, P.M., *Electrophysiological Investigations of Toxic Neuropathies.* Acta. Neurol. Scand. 1982; 66:75.

Lilienthal, H., Winneke G., *Lead Effects on the Brain Stem Auditory Evoked Potential in Monkeys During and After the Treatment Phase.* Neurotoxicol. Teratol. 1996; 18:17-32.

Lipman, J.J., Colowick, S.P., Lawrence, P.L., et al., *Aluminum Induced Encephalopathy in the Rat.* Life. Sci. 1988; 42:863-875.

Maxwell, I.C., LaQuesne, P.M., *Conduction Velocity in Hexachlorophene Neuropathy; Correlation Between Electrophysiological and Histological Findings.* J. Neurol. Sci. 1979; 43:95.

Mayersdorf, A., Israeli, R., *Toxic Effects of Chlorinated Hydrocarbon Insecticides on the Human Electroencephalogram.* Arch. Environ. Health. 1974; 28:159-163.

McBride, M. et al., *Benefits of Special Temporal Lobe Protocol MRI.* Arch. Neurol. 1998; 55:346-8.

Melgaard, B., Alien-Soborg, P., Bruhn, P., *Chronic Toxic Encephalopathy in Styrene Exposed Workers.* Presented at the Third Industrial and Environmental Neurology Congress, Prague, 1979.

Mellerio, F., Kubicki, S., *Encephalopathy Due to Poisoning.* In: A Remond (ed.), Handbook of Electroencephalography and Clinical Neurophysiology, Vol. 15A. Amsterdam: Elsevier, 1977: 108-135.

Murai, Y., Shiraishi, S., Yamashita, Y., et al., *Neurophysiological Effects of Methyl Mercury on the Nervous System.* In: P. Buser, W. Cobb, T. Ohuma. (eds.), Kyoto Symposia (EEG Suppl. 36). Amsterdam: Elsevier, 1982: 682-687.

Mutti, A., Cavatorta, A., Lucertini, S., et al., *Neurophysiological Changes in Workers Exposed to Organic Solvents in a Shoe Factory.* Scand. J. Work Environ. Health 1982; 8:136.

Oken, B., Chiappa, K., *Short-Term Variability in EEG Frequency Analysis.* Clin. Neurophysiol. 1988; 69:169-198.

Otto, B.A., Beningus V.A., Muller, K.E., et al., *Effects of Age and Body Lead Burden on CNS Function in Young Children. I. Slow Cortical Potentials.* Electroencephalogr. Clin. Neurophysiol. 1981; 52:229-39.

Passero, S.M., Battisini, N., Cloni, et al., *Toxic Polyneuropathy of Shoe Workers in Italy. A Clinical, Neurophysiological and Follow-up Study.* Ital. J. Neurol. Sci. 1983; 4:463.

Prick, J.J.G., *Thallium Poisoning.* In: P.J. Vinken, G.W. Bruyn (eds.), Handbook of Neurology. Amsterdam: North Holland, 1979: 239-278.

Preda, H., Mooraru, L., Malonescu, A., Radovici, L., et al., *Aspects Morphologiques de L'intoxication Aigue par L'aldrine.* Ann Méd Lég. 1963; 45:483-485.

Prüll, G., Rompel, K., *EEG Changes in Acute Poisoning with Organic Tin Compounds*. Electroencephalogr. Clin. Neurophysiol. 1970; 29:215 (abstract).

Punkas, G., Rusnak, C., *Certain Encephalographic Aspects in Accidental Poisoning with Ecatox in Children*. Electroencephalogr. Clin. Neurophysiol. 1969; 27:27 (630).

Rosën, I., Haeger-Aronsen, B, Rehnström, S., *Neurophysiological Observations After Chronic Styrene Exposure*. Scand. J. Work Environ. Health. 1978; 4(Suppl. 2):184-194.

Rosenberg, N.L., Spitz, M.C., Filley, C.M., et al., *Central Nervous System Effects of Chronic Toluene Abuse — Clinical, Brainstem, Evoked Response, and Magnetic Resonance Imaging Studies*. Neurotoxicol Teratol. 1988; 10:489.

Sansone, M.E.G., Ziegler, D.K., *Lithium Toxicity: A Review of Neurologic Complications*. Clin. Neuropharmacol. 1985; 8:242-248.

Sax, D.S., Kovacs, Z.L., Johnson, T.L., Feldman, R.G., *Clinical Applications of the Estimation of Nerve Conduction Velocity Distributions*. Prog. Clin. Biol. Res. 1981; 52:113.

Seppäläinen, A.M.H., Hernberg, S., *Sensitive Technique for Detecting Subclinical Lead Neuropathy*. Br. J. Ind. Med. 1972; 29:443.

Seppäläinen, A.M.H., *Neurophysiological Approaches to the Detection of Neurotoxicity in Humans*. CRC Crit. Rev. Toxicol. 1981; 18:245.

Seppäläinen, A.M.H., *Neurophysiological Findings Among Workers Exposed to Organic Solvents*. Neurotoxicology. 1981; 7:29.

Seppäläinen, A.M.H., Raitta, C., Huuskonen, M.S., *n-Hexane-Induced Changes in Visual Evoked Potentials and Electroretinograms of Industrial Workers*. Electroencephalogr. Clin. Neurophysiol. 1979; 47:492.

Small, J.G., *EEG and Lithium CNS Toxicity*. Am. J. EEG Technol. 1986; 26:225-239.

Smith, S.J.M., Kocen, R.S., *A Creutzfeldt-Jakob-Like Syndrome Due to Lithium Toxicity*. J. Neurol. Neurosurg. Psychiatry 1988; 51:120-123.

Spatz, R., Kugler, J., Greil, W., Lorenzi, E., *Das Elektroenzephalogram bei den Lithium-Intoxikation*. Nervenarzt. 1978; 49:539-542.

Stone, J.L., Ghaly, R.F., Hughes, J.R., *Evoked Potentials in Head Injury and States of Increased Intracranial Pressure.* J. Clin. Neurophysiol. 1988; 5:131-161.

Van Sweden, B., Niedermeyer, E., *Toxic Encephalopathies* In: E. Niedermeyer, F. Lopes da Silva (eds.), Electroencephalography. Baltimore: William and Wilkins, 1993: 643-652.

Vinken, P.J., Bruyn, G.W., Klawans, H.L., Handbook of Clinical Neurology, Vol 51. Amsterdam: Elsevier Science Publishers. 1987; 4-7:85-142.

Vrca, A., Kara.i. V., Bo.i.evi., D., et al., *Brainstem Auditory Evoked Potentials in Individuals Exposed to Long-Term Low Concentrations of Toluene.* Am. J. Indust. Med. 1996; 30:62-66.

Wills, M.R., Savory J., *Aluminum Poisoning: Dialysis Encephalopathy, Osteomalacia and Anaemia.* Lancet 1983; 2:29-34.

Chapter 7

VOLATILE SOLVENTS

Solvents are a large number of chemical compounds having the common ability to dissolve and readily disburse fats, oils, waxes, paints, pigments, varnishes, rubber and many other materials.

—R. Lilis, *Maxcy & Rosenau Public Health and Preventive Medicine* (1986).

§ 7-1. Overview.

Volatile organic solvents have been used in industry for at least 150 years. Carbon disulfide was used in the 1840s in an early rubber vulcanization process. Neuropsychiatric symptoms in workers exposed to carbon disulfide were reported in the 1860s. By the turn of the century, the acute and chronic effects of carbon disulfide and several chlorinated and aromatic hydrocarbons were well-known and documented. Recent advances in technology have increased the use of organic solvents. The rapid expansion of the microelectronics industry and the increased use of synthetic instead of natural materials in a wide range of industries have contributed to an increased use of organic solvents.

The existence of the acute effects of solvents on the central nervous system was known soon after the introduction of these chemicals into industrial processes and into occupations such as painting. There was, however, very little investigation into the chronic effects of long-term exposure to solvents at concentrations low in comparison to those involved in acute exposure. This situation has changed dramatically in recent years. Several studies in the 1970s, mostly from Scandinavian countries, yielded data suggesting that long-term, relatively low-level exposure to several industrial solvents and their mixtures could result in chronic toxic encephalopathy (Axelson, 1980; WHO, 1985; Hänninen, 1971; Seppäläinen, 1974, Knave; 1974) From 1961 to 1980, 129 cases of exposure effects to methylene chloride, toluene, xylene, and styrene were reported. Fifty-three patients, most of whom had been working in confined spaces, lost consciousness. Four deaths were recorded. Gastrointestinal effects were also seen.

One of the earliest described effects of chronic exposure to solvents was a condition referred to as chronic painter's syndrome. Also known as neurasthenia or psycho-organic syndrome, the syndrome consists of headache, fatigue, concentration difficulties, problems with short-term memory, irritability, depression, and alcohol intolerance (Bolla, 1990). Several studies of chronic painter's syndrome were carried out in the 1970s and later (Bolla, 1990; Arlien-Soborg, 1979; Van Vliet, 1989; Sandmark,1989; Hane, 1976; Mikkelson, 1980; Cherry, 1985). While some of these investigations — particularly the 1979 Arlien-Soborg study — tended to corroborate the existence of chronic painter's syndrome, others yielded data that led some investigators to doubt its delineation as a clinical entity.

Chronic painter's syndrome is recognized as an occupational disease and is a criterion for disability retirement in the Scandinavian countries. Nevertheless, its existence has been challenged on the basis that investigators have failed to account for confounding variables such as sex, age, intelligence, education, exposure to other neurotoxins, and general health status. A number of investigators have found that in some of the studies identifying chronic painter's syndrome, no dose-related chronic neurotoxic effects from low-level exposure were found when the confounding variables were accounted for (Maizlish, 1987; Cherry, 1985; Gade, 1988; Bolla, 1990). Maizlish, however, did find two point discrimination deficits in the foot (Maizlish, 1987). Bolla, et al. (Bolla 1990) conducted a study of 187 workers at two paint manufacturing plants in the United States. The workers were assessed for symptoms of painter's syndrome using the Zung Depression Index, Scandinavian Questionnaire 16, the Present State Exam, and psychiatric, peripheral sensory, and neuropsychological testing. Some characteristics of depression were noted, but the investigators did not consider these observations to be clinically relevant. They concluded that their results did not support the association of painter's syndrome with the solvent levels found in American paint manufacturing facilities.

This clinical experience worldwide, however, suggests that a "chronic painter's syndrome" does exist and has been seen over the last fifteen years. After using trichloroethylene, workers have also developed a "degreaser's syndrome," not unlike the effect of medications used to treat chronic alcoholics (i.e., antabuse), which usually make the individuals experience nausea and other gastrointestinal symptoms after exposure to alcohol.

§ 7-2. General Neurotoxic Effects of Organic Solvents.

Organic solvents affect both the central and peripheral nervous systems. The effects can be transient or persistent. Transient effects are apparently mediated by the pharmacologic action of solvents within the central nervous system, and are directly related to the measured concentration of solvents in the brain. Persistent neurologic effects are generally associated with histopathological changes in nervous system tissues. Several large epidemiologic studies have evaluated the acute and chronic effects of solvent exposure on the central and peripheral nervous systems.

§ 7-2(a). Peripheral Nervous System.

Among the major effects on the peripheral nervous system (PNS) is axonal degeneration accompanied by characteristic symptoms and signs of a distal, symmetrical, sensorimotor peripheral neuropathy observed in workers exposed to various solvents including n-hexane, methyl *n*-butyl ketone, and carbon disulfide. The disorder has predictable, dose-response relationships, known clinical-pathologic correlates, and a generally consistent clinical course. While the evidence for peripheral nervous system disorders in association with individual solvents is extensive, it is less convincing for mixed solvents. Except when the solvent mixture contains a known neurotoxic agent, evidence for clinically significant peripheral nerve disorders in association with mixed solvents is lacking. Solvent mixtures, rather than individual solvents, are the usual source of exposure for painters. While epidemiologic studies have shown increased rates of adverse PNS symptoms and electrophysiologic abnormalities (Baker, 1994), the association of these disorders with individual solvents has not been demonstrated conclusively in these patients. Also, clear distinctions between clinical and subclinical neuropathies were not made in all studies (Baker, 1994).

In a study by Ørbæk, neurologic testing was carried out on thirty-two patients with solvent-induced chronic toxic encephalopathy (Ørbæk, 1988). The testing revealed slowing of motor conduction velocity in the median nerve that was more severe in follow-up testing done twenty-two to seventy-two months later. Also observed was slowing in peroneal nerve conduction velocity at follow-up, and reduced amplitude in median and sural nerves with prolongation of the action potential. Decrements in temperature sensation between the patients and the control group were also noted. These findings suggest that exposure to solvent mixtures can result in a mild sensory neuropathy that is partially reversible after removal from exposure (Ørbæk, 1988). Using standardized tests of vibration and temperature perception, Bove evaluated peripheral nervous system function in construction painters exposed to solvents (Bove, 1989). The threshold for perception of vibration in the lower extremities was found to be raised in proportion to two indices of exposure to solvent over the year prior to the study. Temperature sensitivity was also depressed (Bove, 1989). Similar deficits were observed by Demers (Demers, 1991) and Bleecker (Bleecker, 1991). The data from these studies suggest that mild subclinical disruption of peripheral nervous system function can occur in workers exposed to solvent mixtures.

§ 7-2(b). Central Nervous System.

Chronic encephalopathy is a major central nervous system disorder frequently associated with exposure to organic solvents. The effects can persist after the immediate exposure period. Neuropsychiatric conditions, including dementia, have also been associated with exposure to solvents. While PNS disorders associated with solvents are well-documented, there is much disagreement and controversy over central nervous system (CNS) effects of solvent neurotoxicity. In 1985, the World Health Organization (WHO) proposed a classification for acute and chronic CNS conditions believed to be caused by exposure to toxic chemicals in the workplace.

Acute CNS effects of organic solvent intoxication are generally well-recognized. Symptoms include dizziness, lightheadedness, in coordination, and transient psychomotor impairment. With the exception of reaction time, effects on psychomotor function are not consistent below permissible exposure limits (PEL). After the individual is removed from exposure, there is usually complete return of function and loss of symptoms.

The controversy over the classification of chronic CNS effects stems from the complexity of the CNS and the variability of solvents, circumstances of exposure, and the metabolism of patients. The World Health Organization (WHO, 1990) proposed three chronic conditions associated with exposure to solvents:

- Organic affective syndrome;
- Mild chronic toxic encephalopathy; and
- Severe chronic toxic encephalopathy.

Organic affective syndrome is a reversible mood disorder occurring in individuals with chronic exposure to solvents (WHO, 1990). Symptoms include irritability, increased fatigue, depression and loss of interest in day-to-day activities. While these symptoms are general in nature, the syndrome does have clinical features that allow the identification of affected individuals. The most significant of these are the temporal relationship of the symptoms to sustained organic solvent exposure and the consistent pattern of symptoms among patients with this condition.

Mild chronic toxic encephalopathy is generally characterized by cognitive and mood disturbances, fatigue, memory and attention deficits. In some cases, there is functional impairment, particularly reductions in psychomotor abilities and short-term memory. The course of the disease is insidious, and the duration is generally days to weeks. There are usually no sequelae.

Severe chronic toxic encephalopathy is considered to be a separate condition, although there is no clear-cut demarcation between the severe and mild forms of the disease. As is the case with the mild disease, the course of the severe disease is insidious and the pathophysiology is not well known. The severe disease is, however, often associated with structural CNS damage. The duration of the disease is indefinite and the effects are usually irreversible. Results of studies strongly suggest that as the severity of the disease increases, reversibility becomes less likely, and structural abnormalities become more likely. The clinical manifestations are similar to those of the mild disease, but the functional deficits are more pronounced and pervasive. Clinical manifestations include loss of personality changes, intellectual abilities, and impairment of memory, abstract thinking, and judgment. Results of some neurophysiologic and neuroradiologic tests are abnormal in patients with this disease. Much of what is known about severe toxic encephalopathy has come from studies of individuals who have abused products containing solvents, rather than from exposures in the workplace. CNS damage has been demonstrated in encephalopathy associated with abuse of solvents.

A modification of this classification scheme was proposed at a later international conference (Baker, 1994). The terminology "organic affective syndrome" was changed to "central nervous system symptoms." Mild toxic encephalopathy was classified into two subtypes based on the predominant neurobehavioral deficit: sustained mood or personality change, called type 2A, or intellectual impairment, called type 2B. Severe chronic toxic encephalopathy, called type 3, was defined as having features characteristic of dementia as defined in *Diagnostic and Statistical Manual of Mental Disorders* (DSM-IV).

Tests of neurobehavioral function have been used to assess both short-term and long-term effects of solvent exposure on behavior. In one study (Cherry, 1980), the effect of styrene on workers employed in the manufacture of fiberglass boats was investigated. Reaction time, vigilance, and other measures of psychomotor function and mood were tested before and after the workday. Compared to a control group, the exposed workers demonstrated a greater degree of mood change and fatigue. Later assessment revealed that workers with slow clearance of styrene had slower reaction time than workers with normal metabolic rates.

The general pattern of results obtained in neurobehavioral studies has been characterized by poor performance in memory functions — particularly short-term memory — in workers exposed to solvents compared to subjects not exposed. Another pattern is a general positive correlation between the duration of exposure and the severity of symptoms. In most studies, a clear dose-response relationship has been demonstrated. Increased levels of cumulative exposure were associated with performance decrements (Baker, 1994). Improvement has been noted in most patients after removal from exposure to solvents or after significant reduction in the level of exposure. However, persistent adverse effects on neurobehavioral function are seen in patients with severe initial impairment even in the complete absence of additional exposure (Baker, 1994). In most studies, a dose-response relationship was evident (Baker, 1994).

A variety of factors — such as age, education, and the general health of the individual, as well as the properties of the individual solvents and the nature of the exposure — can affect the results of neurobehavioral studies. Attempts to account for these factors have not always been successful. In one study (Maizlish, 1987), the investigators developed an exposure index based on duration of employment, airborne exposure limits at the time of testing, and the relative toxicity of the solvents involved. Unfortunately, the observed decrements did not correlate with the exposure index. Indices of exposure were correlated with results, however, in a study of 186 construction painters conducted in 1988 (Baker, 1988). Decrements which correlated with the intensity of exposure included impaired psychomotor function, forgetfulness, disorientation, lassitude and difficulty falling asleep. A controversial reanalysis of neurobehavioral test data, using statistical techniques based on age, education and verbal intelligence, yielded results suggesting that previous diagnoses of solvent-associated encephalopathy in 20 exposed workers were invalid (Gade, 1988).

In a study of two groups of brush painters with long-term exposure to solvents and a heterogeneous group of workers exposed to solvents, it was found that decrements in performance on tests of psychomotor function and short-term memory correlated with indices of exposure derived from history. Workers with exposures exceeding ten years performed particularly poorly on memory tests (Spurgeon, 1992). Hänninen, in a study of monozygotic twins with a history of discordant solvent exposure, found greater performance decrements in those with moderate exposure compared to those with low exposure (Hänninen, 1991). Mikkelsen noted changes in neurobehavioral function in association with solvent exposure (Mikkelsen, 1980). Cerebral atrophy was observed in some patients. However, the investigators noted little risk of organic brain damage in persons with less than thirteen years' exposure, which was calculated to be the equivalent of a TWA of 40 ppm of whiter spirit, a solvent mixture commonly used in Europe.

§ 7-3. Absorption and Metabolism.

Solvents enter the body by three major routes: absorption through the skin, ingestion, and inhalation. Skin exposure most commonly occurs because of spills, manual use of solvents for cleaning and other tasks, misting, and immersion of hands and arms directly into the solvent. Gloves may or may not provide protection. Some solvents can penetrate gloves not specifically designed to protect against the solvent in question.

Inhalation can occur when the breathing zone is contaminated by evaporation of solvents from open surfaces, spills, and open containers. Both inhalation and percutaneous absorption can occur when solvents are used for cleaning. Contamination also occurs with paint spraying. The level of contamination varies with the work setting, the industrial operation, and air movement. A particular job may involve brief periods of high exposure, and longer periods of little or no exposure. Because of the variability in atmospheric conditions, absorption rates and other factors, the assessment of an individual's risk and actual intake of solvents is difficult. Some workers in a plant may be at high risk, while others may have minimal risk. In evaluating overall risk in a particular facility, average exposure level and the range of individual exposure must be considered.

Solvents are taken up into the peripheral blood stream within minutes of exposure by both percutaneous absorption or inhalation (Engstrom, 1978; Riihimäki, 1979). The rate of intake increases with physical exercise, which increases pulmonary capillary blood flow. Uptake in a worker carrying out a strenuous job may increase by a factor of two to three times the baseline (Riihimäki, 1979). Respiratory uptake varies in individuals because of physiologic factors, such as specific air/blood partition coefficients, which are effected by variations in alveolo-capillary membrane permeability and blood solubility. Percutaneous absorption varies with variations in skin thickness, skin perfusion, and the presence of cuts or other breaks in the skin (Rhiimäki, 1978; Bird, 1981).

Tissue concentrations of organic solvents can be estimated with biomathematical compartment models. Fernandez, 1977; Sato, 1977). In this method, organs are grouped on the basis of their infusion rate and lipid contents. Brain, liver, kidneys, spleen, and spinal cord comprise the *vessel-rich group*, characterized by rapid uptake after exposure to organic solvents such as xylene. An individual exposed to a high concentration of a lipophilic solvent for a period as brief as ten to fifteen minutes could receive a high concentration of the solvent in the central nervous system.

Most strategies for evaluating exposure risk do not consider short-term variations in solvent concentrations, but focus instead on full-shift time-weight average (TWA) measurements. This approach can provide useful information only if the air concentrations of the solvent are fairly constant over the time of a work shift. If, for example, the job requires tasks that involve skin exposure such as dipping the hands into the solvent, the individual's risk could be higher than that suggested by TWA measurements.

§ 7-4. Assays for Monitoring Solvent Concentration.

A number of assays are available for monitoring solvent concentration in blood, urine, exhaled air, and fat. These tests can measure uptake resulting from both inhalation and percutaneous absorption. Generally, urinary and fat assays are more useful for determinations of cumulative exposure than are blood and exhaled air assays. Fat assays continue to be useful years after the individual has been removed from the source of exposure. In contrast, blood and air assays are usually useful only during the immediate exposure period because of the short half-life of organic solvents in blood. The usefulness of a specific urine determination varies with the pharmacokinetics and metabolism of the solvent and with its route of excretion.

§ 7-5. Individual Solvents.

Table 7.1
Industrial Uses of Organic Solvents

Solvent	Industrial Use(s)
Ethyl benzene	Manufacture of cellulose acetate, styrene, synthetic rubber; component of gasolines.
Styrene	Manufacture of plastics, rubber, pharmaceuticals.
Toluene	Manufacture of plastics, rubber, gasolines.
Trichloroethylene (TCE)	Manufacture of pesticides, resins, paints, varnishes, cleaning fluids; solvent in vapor degreasing; extraction of caffeine from coffee.
Xylene	Manufacture of paints, lacquers, varnishes, inks, dyes, adhesives, cements, cleaning fluids, perfumes, insect repellents, pharmaceuticals.

§ 7-5(a). Trichloroethylene.

Empirical formula:	C_2HCl_3.
Description:	Colorless liquid.
Synonyms:	Ethylene trichloride, ethinyl trichloride, acetylene trichloride, 1,1,-trichloroethylene, trilene.
Uses:	Degreasing, dry cleaning, adhesives, paint removers, extraction of caffeine from coffee.

Air Limit:*	100 ppm.
Water Limit:*	Fresh water: 45,000 μg/L; salt water: 2,000 μg/L; to protect human health: preferably zero.

*All of these values are subject to change.

Trichloroethylene (TCE) is widely used in industry as a degreaser and solvent and, in the leather industry, as an adhesive. It is used in cleaning fluids, decaffeination of coffee, and the extraction of various plant oils. It is also used as an inhalation anesthetic in obstetrics and for short surgical procedures. Consequently, some industrial workers, operating room personnel, and dentists and dental assistants may be regularly exposed to TCE. Deliberate inhalation produces a state of euphoria, and many industrial workers have become addicted.

§ 7-5(a)(1). Exposure Limits.

The NIOSH standard for workroom air is 1000 ppm for 8 hours. Permissible exposure limit (PEL) was set at 25 ppm in 1987, reduced from 100 ppm. Threshold limit value (TLV) set by the ACGI is 50 ppm. However, these values are subject to change annually, and the revision is usually downward. (See Chapter 1.)

§ 7-5(a)(2). Neurotoxic Effects.

Cranial and peripheral neuropathies in cases of TCE exposure are frequent and striking. Involvement of the trigeminal and facial nerves, both motor and sensory, is frequent (Feldman, 1979). Electromyographic evidence of other nerve injury has also been detected. Visual evoked changes were seen in four of six patients exposed to 100 ppm over a 7.5-hour period. Long-term exposure or acute high-level exposure has been associated with memory disturbances. Decrements in concentration and neuropsychological tasks have been associated with concentrations of 500 ppm. A history of possible TCE exposure should be sought in any patient with a trigeminal neuralgia or trigeminal dysfunction (Feldman, 1979). Neuro-ophthalmologic complications are also seen. These include retrobulbar neuropathy, optic atrophy and oculomotor disturbances associated with industrial exposure to TCE (Lawrence, 1981).

Peripheral neuropathies, sensory and motor, and predominantly distal, are common. Less common disturbances include ataxia, tremor, cerebellar and extrapyramidal dysfunction, dysphagia and other bulbar symptoms (Lawrence, 1981). Examination of nerves from individuals exposed to TCE frequently shows extensive myelin and axon degeneration. Because of its lipid solvent qualities, TCE may act as a demyelinating agent. Animal studies have shown that TCE interferes with miniature end plate potential generation at the neuromuscular junction.

§ 7-5(a)(3). Acute Effects.

Salvini carried out a study in which 6 volunteers aged 20 to 22 years were exposed to TCE at 110 ppm for 2 4-hour periods separated by a break of 1.5 hours (Salvini, 1971). Declines in performance of perception, complex reaction times, manual dexterity and memory were observed. Similar results were obtained when the experiment was repeated with 6 workers who were frequently exposed to TCE. In a follow-up to the Salvini study, Stewart exposed 9 volunteers to TCE at 0, 50, and 110 ppm for 4-hour intervals separated by a 1.5-hour exposure-free break (Stewart, 1974). In addition to the psychological tests used by Salvini, the Flanagan coordination test and digit inspection test were administered. However, Salvini's results were not reproduced in Stewart's study. Test performances were not related to TCE exposure. In another study by Stewart, subjects were exposed to TCE at 200 ppm for 7 hours daily for a period of 1 to 5 days (Stewart, 1970). In addition, 2 subjects were exposed to 100 or 200 ppm for 1, 3.5, or 4 hours. Subjects detected a moderately strong odor for the first 5 minutes of exposure until adaptation occurred. Performance in psychomotor tests, including Crawford manual dexterity, was unchanged, but more effort was required for the Romberg test. On repeated exposure, some subjects experienced headache, light-headedness, and irritation of mucous membranes. More subjects reported torpor after 4 or 5 days of exposure.

In a study by Ferguson and Vernon, volunteers were exposed to TCE at 0, 300, and 1000 ppm for 2 hours at each level of exposure (Ferguson, 1970). The TCE was combined with a placebo which was either 50 mg of an antihistamine or 800 mg meprobromate. As the concentration of TCE was increased, more errors in testing were seen but they were not significant. At the highest concentration, however, there was significant impairment in depth perception, steadiness, and Purdue pegboard tests. The impairment of scores was not affected by the addition of the antihistamine or meprobromate. The decline in performance induced by TCE at levels of 300 and 1000 ppm was enhanced by low blood-alcohol concentrations. Reactions to mental strain after combined administration of TCE and alcohol were investigated by Windemuller (Windemuller, 1978). Heart rate, sinus arrhythmia, and respiration rate were monitored during the visual binary choice task and pursuit-rotor test. The suppression of arrhythmia and the increase in respiration rate was greater with combined TCE and alcohol than with either agent alone or than in the control groups.

In a study by Stewart, 20 subjects (10 males and 10 females) were exposed to 20, 100, and 200 ppm TCE for 1.3 or 7.5 hours daily (Stewart, 1974). Among the females, the visual evoked responses (VER) were changed at 100 ppm, and to a greater degree after 7.5 hours exposure. The females also experienced fatigue and had an increased need for sleep. VER was changed in only one male. Another male demonstrated EEG changes at 200 ppm. Although Flanagan coordination and random number inspection were impaired, no dose-response relationship was established.

§ 7-5(a)(4). Chronic Effects.

In a study of metal workers in Denmark, metal degreasers who had worked during the preceding year with either TCE or fluorocarbon (CFC) were invited to participate in a one-day clinical examination. Of 116 qualified workers, 109 participated, seventy had been exposed to TCE for a mean duration of 7.1 years, at a rate of 25 hours a week. Another 25 had been exposed (mostly to CFC) for an average of 4.2 years, at a rate of 15.1 hours a week. A cumulative exposure index was established based on the number of hours spent degreasing each week multiplied by the number of years of exposure multiplied by the number of exposure weeks a year (45). Three exposure groups were established: 0.5 (low), 2.1 (medium) and 11.0 (high) years' mean full-time exposure. An odds ratio for developing intellectual impairment was established for each exposure group, taking into account various confounding variables including age, arteriosclerotic condition, alcohol abuse, present exposure to solvents, preexisting intellectual level, and neurologic and psychiatric disease. The odds ratios for the medium and high exposure groups were 5.9 and 13.7, respectively.

A number of field studies have been carried out to assess the health conditions of workers exposed to TCE. In a study by Grandjean, 80 workers from 10 factories in the mechanical engineering industry were investigated (Grandjean, 1955). These men were employed as degreasers and worked close to open and closed tanks of TCE heated to 70-80. C. Air concentrations of TCE near the tanks and the center of the working space ranged from 20 to 40 ppm. Medical histories taken from 50 workers with a mean age of 43 years and exposure durations from 1 month to 15 years (with a mean of 3.75 years) revealed that all but 2 workers had a variety of symptoms and complaints. About 38% of the workers had seen their physicians because of symptoms possibly related to TCE exposure. The most frequent complaints included: alcohol intolerance — 38%; cardiac symptoms — 18%; dizziness — 50%; emotional lability — 20%; fatigue — 44%; gastrointestinal symptoms — 28%; headache — 32%; and respiratory symptoms — 24%. Further examination revealed neurologic changes in 28% of the workers, signs indicating autonomic nervous system impairment in 36% of the workers, and mild or moderate psycho organic syndrome in 34% of the workers. Urinary trichloroacetic acid ranged from 8 to 144 mg/ml (with a mean of 86.7 mg/ml). The relationship between trichloroacetic acid excretion and exposure was linear. The ratio of trichloroacetic acid excretion to exposure was in the range of 4:1 to 2:1, with the higher values in the younger workers.

Various neurologic symptoms were found in studies of workers carried out in the 1980s (Barrett, 1987; Landrigan, 1987). Reports of impairment of cranial nerves, particularly the fifth, encouraged a number of studies investigating trigeminal somatosensory evoked potentials (TSEP). Barrett investigated 104 degreasers, aged from 18 to 62 years (with a mean of 41.6 years), who were chronically exposed to TCE (Barrett, 1987). Exposure durations ranged from 1 to 28 years (with a mean of 8.23 years) at an average daily exposure of 7 hours. Fifty-two healthy non-exposed individuals served as the control group. Trigeminal nerve symptoms were seen in 18 workers (17.3%). Workers with trigeminal symptoms tended to be older than those who were symptom-free. However, they did not differ in excretion of urinary trichloroethanol and trichloroacetic acid. Forty workers (38.4%) demonstrated abnormal TSEPs with an increase in latency or amplitude. Abnormal trigeminal function was found in 6 of 64 workers with normal TSEPs. If latencies only are considered, the specificity and sensitivity of the tests were 79% and 50% respectively, an indication that this test may be suitable for screening. One or more of the following symptoms were present in half of the workers: asthenia, dizziness, headache, and some neuropsychiatric manifestations.

Landrigan investigated degreasers exposed to TCE at a TWA of 117 to 357 mg/m^3 (Landrigan, 1987). However, peak values over 5 to 15 minutes were 413 to 2000 mg/m^3. Acute symptoms were seen in 77.8% of the workers investigated. Those with the highest exposure had a mean of 4.25 symptoms. After conditions at the plant were improved, resulting in lower TWAs, the mean declined to 1.5 symptoms. Fatigue and sleepiness persisted, however. Mean urinary trichloroacetic acid excretion went down from 500 mg/l to less than 100 mg/l at the end of the workday, also after the improvement of work conditions.

Exposure levels for 31 workers in a printing plant who had been exposed to TCE for a mean duration of 16 years fell as conditions were improved over the years, but remained at a range of 17 to 70 ppm. Workers exhibited a minor slowing of sensory nerve conduction velocity and increased latency of the masseter reflex. Other parameters, including motor conduction velocity, blink reflex latency, and autonomic nerve tests, were normal. However, in a study of 31 workers exposed to TCE for a mean duration of 7 years, Triebig found no difference between the exposed workers and controls in their motor or sensory conduction velocities (Triebig, 1982).

§ 7-5(a)(5). Pharmacokinetics and Metabolism.

Trichloroethylene most often enters the body through inhalation. Exercise has a profound effect on the alveolar and blood concentrations resulting from exposure to TCE. Åstrand and Övrum exposed 15 young males (ranging in age from 22 to 29 years) to TCE air concentrations of 100 and 200 ppm at rest and during light, moderate, and heavy exercise (Åstrand, 1976). Four successive 30-minute exposure sessions were carried out a day. An exposure of 100 ppm (540 mg/m^3) at rest resulted in an alveolar concentration of about 125 mg/m^3, an arterial blood concentration of about 1.2 mg/kg, and a venous blood concentration of 0.6 mg/kg. The relationship between alveolar and blood concentrations of TCE was linear. The relatively high alveolar concentration, which increased with work, may have been due to the poor solubility of TCE in blood. With light work, the alveolar concentration almost doubled, and the arterial concentration more than doubled. At rest, the uptake was 53% of the administered dose. With light work, the uptake decreased to 40% of the administered dose. However, the absolute amount taken up rose after 30 minutes of exposure, and declined further at 90 minutes of exposure. Heavy exercise was associated with a decline in percentage uptake to 25%.

Although TCE can cause dermatitis on prolonged contact, absorption through the skin does not result in significant systemic uptake. In a study carried out by Stewart and Dodd, the thumb was immersed in liquid TCE for 30 minutes (Stewart, 1964). The resulting peak concentration in breath was 0.5%.

With low-temperature radiography, Bergman demonstrated that a very high concentration of TCE was attained in a rat brain immediately after a 10-minute inhalation (Bergman, 1979). After 30 minutes, however, only TCE concentration in the brain was obtained. After eight hours, however, TCE was still detectable, and the highest levels were found in the liver. Savolainen found high concentrations in perineal fat, and concentrations in several organs that exceeded blood levels (Savolainen, 1977).

Approximately 75% of absorbed TCE is metabolized. Absorbed TCE may be oxidized to epoxide, which is converted to chloral hydrate, which is reduced in turn to trichloroethanol by liver dehydrogenase. Chloral hydrate may also be oxidized to trichloroacetic acid by chloral hydrate dehydrogenase. Both trichloroacetic acid and trichloroethanol are excreted in the urine. Trichloroethanol is conjugated with glucoronic acid (Bartonicek, 1962).

Some data suggest that TCE and trichloroethanol accumulate in tissue and are slowly released. Müller found that following intake of trichloroethanol, trichloroacetic acid, or chloral hydrate, the decline in concentration of trichloroethanol in the blood ran parallel to the other chemicals (Müller, 1974). The half-life for trichloroethanol was approximately 100 hours following intake of TCE, 65 hours following intake of chloral hydrate and trichloroethanol, and 50 hours following intake of trichloroacetic acid.

Because of the long-lasting excretion of the metabolites of TCE, the amount of TCE taken up and exhaled unchanged is difficult to evaluate in any great detail. Data suggest that the amount of exhaled, unchanged TCE depends on the exposure.

There is controversy over the value of urinary excretion of trichloro compounds for biological monitoring. Great interpersonal variations in urinary excretion have been observed. Some investigators have found a good correlation between exposure and excretion of trichloroethanol or trichloroacetic acid. Inoue used a diffuse sampling method to evaluate the TWA. The metabolite level in urine collected at the end of a shift was measured in 140 workers exposed to TCE and in

114 non-exposed control subjects. A linear correlation was found between exposure and the urinary excretion of TCE, trichloroethanol, and trichloroacetic acid, and total excreted trichloro compounds. Stewart, however, found no correlation (Stewart, 1970).

§ 7-5(b). Benzene.

Empirical formula:	C_6H_6.
Description:	Clear, volatile flammable liquid.
Synonyms:	Benzol, phenyl hydride, cyclohexatrine.
Uses:	Rubber processing, munitions, dyes, leather.
Air Limit:	10 ppm.
Water Limit:	Fresh water: 5300 μg/L; salt water: 5100 μg/L; to protect human health: preferably zero.

Although its use has been curtailed because of its toxic reactions, benzene is still used in many industrial processes. It is utilized in the production of motor fuels, rubber, dyes, leather, munitions, and electric fittings. Workers in chemistry laboratories and coal tar distilleries can be at risk of exposure to benzene. Acute intoxication has occurred in workers cleaning or repairing benzene tanks. Excessive inhalation is often associated with a euphoria and alcohol-like intoxication frequently accompanied by drowsiness, giddiness, ataxic gait, tinnitus, headache, sensations of tightness in the chest, nausea and vomiting. Severe intoxication may be associated with muscular twitching, followed by convulsive seizures, paralysis, and loss of consciousness. In cases of very severe intoxication there may be an immediate loss of consciousness followed by fatal respiratory failure. In patients who survive the acute effects of benzene, recovery is usually complete, although some symptoms such as headache, chest pain, shortness of breath, anorexia, nausea, and vomiting may persist for a short period (Goetz, 1985).

§ 7-5(b)(1). Exposure Limits.

In mid-1978, NIOSH recommended adherence to an existing federal standard of 10 ppm (30 mg/m^3) as a time-weighted average, with a ceiling of 25 ppm.

§ 7-5(b)(2). Neurotoxic Effects.

Central and peripheral nervous system damage has been observed in patients exposed to benzene. Pyramidal tract involvement, paresthesia, hypesthesia, paraplegia, retrobulbar neuritis, median nerve lesions and convulsive disorders have been observed in association with benzene exposure and with the use of benzene as therapy for leukemia. Benzene is only rarely used for leukemia therapy today (Goetz, 1985). Peripheral neuropathy possibly associated with benzene has been studied extensively. Since toluene is often mixed with benzene in industrial processes, it is often difficult to determine which solvent may be the causative factor. In one study, leather workers exposed to benzene demonstrated slowed conductance velocities, and other signs of denervation and clinical atrophy (Baslo, 1982). Animal studies have shown that both acute and chronic benzene intoxication alter the gamma-aminobutyric acid (GABA) system. GABA levels can increase to 5 to 6 times the normal level in the cerebellum and pons. With prolonged exposure, however, GABA levels return toward normal.

§ 7-5(b)(3). Metabolism of Benzene.

Low molecular weight organic chemicals that volatilize at room temperature are called volatile organic compounds. Benzene is one such compound. There are hundreds of other volatile organic compounds. Only a few, such as the aromatics, aliphatics, and the chlorinated aliphatics, are of sufficient importance to mention.

The most widespread aromatics are benzene, toluene and xylene. These are referred to collectively as BTX and are used as solvents and degreasers. Most non-essential uses of benzene have been curtailed in industrial countries. Depending on its source, there may be trace amounts of benzene in toluene, and to a lesser extent in xylene. The level of this contamination has been reduced with improved manufacturing quality control. BTX are acutely neurotoxic at high doses. Headaches and lightheadedness are the earliest signs of exposure, followed by confusion, seizures, coma and death. BTX are readily absorbed by the lungs, intestine and skin. The skin serves as a target organ and becomes defatting. A chronic dermatitis develops in exposed workers. Exposure in the home and community may occur when high levels of solvent vapors are inhaled during showering with contaminated water. Homes may also be contaminated (especially basements) from leaking underground storage tanks. The extent of benzene toxicity in the workplace is dependent on many factors, but ultimately the air concentration of benzene is the single most important factor. Other factors are duration of exposure and the nature of the job. At low concentrations, benzene may be detected because of its odor. As the concentration increases, itching and tingling are sensed, followed by irritability, headache and behavioral changes (Molhave, 1992). Benzene is metabolized differently from toluene and xylene, with which it shares acute neurotoxic properties, acting as a central nervous system depressant.

Benzene is used for many purposes in chemical synthesis, but primarily for the production of polystyrene plastics. Many other industries use benzene as a starting substance for chemical production. Benzene continues to play a major role as a solvent on a worldwide basis, although there are other less toxic solvents available. Benzene is the simplest aromatic and the most carcinogenic. Liver and kidney toxicity is not a prominent finding, but leukemia is. Do not confuse it with benzine, which is a mixture of organic solvents containing little benzene. The word "benzine" is used interchangeably with the word "gasoline" in some foreign countries.

For the average citizen, the two most common means of exposure are adding gasoline to fuel tanks and smoking cigarettes. Recent pre-clinical studies suggest that smoking during pregnancy is linked to increased rates of attention deficit hyperactivity disorder (ADHD) in male offspring. It is possible that the presence of benzene in the inhaled smoke is a contributing factor to the neurobehavioral difficulties in the children. The association of benzene and aplastic anemia was established at the beginning of this century (Santesson 1897; Selling, 1917). An important factor to consider is individual susceptibility. It is not possible to predict which individuals will be susceptible to aplastic anemia or leukemia. Studies are underway to develop biomarkers to identify individuals at risk.

The mechanism by which benzene produces bone marrow suppression is complex. It involves several metabolites of benzene, their transport from liver to bone marrow, and further metabolism in more than one target in the bone marrow. Benzene is converted to benzene oxide, which is in equilibrium with its oxepin. Cytochrome P450 2E1 appears to be most active in catalyzing this reaction. Further metabolism of benzene occurs, yielding phenol, which can be further hydroxilated to hydroquinone and catechol. Further hydroxylation may yield 1,2,4-trihydroxy benzene. The phenolic compounds may be conjugated with etheral sulfate or acid. The resulting glucoronic acid detoxifies the benzene from the body. Other metabolites that may be formed from benzene via the epoxide-oxepin pathway are premercapturic acid (which results from the conjugation of glutathione with the epoxide) and benzene dihydrodiol (which is mediated by the enzyme epoxide hydrolase). It appears that the mechanism by which benzene produces aplastic anemia involves inhibition of stem cell and early blast cell maturation (Brooks, 1995; Ballantyne, 1993).

§ 7-5(c). Toluene.

Empirical formula:	$C_6H_5CH_3$.
Description:	Clear, colorless, non-corrosive liquid with a sweet, pungent, benzene-like odor.
Synonyms:	Toluol, methylbenzene, phenylmethane, methylbenzol.
Uses:	Used in the manufacture of benzene and as a chemical feed for toluene disocyanate, phenol benzyl and benzyl derivatives, benzoic acid, toluene sulfonates, nitrotoluenes, vinyltoluene, and saccharin. Also used as a solvent for paints and coatings, and as a component of automobile and aviation fuels.
Air Limit:	200 ppm.
Water Limit:	No adverse level in drinking water has been established.

One of the most widely used organic solvents, toluene is an ingredient of paint and lacquer thinners, cleaning agents, dyes, and engine fuels. It is also a constituent of many of the glues associated with the neurotoxic syndrome seen in glue sniffers. Glue sniffing can result in psychotic behavior, unconsciousness, and death. (Winck, 1968). Toluene is used in many histological procedures, and workers in histology laboratories may be at risk of exposure. Its toxic effects are similar to those of benzene (Barnes, 1979).

§ 7-5(c)(1). Exposure Limits.

The United States standard is 200 ppm as an 8-hour TWA, with an acceptable ceiling concentration of 300 ppm. Maximum peaks above the 500 ppm ceiling are allowed for10 minutes. NIOSH has recommended a TWA limit of 100 ppm, with a ceiling of 200 ppm for a 10-minute sampling period. ACGIH recommends a TWA of 100 ppm and a STEL of 150 ppm.

§ 7-5(c)(2). Neurotoxic Effects.

Signs of neurologic effects occur after exposure to as little as 200 ppm. At exposures of 800 ppm, signs and symptoms may persist for several days. Early exhilaration occurs with acute exposure, followed by dizziness, ataxia, mild confusion, and fatigue. Chronic exposure has been associated with tremor, unsteadiness, emotional lability, jaw jerk and other primitive reflexes, as well as cerebellar ataxia with and without optic nerve dysfunction (Keane, 1978; Takeuchi, 1981). The acute effects of inhaling toluene are generally reversible. However, the acute effects may be an early sign of central nervous system impairment, which could lead to irreversible losses (Åstrand, 1972; Gamberale, 1972 via Echeverria, 1989). Results of studies of the neurobehavioral effects of inhaling toluene have been mixed. In a study of volunteers, it was found that inhaling toluene at 100 ppm had adverse effects on some aspects of memory and visual perception, but had little effect on most psychomotor skills.

Evidence of permanent central nervous system damage has been obtained with magnetic resonance imaging (MRI).

§ 7-5(c)(3). Acute Effects.

Studies involving controlled exposure have provided data on the acute effects of toluene. In a study by Andersen, 16 healthy volunteers aged 21 to 32 years (with a mean of 24 years) were exposed to toluene at concentrations of 0, 10, 40, and 100 ppm (Andersen, 1983). During the first hour in the exposure chamber, the subjects were not exposed to toluene. For the next 7 hours the subjects were subjected to exposure at the levels specified in the investigation. Various performance tests were carried out before exposure and at 2 and 5 hours following exposure, except for word memory which was done prior to and at the end of the 7-hour exposure period. Included in the test battery were the Bourdon-Wiersma test, five-choice serial reaction time (concentration, vigilance, aiming), Landolt's ring test (visual acuity and perception), multiplication test, rotatory pursuit test (eye-hand coordination), screw-plate test (eye-finger coordination), and word memory. Eye irritation was reported by about 50% of the subjects. A weak correlation was found between toluene exposure and performance on the screw-plate test, Landolt's ring test, and the multiplication test. However, the subjects reported that the tasks seemed to be more strenuous. A few subjects experienced prolonged reaction time at 100 ppm. All subjects were able to smell toluene, but adaptation occurred. The study design did not take into account possible accumulation effects. Also the tests were carried out at rest, perhaps minimizing neurotoxic effects, instead of at various work levels which might have doubled or tripled intake, thereby increasing neurotoxic effects.

Another test with volunteers was carried out by Gamberale and Hultengren (Gamberale, 1972). This test exposed 12 healthy male volunteers, 20 to 35 years old, to 100, 300, 500, and 700 ppm toluene for 20 minutes at each exposure. Several performance tests were used. Two tests (identical numbers, spokes) measured perceptual speed, and two others (simple and choice) measured visual reaction time. An improvement in reaction time due to training, which was seen in the control, was not evident during exposure to toluene. At the higher exposure levels, reaction times were prolonged. Reaction time prolongation was significant at 300 ppm. A training effect in perceptual tasks also declined during exposure to toluene. Significant slowing of perceptual speed was not seen until 700 ppm exposure.

Echeverria conducted a study utilizing 42 volunteers, aged 18 to 35 years (with a mean of 22.5 years), who were exposed to 0, 75, and 150 ppm for 7 hours over 3 days (Echeverria, 1989). A battery of computer-administered tests were used, including verbal memory, verbal ability, visual memory, perception, visuomotor response, manual dexterity, fatigue and mood profile. At 150 ppm, results included decreases of 6% in digit span, 9.4% in pattern memory, and 6.5% for both the pin number and moving pins phases of the manual dexterity test. Pattern recognition increased in latency by 12.1%. At 75 ppm, most test performances were also reduced, but to a lesser extent. Headache, mucosal irritation, and other symptoms increased in a dose-dependent manner. In general, the test results suggest that neurotoxic effects associated with toluene begin to occur at about the exposure limits specified in the United States and Europe.

In a study conducted by Dick, 144 volunteers aged 18 to 38 years were exposed to toluene 100 ppm for 4 hours at rest (Dick, 1984). Tests included choice reaction time, visual-vigilance task, and pattern recognition task. Significant impairment in hits for the visual-vigilance task were seen after a 2-hour exposure. During the last hours of exposure, however, the impairment was not significant. Choice reaction time was not affected, and changes in pattern recognition were not significant. These adverse effects may have been more severe with exercise.

In a study of 8 volunteers, Cherry investigated the effects of toluene on simple visual reaction time, choice reaction time, visual search, and subject-paced tracking task (Cherry, 1983). While toluene had no significant effects on these tests, when alcohol was administered concomitantly with toluene there was a significant trend toward poorer performance than with alcohol alone. Iregren, however, found no evidence of enhanced effects with combined alcohol/toluene administration (Iregren, 1986). The subjects were 12 healthy volunteers exposed to 300 mg/m^3 by inhalation for 4.5 hours, 15 mmol/kg of body weight of ethanol, or to a combination of both. While inhalation of toluene was associated with headache, irritability, and a slight narcotic effect on heart rate, no effect on test performance (simple reaction time, choice reaction time, color-word vigilance, memory reproduction) was observed. Ethanol alone increased heart rate and had a negative effect on test performance.

Hydén carried out a study in which exercise was a factor (Hydén, 1983). Fifteen healthy volunteers were exposed to toluene at concentrations from 103 to 148 ppm for 70 minutes. Light exercise was done during part of the exposure time. A vestibulooculomotor test battery was administered, measuring visual-vestibular interaction. The results indicated impaired visual suppression of vestibular nystagmus, suggesting an altered function of the brainstem and/or cerebellum.

§ 7-5(c)(4). Abuse.

Investigation of the abuse of toluene has provided useful information on the acute, subchronic, and chronic neurotoxic effects of toluene. Grabski described a 21-year-old man who had been a long-term toluene abuser (Grabski, 1961). The patient demonstrated overt signs of cerebellar dysfunction. Five years later, in a follow-up study of the patient, who had continued his abuse of toluene, it was found that he had increasing tremor, unsteady movements, and impaired memory. Roentgenographic studies showed central and cortical atrophy, particularly in the frontal area (Knox, 1966).

Hormes carried out a study of 20 patients who had abused solvents, primarily toluene, for at least 2 years (Hormes, 1986). Thirteen had neurological impairments, including pyramidal, cognitive, cerebellar and brainstem/cranial nerve abnormalities.

Rosenberg carried out a study of 11 individuals who had abused various solvents, 60% of which contained toluene as the main component (Rosenberg, 1988). The average daily toluene consumption was calculated to be 350 mg. Rosenberg found that several of the patients had cognitive impairment, cerebellar dysfunction, and prolonged latencies of late components of brainstem auditory evoked response. Magnetic resonance imaging (MRI) revealed cerebral atrophy and loss of gray-white matter demarcation.

Chronic depression has been reported in glue sniffers. In an investigation of 27 young glue sniffers by Massengale, chronic depression was found in several patients (Massengale, 1963). Sniffing was apparently reducing anxiety in several patients. However, neuropsychological examination of 16 patients revealed no decline in performance compared with controls.

Fornazzari investigated a group of solvent abusers with a history of abuse of about a year (Fornazzari, 1983). They were acutely intoxicated the day they presented. Six patients had cranial nerve impairment, 5 had impairment of short-term memory, and 11 had cerebellar dysfunction. Patients found to be impaired at the clinical neurological examination demonstrated poor performance in the psychological test battery. Computerized tomography (CT) revealed that these patients had more atrophy of the cerebellum. On reexamination, little improvement was seen in neurological findings or in test results. Fourteen patients had a total daily toluene consumption of 425 mg/day, 9 consumed 160 mg/day, and 1 used 200 mg/day. However, there was no clear correlation between consumption and functional or morphological scores.

Rosenberg reported on 7 individuals who had abused solvents, mainly toluene, at about 350 mg/day, for an average duration of 168 months (Rosenberg, 1988). On examination by a neuropsychologist, 6 scored in the dementia range. Neurological examination of all 7 patients revealed cerebellar dysfunction in 6, and 4 had spasticity. One patient died, apparently from the solvent abuse, but the brain appeared only mildly to moderately abnormal and was without neuronal loss or gliosis. MRI showed increased signal density periventricularly on T_2-weighted images, and indication of increased water content in the white matter. Also shown on MRI were diffuse cortical, cerebral, and cerebellar atrophy, and loss of differentiation between gray and white matter.

Impairments of various parts of the nervous system have been reported in association with toluene abuse. Axonal type neuropathy associated with toluene was first reported in 1974 by Shirabe (Shirabe, 1974). See Table 7.2 for a summary of reported nervous system impairments.

Table 7.2
Nervous System Impairments Associated with Toluene

Impairment	Reference
Equilibrium disorders with diffuse brain atrophy	Sasa, 1978
Optic neuropathy with cerebellar dysfunction	Keane, 1978
Optic neuropathy with sensorineural hearing loss	Ehyai, 1983
Abnormal brainstem auditory evoked potentials with pontomedullary potentials	Metrick, 1982
Long-lasting visual hallucinations	Channer, 1983
Subclinical sensory neuropathy	Ehyai, 1983
Status epilepticus	Allister, 1981
Respiratory arrest	Cronk, 1985
Schizophrenic type disorder	Tarsh, 1979; Weisenberger, 1977
Death	Edh, 1973; Bass, 1970; Ramsey, 1989 (207)

In some investigations, no association between toluene and neurotoxic effects was detected, or patients recovered. In a study of young glue sniffers, no significant differences were found in test performances between the sniffers and the controls. However, a study by Mahmood revealed that, over a period of toluene abuse of 6 years, an 18-year-old girl developed ataxia, spontaneous nystagmus, pyramidal signs, visual impairment, and cognitive dysfunction. With abstinence, she improved and eventually recovered. Another investigation of 28 young patients with a history of solvent abuse from 3 to 18 months also revealed no difference from controls in potential abilities (Mahmood, 1983). However, their performance was poorer in tests of acquired abilities. King investigated a group of 10 patients aged 8 to 14 years who had been referred because of various symptoms, including euphoria, hallucinations, ataxia, convulsions, diplopia, behavioral changes, and coma (King, 1981). Thirteen of the patients improved.

§ 7-5(c)(5). Chronic Effects.

Several cross-sectional studies and evaluations of the health of workers have provided information on the chronic effects of exposure to toluene. Matushita investigated the health conditions of 38 female workers exposed to toluene-containing glues used in the manufacture of shoes (Matushita, 1975). Controls were 16 female workers employed in the same plant, but who were not exposed. The average duration of exposure was 3.5 years. Mean toluene concentrations ranged from 60 to 100 ppm. The exposed workers complained of hand dermatitis, itching, general weakness, and dysmenorrhea. They also expressed an uneasiness over exposure to toluene. Clinical neurological examination revealed reduced gripping power of the hands, and decreased agility and tapping tempo.

Workers in rotogravure printing plants are at risk of long-range exposure to toluene. Larsen studied 22 male rotogravure workers (Larsen, 1988). The ages of the men ranged from 35 to 65 years (with a mean of 44.7), and the mean duration of exposure was 12 years. An organic effective syndrome was found in 7 workers, and signs of mild chronic encephalopathy were observed in 6. No abnormalities were found in the other workers.

In a study by Ørbæk and Nise, 30 male rotogravure workers were investigated for possible neurotoxic effects in association with toluene (Ørbæk, 1989). The median duration of exposure was 29 years, and the average age was 50 years. At the time of investigation, the exposure to toluene was 42 mg/m^3 (TWA) in one plant and 157 mg/m^3 in another. During cleaning operations, however, peaks of 760 mg/m^3 were measured. After a 66-hour period of non-exposure, the blood concentration of toluene was measured on a Monday morning. Blood levels of toluene ranged from less than 0.05 to 0.65 μmol/l (with a median of 0.08 μmol/l). Among the symptoms most frequently reported by the printers were neurasthenic symptoms, including fatigue (60%), impaired memory (60%), impaired concentration ability (40%), irritability (37%), headaches (30%), depression (20%), paresthesia (53%), and mood lability (27%). While paresthesia was reported by more than half of the workers, only 3 showed clinical signs of polyneuropathy. In testing, lower scores were produced by exposed workers in Benton visual retention, synonyms, and in digit symbol. In other tests, no differences were found between exposed workers and controls except for a hand motor test in which exposed workers had higher scores than did controls.

Iregren investigated 34 rotogravure printers with an average exposure time of 16.3 years (Iregren, 1982). They were compared with workers (automobile and industrial spray painters) from an earlier study (Elofsson, 1980) who were exposed to a mixture of solvents. Reaction time in the rotogravure workers was significantly poorer than in the controls. This effect may have been due, in part, to toluene intoxication.

In another study, rotogravure printers had been exposed to solvents, mostly toluene, for a mean duration of 22 years. The level of exposure was approximately 100 ppm, except for the last few years when exposure dropped to about 78 ppm. When the presses were washed, however, the exposure level was quite high. The offset printers had experienced occasional exposure to solvents, primarily isopropyl alcohol, ethyl acetate, and aliphatic hydrocarbons, rather than toluene. The incidence of memory disturbances was significantly higher in the rotogravure printers. However, the offset printers had significantly higher neuropathy scores, more sulcus widening, particularly in the temporal and occipital regions, and larger supravermian cisterns. Psychological test results were slightly abnormal in both groups. The rotogravure printers' visual memory, visual intelligence and eye-hand coordination showed some slight abnormalities. Parameters taken into account in this study included alcohol consumption, autonomic nervous system screening, and results of EEG and neuropsychological examinations. High exposure to toluene was associated with poor performance in visual cognitive functions. High alcohol consumption and toluene exposure, however, were associated with intact performances. These results suggest that inhaled toluene and ingested alcohol may interact in an antagonistic manner. Among the workers exposed to toluene, 42% were heavy drinkers, compared with 3% of the offset printers.

Other workers exposed to toluene include those in the paint, flooring, and adhesive industries. Winchester and Madjan investigated 42 workers, with a mean age of 31.5 years, employed in the paint, adhesive, and printing industries (Winchester, 1986). The workers were exposed to low levels of solvents, mainly toluene, for an average of 6.8 years. Among the more common complaints were headache, eye irritation, nausea, respiratory symptoms, light-headedness, and dizziness. About 31% of the workers believed their general health had deteriorated during their yeas of employment. Other problems associated with solvent exposure included impaired memory and concentration, and slowed reaction times. Slow reaction times were particularly prevalent among younger workers who had greater exposure (80 ppm) than the older workers (40 ppm). Average blood toluene was 0.15 μg/ml. Urinary hippuric acid excretion was 1900 mg/ml compared to 1050 mg/ml in controls.

Ekberg investigated floorers, with an age-matched group of carpenters as a control (Ekberg, 1986). Some floorers had average exposure times of 20 years (high) while others had exposure times of 5 to 10 years (low). Workers with high exposure had a higher rate of depression and poor performance in the visuospatial block test. Workers with low exposure times did poorly in the psychomotor bolt test. Impairment of perceptual functions was associated with exposure to adhesives containing benzene, acetone, and xylene, as well as toluene.

Exposure to glues containing alcohol was associated with visuoanalytical impairment.

Evoked potentials have been used to assess the long-term effects of exposure to toluene. RCA investigated 49 workers employed in a printing plant where toluene had been used as the only organic solvent for more than 30 years (RCA, 1995). The mean length of employment was 21.4 years. Fifty-nine unexposed workers served as a control. N75, P100, and N145 waves of the pattern reversal evoked potentials were analyzed. In the workers exposed to toluene, significantly greater amplitudes were found in all waves, with significantly longer latency of the P100 wave.

Abbate used electrophysiologic techniques to investigate the effects of toluene exposure on the auditory function of 300 rotogravure printers (Abbate, 1993). Forty workers with apparently normal hearing ability were selected from this group for testing. They were examined by means of an adaptation test utilizing the brainstem auditory evoked potential technique with 11 and 90 stimulus repetitions a second. The investigators demonstrated that toluene is able to induce a significant alteration in the electric responses with both 11 and 90 stimulus repetitions. The alteration constitutes an exposure-induced modification of physiologic stimulus conduction mechanisms occurring in the absence of any clinical sign of neuropathy. The modification was observed in the electric responses of the entire auditory system, from peripheral receptors to brainstem nuclei.

§ 7-5(c)(6). Pharmacokinetics and Metabolism.

The lungs and gastrointestinal systems are the major routes of toluene uptake. Skin has a relatively minor role, but under certain conditions it may contribute substantially to total uptake (Sato, 1978). Total uptake is dependent on several factors, including respiratory volume, air concentration, exposure time, blood/air partition coefficient, blood transport, tissue solubility, and metabolic rate (Fiserova-Bergerova, 1985).

Toluene can be detected in blood 10 minutes after exposure. Blood level increases rapidly for 10 to 15 minutes after exposure and reaches a plateau in about 25 minutes (Åstrand, 1972). Wallén found that after a 30-minute exposure to 100 ppm at rest, the concentration of toluene in arterial blood was about 1 ppm; at 200 ppm it was 2.7 ppm (Wallén, 1986). Light work more than doubled the concentration in the same time period and delayed the leveling off. In this study, however, there was no difference in blood levels between workers with and without symptoms.

Absorption from the gastrointestinal tract is almost complete, but maximal blood levels are attained more slowly than after inhalation (Pyykkö, 1977).

Factors influencing the distribution of toluene to various tissues include partition coefficients (tissue/blood), perfusion, duration of exposure, and rate of elimination. Since perfusion in the brain is quite high, brain lipid receives large amounts of toluene. In the case of a worker who was acutely exposed in a confined space and died, the blood concentration of toluene was 48 μg/g, the liver concentration was 65 μg/g, and the brain concentration was 80 μg/g (Takeichi, 1986). It is possible that subcutaneous fat may act as a reservoir for toluene. Pyykkö found that concentration in fat continued to increase a full hour after cessation of exposure (Pyykkö, 1977). Carlsson found that after a 2-hour exposure to 80 ppm at rest, the subcutaneous fat concentration was 0.7 mg/kg, increasing to 9.9 mg/kg when light work was carried out (Carlsson, 1982). In this study, the half-life in adipose tissue was determined to be 0.5 to 2.7 days.

Toluene is metabolized in the liver to benzoic acid (about 80%) by side-chain oxidation via benzyl alcohol and benzaldehyde. Benzoic acid, almost completely conjugated with glycine, is excreted as hippuric acid in the urine. A small amount of benzoic acid is conjugated with glucuronic acid to benzoylglucuronide and excreted in the urine. About 1% is excreted as cresols (Bakke, 1970). There may be ethnic differences in the metabolism of toluene resulting in different amounts of cresol and hippuric acid excreted in the urine (Inoue, 1986).

The urinary excretion of hippuric acid is recommended as a marker of toluene exposure by the World Health Organization (WHO, 1981) and the American Conference of Governmental Industrial Hygienists (ACGIH, 1984). However, because of the possible ethnic differences in hippuric acid excretion, and because of interference by concomitant exposure to other compounds such as styrene, etylebenzene, and benzoic acid, the accuracy of the hippuric acid marker may not be consistent, particularly at low exposure levels (Wilczok, 1978). The excretion of *o*-cresol has been suggested as more specific than that of hippuric acid as a marker. However, it is recognized that *o*-cresol excretion is influenced by sex, body size, age, and use of alcohol and tobacco (Bælum, 1987).

§ 7-5(d). N-hexane.

Empirical Formula:	C_6H_{14}.
Description:	Clear, colorless liquid.
Uses:	Used for oil seed extraction, rubber processing, component of glues, solvent in paints, lacquers, printing ink.
Air Limit:	In the United States the threshold limit is 100 ppm.
Water Limit:	No values set.

When *n*-hexane was first used, it was thought to be harmless. In recent years, however, *n*-hexane has been identified as a significant neurotoxin. Among the more frequent applications of this compound are the extraction of vegetable oils and the printing of laminated products. It is also a component of glues and has become a source of inhalant abuse. Acute exposure, such as occurs with inhalant abuse, induces a euphoric effect, while chronic exposure is associated with pronounced peripheral neuropathy. Many glues contain both toluene and *n*-hexane, and it was not until sniffers started to use glues containing *n*-hexane only that its abuse potential was realized (Towfighi, 1976).

§ 7-5(d)(1). Exposure Limits.

The United States standard is 500 ppm. NIOSH has recommended a TWA of 100 ppm with a 510 ppm ceiling value for 15 minutes exposure. ACGIH (1983/84) proposed a TWA of 50 ppm. N-hexane has been associated with neurologic disease at levels ranging from 20 to 240 ppm. (Goetz, 1985).

§ 7-5(d)(2). Neurotoxicity.

N-hexane apparently does not induce significant signs of encephalopathy. Signs of central nervous system disturbances, such as seizures and significant delirium, are not usually associated with *n*-hexane (Spencer, 1980). Peripheral neuropathy is the nervous system disease most often associated with *n*-hexane. Gradual onset of distal paresthesia and weakness with or without ataxia, often accompanied by weight loss, may suggest toxicity in a patient exposed to *n*-hexane. Spasticity, a sign of upper motor neuron damage, may also occur. Symmetric sensory dysfunction in the hands and feet is a frequent presenting complaint. On examination, pin, vibratory, and thermal sensation are under-active. As the neuropathy progresses, atrophy and weakness may extend from the distal areas proximally. In later stages of the disease, there may be loss of reflexes in the ankles. The disease may develop more rapidly in glue sniffers. While cranial neuropathies are rare, abnormal color vision associated with macula damage has been reported (Prockop, 1974).

Although the neuropathy is predominantly axonal, nerve conduction studies have shown a marked slowing of velocity attributable to the demyelination that occurs with the early swelling of the affected axons. The slowing increases with the intensity of the disease, and in extreme cases, no conduction can be detected (Goetz, 1985). Also seen are symmetric distal fibrillation potentials and positive waves with reduced amplitude of muscle action potentials (Goetz, 1985).

The axonal transport dysfunction seen in association with *n*-hexane neurotoxicity may be due to the actions of 2,5,-hexanedione, a metabolite of *n*-hexane. This metabolite appears to bond with glycolytic enzymes in the nerve fiber, inducing a dose-dependent inhibition of enzyme activity along the length of the fiber. The most distal regions of the axons become enzyme deficient first, with consequent dysfunction of distal axonal transport and nerve fiber degeneration (Spencer, 1980, via Goetz, 1985).

The only treatment for *n*-hexane neuropathy is removal from the source of exposure. Supportive treatment such as steroids and large doses of B-complex vitamins have not been effective. Upon removal from exposure to *n*-hexane, recovery occurs over a period of several weeks. However, transient exacerbation of symptoms may also occur over a period of weeks.

§ 7-5(d)(3). Acute Effects.

Much of what is known about the acute and chronic effects of *n*-hexane has come from examination of abusers, mainly glue sniffers. The first reports of polyneuropathy associated with glue sniffing emerged in the 1970s. Early descriptions of the symptoms associated with the neurotoxic effects of *n*-hexane indicated long-term impairment of the PNS (Gonzales, 1972; Matsumura, 1974; Korobkin, 1975; Shirabe, 1974). Korobkin described a 29-year-old man who had been sniffing vapor from contact cement for 5 years (Korobkin, 1975). The man switched to sniffing another product, and a few months later showed increasing signs and symptoms of polyneuropathy including weakness and ankle atrophy which was more severe distally, peripheral sensory loss, reduced motor nerve conduction velocities, particularly distally, and low amplitude sensory action potentials. He also experienced transiently blurred vision. Tendon reflexes were preserved except for ankle jerks. Neurogenic changes were detected with electromyography. It was determined that the new product contained *n*-hexane. When the man went back to the old product, the symptoms resulting from the new product persisted for a few months and then began to subside. However, the man developed hyperactive tendon reflex and spasticity in the legs. Biopsy of the radial cutaneous nerve showed periodic discontinuous axonal swellings with thinning of the overlying myelin sheaths and patchy demyelination. Electron microscopy showed densely packed whorled masses of neurofilaments.

Other signs and symptoms described by investigators in association with *n*-hexane abuse include sensorimotor neuropathy, reduced conduction velocity, impaired mental function (Towfighi, 1976), paresis, severe muscle atrophy and paresthesias in the feet, ascending to the legs (Altenkirch, 1977). Biopsy findings include focal enlargements of axons with widening at the nodes of Ranvier, fragmentation of myelin, focal thinning, retraction of paranodal myelin, accumulation of neurofilaments in axons, Wallerian-like degeneration (Towfighi, 1976), paranodal axonal swelling with retracted myelin sheaths, and accumulation of neurofilaments in the axons (Altenkirch, 1977).

The general pattern that emerges after cessation of the abuse is slow improvement, but often with periodic recurrence of symptoms, and, in some cases, appearance of new symptoms. Motor nerve conduction velocities improve, but in many cases never return to pre-abuse levels (Korobkin, 1975).

§ 7-5(d)(4). Chronic Effects.

The first report in the United States describing neuropathy associated with long-term occupational exposure to *n*-hexane was published in 1971 (Herskowitz, 1971). It described the development of neuropathy in 3 workers in a furniture factory working in *n*-hexane air concentrations averaging 650 ppm with peaks of 1300 ppm. After 2 to 4 months of exposure, all 3 workers developed symmetrical distal sensory-motor polyneuropathy with reduced nerve conduction velocities, and fibrillations in EMG. Biopsy findings included a mixture of demyelination and axonal degeneration.

Huang studied 4 patients who had been exposed to *n*-hexane in a ball-manufacturing factory (Huang, 1989). Air concentrations of *n*-hexane in the poorly ventilated facility averaged 109 ppm. The duration of exposure for each of the 4 workers was 3, 12, 14, and 108 months, respectively. Symptoms included general malaise, muscle pain, weakness and numbness in the legs, headache, dizziness, weight loss, and anorexia nervosa. Observed signs included weakness and sensory impairment of the upper and lower extremities, and absence of deep tendon reflexes in the upper and lower extremities. The distal and lower limbs were more severely affected. After removal from exposure, recovery was slow, extending over several months to a year. Lower limbs recovered to near normal in a year. Sensory symptoms resolved in 3 to 5 months, and tendon reflexes returned to normal in about a year. Nerve conduction velocity improved slowly. At 15 months, nerve conduction velocity continued to improve, but was still below normal in all limbs.

In the late 1970s and early 1980s, the TLV for *n*-hexane was 500 ppm. In 1981, Ruff reported on an individual who developed symptoms of neuropathy while working in a situation where the mean *n*-hexane air concentration was 325 ppm, with a reported single peak value of 450 ppm (Ruff, 1981). After 4 years of exposure, the patient, a 60-year-old male, began to complain of distal numbness and weakness in the legs. The condition progressed slowly over the next 2 years. In time, sensory nerve response was absent, and motor nerve conduction velocity was reduced. Electromyographic studies revealed denervation. A sural biopsy, done 2 years after retirement when symptoms were still present, revealed reduction in the number of myelinated axons, enlarged axons, and focal axonal swellings. Pronounced accumulation of neurofilaments were shown with electron microscopy. This case demonstrates that long-term exposure to *n*-hexane at low concentrations may cause severe and long-lasting mixed polyneuropathy of the axonal type.

Much of the evidence implicating *n*-hexane in polyneuropathy was obtained in studies of the Italian shoe industry. When reports of neuropathy began to surface, triorthocresylphosphate (TOCP) was first believed to be the causative agent (Buiatti, 1978). TOCP was used in several shoe manufacturing processes, and the symptoms and histopathological changes characteristic of TOCP neuropathy were similar to those of the complaining workers. Evidence suggesting that *n*-hexane may have been involved in the worker's neuropathy was obtained by Abbritti in a study of 122 workers with neuropathy employed in 72 shoe factories in different parts of the country (Abbritti, 1976). Of these, gluing was done by 46%, cleaning by 45%, and other jobs by 29%. The observation that the more serious cases tended to start in the winter and early spring suggested a vapor was involved because factory windows were more likely to be closed at that time. Milder cases, however, started at any time. The solvents used most frequently were paraffin hydrocarbons (pentanes, *n*-hexane, heptane), cyclic hydrocarbons (cyclopentane, cyclohexane), and toluene. Since little or no TOCP was used in the plants investigated, suspicion was directed away from TOCP and toward the paraffin hydrocarbons, which contained high amounts of *n*-hexane. Similarity between the signs and symptoms associated with abuse of *n*-hexane and those observed in the workers strengthened the case against *n*-hexane. Further evidence implicating *n*-hexane came from a small study carried out by Scelsi in which he reported on 3 women with polyneuropathy (Scelsi, 1980). These women were workers employed in the manufacture of raincoats who had been exposed to a glue containing 80% *n*-hexane.

In an epidemiologic study of more than 350 Italian shoe workers, Buiatti demonstrated that polyneuropathy was more frequent among workers exposed to solvents, and that a significantly higher incidence of neuropathy was found in workers who used glue in excess of 1.3 kg a day, and in factories with an air space for each worker of less than 40 square meters (Buiatti, 1978). Polyneuropathy was found in 85 (25%) of the workers, and was more common in workers over 40 years old than in those under 40. The afflicted workers had the characteristic symptoms of polyneuropathy, including lower-limb weakness and pain, upper-limb paresthesias, and muscle spasm. N-hexane was a component of 40% to 99.5% of glues used in the surveyed factories.

Another large study of the Italian shoe industry was reported in 1983 (Passero, 1983). A total of 654 workers participated in this extended evaluation of the prevalence of neuropathy, which demonstrated that although neuropathy associated with exposure to solvents usually resolves, it can persist. Workers with positive findings presented for follow-up every 3 months for a year, and then once a year from 1973 to 1981. Neurologic and neurophysiologic abnormalities were found in 184 workers, but only 98 of these were found to have toxic neuropathy. Of these 37 were minimally affected, 45 had mild symptoms, and 16 had moderate to severe impairment. The most severe disease was found among workers employed in gluing and cleaning. Severe cases were frequent in small factories with poor exposure standards and among those patients who worked at home. Frequently reported signs and symptoms included sensorimotor distal neuropathy, epigastric pain, headache, insomnia, irritability, nausea and vomiting. Two workers had paresis of respiratory muscles and died from either pulmonary or cardiac failure. EMG findings, such as fibrillations, enervation, and differing intensities of abnormal motor unit potentials, generally correlated with severity of disease. While most patients improved, residual signs were noted in about 50% and persisted in 6 of 7 of the workers most severely affected. Paresthesias and cramping pain persisted even in patients with improved motor conduction velocity. Hyperreflexia or spasticity — signs of possible CNS impairment — were seen in 13 of 39 workers reexamined a year after onset. MCV returned to normal over 12 to 36 months in some patients; and in 6 to 24 months in mild cases. However, in some patients MCV was still below normal 8 years after onset. Commercial *n*-hexane was found in 82.5% of the glue and solvent samples from the factories.

Oge carried out a study of 27 workers with polyneuropathy associated with exposure to *n*-hexane (Oge, 1994). This study demonstrated two electrophysiologic correlates of the pathologic changes characteristic of *n*-hexane neuropathy. One is the data from motor nerve conduction studies which reflect the distal axonopathy process. The other is involvement of the central motor pathways. The subjects had worked in the production of shoes and leather coats for periods ranging from 4 months to 20 years, with a mean of 4.4 years. Duration of exposure to glues containing high percentages of *n*-hexane ranged from 4 months to 2 years. These men worked in small, poorly ventilated shops in Turkey. Recorded TWAs in these shops were between 60 and 810 ppm. The onset of symptoms of polyneuropathy was between April of 1991 and April of 1992. All patients claimed to have removed themselves from exposure when they noticed symptoms, which included muscle weakness, paresthesias, pain, and cramping. Electrophysiologic studies (nerve conduction, needle electromyography) and magnetic stimulation studies (cervical magnetic stimulation, transcranial magnetic stimulation) were done, and the results were as follows:

- *Sensory nerve conduction:* The recorded potentials in the upper and lower extremities of exposed patients had lower amplitudes and longer latencies than those of the controls.
- *Motor nerve conduction:* Distal motor latencies were significantly longer, and motor conduction velocities were significantly slower in the exposed patients than in the controls. Motor conduction velocities of the ulnar nerves increased steadily from the forearms to the proximal segments, lowering the difference between exposed patients and controls at the most proximal regions. A similar pattern was seen in arm segments of median nerves. In the exposed patients, compound muscle action potentials elicited with wrist or ankle stimulation of nerves were low in amplitude compared with the controls.
- *Cervical magnetic stimulation:* The increase of motor conduction velocities in the proximal ulnar nerve segments of exposed patients was close to normal values. Latencies of

maximal muscle response (MMR) were significantly longer than in the controls, as was the neck-to-axilla conduction time. The long MMR latencies were probably due to the slowed conduction in the distal regions of the ulnar nerve.

- *Transcranial magnetic stimulation (central conduction time):* The central conduction times (CCT) of the exposed patients were longer than those of the controls.

Many exposed workers met the specified mandatory electrophysiologic criteria of *Research Criteria for Diagnosis of Chronic Inflammatory Demyelinating Polyneuropathy,* set by the American Academy of Neurology Task Force in 1991, for segmental demyelination in the peripheral nerves (Oge, 1994). Eighteen patients demonstrated reduction in conduction velocity in two or more motor nerves, 20 demonstrated partial conduction block of abnormal temporal dispersion in one or more motor nerves, 21 showed prolonged distal latencies in 2 or more motor nerves, and 16 showed absent or prolonged minimum F wave latencies in two or more motor nerves.

§ 7-5(d)(5). Metabolism.

The lungs are the major route of absorption for *n*-hexane. A linear relationship exists between the concentration in alveolar air and in venous blood (Brugnone, 1978). Retention in the lungs has been calculated at 15% to 28% (Brugnone, 1978; Veulemans, 1982; Mutti, 1984; Nomiyama, 1974). Veulemans calculated 24% retention after exposure to 360 or 720 mg/m^3 (Veulemans, 1982). Retention has been shown to go down from 23% to 16% during work (Veulemans, 1982). Absorption from the gastrointestinal tract is minimal. N-hexane has been shown to penetrate excised human skin at the rate of 0.83 μg/cm^2 per hour (Lodén, 1986).

The distribution of *n*-hexane in humans is not well-known. Baker and Rickert exposed rats to *n*-hexane at different levels and measured resulting levels in blood, sciatic nerve tissue, and brain tissue (Baker, 1981). Results were as follows:

ppm	Blood (mg/l)	Sciatic nerve (mg/kg)	Brain (mg/kg)
500	1.3	12.0	1.8
1000	2.2	48.0	19.7
10,000	20.9	430.5	54.2

N-hexane is metabolized mainly in the liver, first to 2-hexanol, which is transformed to either 2-hexanone (methyl butyl ketone) or 2,5-hexanediol. Both of these may be transformed to 2,5-hexanedione, which is thought to be the main metabolite excreted in the urine (Governa, 1987). Good correlation has been demonstrated between the concentration in the breathing zones in the workplace and excretion of metabolites in the urine. The best correlations have been found for 2-hexanol and 2,5-hexanedione. Unmetabolized *n*-hexane is excreted in small amounts in the urine and is well-correlated with ambient air concentration. It may thus be used for biological monitoring (Imbriani, 1984).

§ 7-5(e). Methyl Alcohol (Methanol).

Empirical formula:	CH_3OH.
Description:	Colorless, volatile liquid with a mild odor.
Synonyms:	Methanol, wood alcohol, wood spirit, carbinol.
Uses:	Industrial solvent for inks, resins, and other materials, paint and varnish removers, antifreeze, plastics.
Air Limit:	200 ppm.
Water Limit:	No criteria set.

Methyl alcohol has a wide range of uses, including solvent, antifreeze, combustible, and as an adulterant of ethyl alcohol. Methyl alcohol neurotoxicity is usually associated with ingestion rather than inhalation of its vapors. While methyl alcohol itself is only mildly toxic, the oxidation products resulting from its metabolism, formaldehyde and formic acid, induce a severe acidosis and a variety of neurotoxic effects (Roe, 1969).

§ 7-5(e)(1). Exposure Limits.

The United States standard is 200 ppm, as is the 1983/1984 ACGIH TWA value. The NIOSH recommendation is adherence to the United States standard of 200 ppm, or 262 mg/m^3, as a TWA for a 10-hour workday and 40-hour week.

§ 7-5(e)(2). Neurotoxic Effects.

In addition to the central nervous system, early toxic symptoms may involve the gastrointestinal and respiratory systems, as well as the visual apparatus. Clinical toxicity is induced by metabolic acidosis as well as by the direct effects of accumulated toxic products. Because of the slow oxidation and excretion of methyl alcohol, toxic symptoms do not usually appear until 12 to 48 hours after ingestion and may last for several days. Central nervous system symptoms similar to intoxication with ethyl alcohol may appear at first. These may include restlessness, in coordination, delirium, and hallucinations. Memory defects and confusion are also seen. As the severity of the toxicity increases, serious, possibly life-threatening symptoms may occur. These include stupor, coma, tonic muscle contractions, opisthonos, hyperactive reflexes, and convulsions. Less frequent symptoms include, dysdiadochkinesis, hyosmia, and involvement of the sixth, seventh, and eighth cranial nerves. Respiratory failure is the usual cause of death in fatal cases of methanol poisoning (Goetz, 1985).

Visual disturbances and various ocular manifestations are frequently associated with methanol poisoning. Amblyopia, scotomas, and even total blindness may occur from a few hours to several days after consumption of methanol. Other manifestations include dilated pupils non-reactive to light and ocular pain. Vision may improve as the patient recovers from acute intoxication, but permanent central scotomas or complete blindness may occur as sequelae. Severe nuchal rigidity, accompanied by coma, may also occur. Another sequela is a Parkinson-like extrapyramidal syndrome characterized by bradykinesia, low voice volume, mixed facies, mild tremor, and rigidity. Upper motor neuron disease (increased reflexes) or lower motor neuron disease (decreased reflexes) and dementia may also be seen (Goetz, 1985).

§ 7-5(e)(3). Metabolism.

Metabolic events may determine the severity of methanol poisoning. Both methyl alcohol and ethyl alcohol share the same degrading enzyme, alcohol dehydrogenase. If both alcohols are consumed together, they will compete for the enzyme, thus reducing the amount of methanol metabolized to toxic formaldehyde and formic acid.

§ 7-5(f). Methyl-N-Butyl Ketone (MBK).

Empirical formula:	$CH_3CO(CH_2)_3CH_3$.
Description:	Colorless liquid with a characteristic odor.
Synonyms:	2-hexanone, MBK, butyl methyl ketone.
Uses:	Used primarily as a solvent, paint thinner.
Air Limit:	100 ppm.
Water limit	No standards set.

This solvent was not widely used until the 1970s, when its use as a paint thinner, solvent for dye printing, and cleaning agent increased. The number of cases of chronic toxicity associated with this solvent increased as its use increased. Inhalation is the usual means of exposure, but oral exposure stemming from contaminated food and cutaneous contact has occurred.

§ 7-5(f)(1). Exposure Limits.

The present threshold limit air value (TLV) in the United States is 25 ppm. Because of concern over the neurotoxic potential of MBK, the United States National Institute for Occupational Safety and Health has recommended a limit of 1 ppm. The ACGIH had stated a TWA of 5 ppm.

§ 7-5(f)(2). Neurotoxic Effects.

Sensorimotor polyneuropathy has been associated with exposure to MBK. The development of the disease is slow and painless, progressing over a period of several months after chronic exposure. Dissociations of compromised sensory modalities have been reported. Light touch, pin prick, and temperature discrimination are often impaired, while vibratory and position senses and C-fiber deep pain awareness are not affected (Spencer, 1980). Multifocal axonal degeneration involving swelling and neurofilamentous accumulations at paranodal areas is seen early in the course of the disease. Severe myelin thinning overlying the axonal swelling is also seen, as is distal axonal degeneration occurring in later stages of the disease. The axonal degeneration resembles terminal axonal neuropathy, also referred to as "dying back" (Mendell, 1977).

§ 7-5(f)(3). Pharmacokinetics and Metabolism.

Absorption of MBK takes place by means of inhalation, and through the gastrointestinal tract and the skin. In one study, healthy volunteers were exposed at rest to MBK at 100 ppm for 4 hours, or at 10 to 50 ppm for 7.5 hours (DiVincenzo, 1978). Resulting breath concentrations were 1.4 and 3.3 ppm respectively. Blood concentrations were measurable only after the highest exposure level and did not exceed 1.2 μg/ml. Lung retention was, respectively, 75% and 92% of the inhaled amount. Skin exposure can result in considerable absorption. The skin exposure of volunteers resulted in an uptake of 4.8 to 8.0 μg per minute per square centimeter of skin surface. It was calculated that if a hand were immersed in liquid MBK for 1 hour at a skin absorption rate of 5 μg per minute per square centimeter of skin surface, about 220 mg would be absorbed. This would be more than twice the amount taken up by inhalation at 25 ppm for 1 hour. Little is known about the distribution of MBK in humans.

The metabolism of MBK has been investigated in animal studies. In rats, MBK has been shown to metabolize to 2-hexanol and 2,5-hexanedione (2,5-HD) (Katz, 1980). It has been suggested that the metabolites become neurotoxic when they are converted to 2,5-HD. It is thought that the same metabolic pathways may be active in humans (DiVincenzo, 1978).

§ 7-5(g). 1,1,1-Trichloroethane.

Empirical formula:	CH_3CCl_3.
Description:	Colorless, nonflammable liquid with an odor similar to chloroform.
Synonyms:	Methyl chloroform.
Uses:	Degreasing, dip-cleaning metals, dry cleaning, propellant.
Air Limit:	350 ppm.
Water Limit:	Fresh water: 18,000 μg/L; salt water, 31,200 μg/L; to protect human health: 1,030,000 μg/L.

In recent years, this compound has come to be used in many processes that formerly utilized carbon tetrachloride. In its liquid form, it is used as degreaser and for cold cleaning, dip-cleaning and bucket cleaning of metals. It is also used for dry cleaning, vapor degreasing, and as a propellant. The major route of entry is inhalation. Some entry occurs through skin absorption, and there have been some instances of ingestion.

§ 7-5(g)(1). Exposure Limits.

In 1983/84, the Federal standard and the ACGIH TWA value were set at 350 ppm. Previously, NIOSH had recommended a standard of 350 ppm for occupational exposure, but altered its recommendation in 1983 to 200 ppm. A STEL of 450 PPM was set by the ACGIH in 1983.

§ 7-5(g)(2). Neurotoxicity.

Peripheral neuropathy has been reported in workers exposed to 1,1,1-trichloroethylene.

Two women working as degreasers at a plant manufacturing electric motors reported numbness in the hands and other neurologic symptoms. Both worked at jobs requiring immersion of the hands into the solvent over the course of a work shift of several hours.

> *Case 1:* A 25-year-old woman presented with complaints of numbness and disturbance of sensation in both hands beginning after working three months as a degreaser. She had worked six years previously in a different department with no problems. On examination, she was found to have hypoactive reflexes and minimal blunting of sensation in the right hand. Nerve conduction studies showed low median and ulnar sensory action potential amplitudes with normal ulnar motor and distal sensory latencies. Four years later, distal sensory latencies were found to be prolonged.
>
> *Case 2:* A 40-year-old woman presented to the same neurologist six months after starting the degreasing job. After four weeks on the job, she developed dizziness and complained of numbness in the hands and cheeks. Blunting to pinprick in a

stocking/glove distribution was found to be more marked in the hands.

The neurologist considered that the symptoms were consistent with preponderantly distal sensory neuropathy. Neither patient had evidence of underlying metabolic disease or exposure to other toxins, including alcohol. Case 1 was transferred to another department and began to improve, but symptoms recurred three years after leaving the plant. Case 2 remained at the plant and continued to have symptoms, including impaired sensation in the hands and feet. Sural nerve biopsies showed chronic ongoing neuropathy (axonopathy and myelinopathy).

Air sampling showed that levels of 1,1,1-trichloroethylene were well below the exposure limit of 350 ppm. Analysis of the solvent, carried out after the patients presented, did not detect known neurotoxins. No previous association of peripheral neuropathy with 1,1,1-trichloroethylene had been reported. The patients' complaints of hand numbness at presentation were atypical for occupational toxic neuropathies, which usually affect the longer nerves in the lower extremities earlier and more prominently than the upper extremities.

At the time, there were insufficient data to conclusively implicate 1,1,1-trichloroethane. Other possibilities include other workplace toxins, toxins unrelated to the workplace, and contamination of the degreaser batch with a neurotoxin.

§ 7-5(h). Xylene.

Empirical Formula: $C_6H_4(CH_3)_2$.

Description: Exists in three isometric forms: ortho-, meta-, and para-xylene. Meta-xylene and ortho-xylene are mobile, colorless, flammable liquids. M-xylene is the major constituent of commercial xylene, which usually includes the other isomers as well as

	ethylbenzene and small amounts of other compounds.
Synonyms:	Xylol, dimethylbenzene.
Uses:	Solvent; ingredient of paints, lacquers, varnishes, inks, dyes, adhesives, cements, cleaning fluids; chemical feedstock for xylidines, benzoic acid, phthalic anhydride, isophthalic and terephthalic acids, as well as their esters; used in manufacture of quartz crystal oscillators, hydrogen peroxide, perfumes, insect repellents, epoxy resins, leather, pharmaceuticals.
Air limit:	100 ppm.
Water limit:	No adverse level in water has been calculated.
Points of attack:	Central nervous system, eyes, gastrointestinal tract, blood, liver, kidneys, and skin.

Xylene is widely used in the synthesis of other chemicals such as polyester, and as a solvent in adhesives, paints, and lacquers. It is a component of gasoline and paint thinners. Workers at risk include those in the photogravure, leather, rubber, and plastics industries. Workers in histology laboratories are also at risk of exposure. Formerly obtained through the distillation of coal tar, xylene is now produced by catalytic reforming of petroleum. Most commercial xylene is a mixture of isomers. A typical commercial xylene may contain about 44% m-xylene, 20% *o*-xylene, and 15% ethylbenzene. The types and degrees of neurotoxic effects can vary with different isomers of xylene.

§ 7-5(h)(1). Exposure Limits.

The United States and ACGIH TWA standard for all isomers is 100 ppm. NIOSH also recommends a ceiling concentration of 200 ppm as determined by a sampling period of 10 minutes.

§ 7-5(h)(2). Neurotoxic Effects.

Acute exposure to xylene vapor may cause central nervous system depression and minor reversible effects on liver and kidneys. At high concentrations, xylene vapor may cause dizziness, staggering, drowsiness, and unconsciousness. At very high concentrations, xylene vapor may cause pulmonary edema, anorexia, nausea, vomiting, and abdominal pain. Liquid xylene is irritating to the eyes and mucous membranes. Aspiration of a few milliliters may cause chemical pneumonitis, pulmonary edema, and hemorrhage.

Early incidents of neurotoxic effects of xylene include a 1902 report of a 25-year-old man who developed symptoms after heavy exposure in a poorly ventilated room. At first he had a feeling of euphoria, followed by dyscoordination, paresthesias, tremor and anxiety. A chronic neurasthenic syndrome developed later (Rosenblath, 1902).

§ 7-5(h)(3). Acute Effects.

Studies involving controlled exposures have provided information on the acute neurotoxic effects of xylene. In one study, volunteers were exposed in an exposure chamber to concentrations varying from 110 to 660 ppm for 15-minute periods (Carpenter, 1975). Effects were limited to one subject who reported sleepiness at 230 ppm and to another who reported dizziness at 460 ppm. Gamberale, et al., used psychological tests to determine the effects of xylene exposure in an exposure chamber on 15 healthy male volunteers, aged 21 to 23 years, at the following concentrations:

435 mg/m^3 for 70 minutes at rest;

1300 mg/m^3 for 70 minutes at rest; and

1300 mg/m^3 for 30 minutes at moderate exercise followed by 40 minutes at rest (Gamberale, 1978).

Tests included various reaction time measurements, short-term memory, and critical flicker fusion. Significant impairment in reaction time and short-term memory was found at the highest exposure level. The effects appeared to be more closely related to the level of absorption of xylene rather than to its concentration in the air. The absorption of xylene corresponded to a biological limit value between 600 and 1000 mg.

Evoked potentials have also been used to assess the effects of controlled exposure to xylene. In a study of healthy young volunteers Seppäläinen, et al., investigated the effect of xylene and ethanol on visual evoked potentials (VEP) and somatosensory evoked potentials (SEP) (Seppäläinen, 1981). At an exposure of 4 hours to 700 or 1200 mg/m^3 of m-xylene, no significant effects on latencies or amplitude of SEPs or VEPs were observed. Ethanol combined with xylene at 1200 mg/m^3 was associated with a decreased amplitude of N60-P115, while ethanol alone increased latencies of P50. N60, P115, and N155. No effect on amplitude was observed.

Savolainen and colleagues carried out a series of investigations on the effects of xylene on the sense of balance, reaction time, and various psychophysiological functions. In one study, volunteers exposed for 6 consecutive days to fluctuating levels and stable levels of xylene at 100 to 200 ppm exhibited impairment of choice reaction time in the afternoon of the first exposure day. In the subsequent days, reaction time was normal. Impairment of reaction time appeared to be related to the blood xylene level (Savolainen, 1979).

Another study of the effects of xylene and ethanol, administered both alone and in combination, on simple and choice reaction time, also demonstrated minimal results (Savolainen, 1980). Both choice and simple reaction times were unaffected by 4 hours of exposure to xylene at 150 ppm or to ethanol at 0.4g/kg. Slight, statistically insignificant impairment of choice reaction time was seen at a xylene concentration of 280 ppm. Greater impairment was obtained with ethanol.

Investigating the effects of xylene on equilibrium, Savolainen conducted a study in which the levels of exposure to xylene differed through the day in an attempt to simulate industrial conditions (Savolainen, 1979). Exposures were as follows:

> Morning exposure: 3 hours at slightly less than 100 ppm of m-xylene (4.1 μmol/l) with short peaks of 200 ppm corresponding to a TWA of 100 ppm;
>
> One-hour lunch break; and
>
> Afternoon exposure: 3 hours at a TWA of 200 ppm with peaks of 400 ppm.

Impaired balance was associated with the afternoon exposure. The greatest degree of impairment was seen in the anterior-posterior axis with the eyes closed, and in the lateral axis with the eyes closed. Peak impairment was seen at a venous blood xylene level of 29.1 μmol/l. In a similar study, Savolainen observed a slight impairment of equilibrium associated with a few days of low-level exposure, followed by normalization (Savolainen, 1979). At peak levels, however, impairment of balance was again observed, suggesting that tolerance may have developed. In another study, body sway improved with exercise, possibly because of increased arousal (Savolainen, 1985).

In a study of the effects of xylene and ethanol on equilibrium, xylene at 155 ppm administered for 4 hours had a slight adverse effect on balance at the anterior-posterior axis (Savolainen, 1980). At 300 ppm, slight impairment was seen both at the anterior-posterior and lateral planes. When ethanol was co-administered with xylene at low doses, an additive effect was seen. However, when the two substances were given concomitantly at higher doses, an antagonistic effect was seen.

§ 7-5(h)(4). Acute Industrial and Accidental Exposure.

In 1970, three workers painting the interior of a storage tank were overcome by vapors of xylene and other solvents. The paint was 34%

solvent of which 90% was xylene. The estimated xylene concentration in the tank was 10,000 ppm. One worker died and an autopsy revealed petechial hemorrhages in the gray and white matter of the brain, as well as anoxic neuronal changes with swelling and loss of Nissl substance. The two survivors appeared to be confused after regaining consciousness. One demonstrated ataxia and slurred speech. Both had transient hepatic impairment, and one had slight impairment of renal function (Morley, 1970).

Mass acute exposures have also been reported. In 1980, a number of patients and employees at a hospital developed headache, dizziness, irritation of mucous membranes, nausea, and vomiting, all within 30 minutes. The symptoms persisted from 2 to 48 hours. An investigation revealed that a liter of xylene had been discarded by pouring the liquid out of the container. The hospital's ventilation system then distributed the xylene to several rooms (Klaucke, 1982). A 1960 report describes an incident in which 8 spray painters working in a confined space experienced acute symptoms, including dizziness, headache, a feeling of drunkenness, and gastric distress (Goldie, 1960). One worker had epileptic seizures, although his EEG was normal.

§ 7-5(h)(5). Chronic Exposure.

Chronic effects, primarily neuropsychiatric symptoms, have been reported in subjects exposed to solvents in several industries, including photogravure, ink manufacturing, flooring, and histology laboratories. In most reports, exposure has been to mixtures of solvents rather than to xylene alone.

Histology technicians are exposed to a variety of solvents and other chemicals in addition to xylene, including formaldehyde, ethanol vapor, and toluene. It has been shown that the technicians exhibit more neuropsychiatric symptoms than secretarial and clerical workers in the same establishments (Kilburn, 1985). The technicians complained of concentration problems, memory impairment, mood swings, impaired balance, and sleep problems. The symptoms, however, did not correlate with concentration levels of the solvents. A later and larger study of histology technicians also failed to correlate symptoms with solvent levels (Kilburn, 1989). Age was determined to be a significant factor in this study. Formaldehyde was associated with reduced performance on visual memory, story memory, digit scan, and pegboard tests. Solvent exposure was associated with impaired story recall in other studies (Kilburn, 1985; Kilburn, 1989).

Following exposure to solvent mixtures of which xylene forms a major part (43.6%), symmetrical ascending motor polyneuropathy with accompanying sensory disturbances have been reported. In one patient, autopsy revealed chromatolysis of perikaryons in anterior horn cells with apparent loss of neurons (Means, 1976).

§ 7-5(h)(6). Metabolism and Pharmacokinetics.

Xylene is readily absorbed in the lungs and to a much lesser extent through the skin and gastrointestinal tract. Retention of the various isomers of xylene varies from about 60% to 65% (Sedivec, 1976). The amount taken up also varies with exposure level and physical effort. In one investigation, retention was shown to be about 65% during rest and light work, decreasing to about 50% during heavy work (Åstrand, 1978).

Evidence that lung retention depends on exposure level as well as duration of exposure was provided by Senczuk and Orlowski (Senczuk, 1978). Subjects in their study were exposed to xylene at 100, 300, and 600 mg/m^3. Results were as follows:

100 mg/m^3: 87% retained initially; 84% at end of session (mean = 5%);

300 mg/m^3: 83% retained initially; 67% at end of session (mean = 75%);

600 mg/m^3: 78% retained initially; 65% at end of session (mean = 71%).

Exercise is positively correlated with the uptake of xylene. Åstrand exposed healthy males to 435 mg/m^3 for 30 minutes during rest, and light, moderate, and heavy work (Åstrand, 1978). The mean uptake at rest was 79 mg. The uptake increased to 219 mg, 301 mg, and 392 mg during light, moderate, and heavy work, respectively. Åstrand also found that alveolar concentration was affected by exercise. At rest, the alveolar concentration was 15% of the environmental concentration, increasing to 20% and 30% at light and moderate work, respectively. Arterial and venous blood concentration also increased during exposure. The increase was particularly rapid during the first few minutes of exposure and increased further with work. As work proceeded, however, the blood concentrations leveled off. At rest, at an exposure of 100 ppm, the arterial blood concentration was 0.9 mg/kg, increasing to 1.6 mg/kg at 200 ppm.

Moderately heavy work at 100 ppm resulted in an arterial concentration of 6.8 mg/kg. Venous blood concentrations paralleled arterial concentrations at lower levels. Ramsey investigated workers in a histology laboratory exposed to mixed xylene at concentrations of 34 to 68 ppm (Ramsey, 1978). At the end of a working day, blood concentration ranged from 1.65 to 2.47 mg/l.

Absorption through the skin has not been found to be a major entry route for xylene. In one study, hands were immersed in liquid xylene for 15 minutes resulting in an uptake of 35 mg, which was equal to the amount taken up by the lungs at an exposure of 100 ppm for a similar time period (Riihimäki, 1978).

Animal studies have shown that inhaled xylene is rapidly taken up by body fat, and by various parts of the nervous system. It has been found still to be present in nervous tissue one hour after exposure (Bergman, 1979). In another animal study, Carlsson found rapid absorption in fat (Carlsson, 1981). After eight hours of exposure, the concentration in fat was about ten times the blood concentration. At the same time, the concentration in the cerebrum and cerebellum was about 40% of that in the blood. The concentration in the sciatic nerve, however, was twice the blood level. Fabre found that chronic intoxication resulted in concentrations of 148 μg/g in the adrenal glands,

130 μg/g in bone marrow, 100 μg/g in the brain, and 91 μg/g I blood (Fabre, 1960).

Engström and Bjurström exposed volunteers to 100 and 220 ppm for two hours (Engstöm, 1978). Biopsies of subcutaneous fat revealed no significant difference in concentration at 2 and 22 hours after exposure. Concentrations in adipose tissue ranged from 4 to 8 mg/kg.

Ramsey exposed subjects to xylene for 2 hours at 100 and 200 ppm (Ramsey, 1984). Resulting mean adipose tissue concentrations were 6 and 9 mg/kg in adipose tissue at 100 and 200 ppm, respectively. The relatively high concentration in adipose tissue is thought to be due to xylene's moderate solubility in blood and high tissue solubility.

Xylene is metabolized by oxidation to methyl benzyl alcohol and methyl benzoic acid. It is conjugated with glycine, and excreted in the urine as methyl hippuric acid. Reported percentages of xylene excreted as methyl hippuric acid vary widely. Sedivec and Flek reported 95% to 99% (Sedivec, 1976), Engström reported 80% to 90% (Engström, 1977), and Ogata reported 72% (Ogata, 1970). Xylenols resulting from aromatic hydroxylation accounts for less than 1% to 2% in urine (Bakke, 1970).

§ 7-5(i). Styrene.

Empirical Formula: $C_6H_5CH{=}CH_2$.

Description: Colorless to yellowish, very refractive, oily liquid with a penetrating odor.

Synonyms: Cinnamene, cinnamol, phenythylene, phenylethylene, styrene monomer, styrol, styrolene, vinylbenzene.

Uses: Upon heating to 200° C, styrene polymerizes to form the plastic polystyrene. It is used in combination with 1,3-butadiene or acrylonitrile to form copolymer elastomers, butadiene-

	styrene rubber, and acrylonitrile-butadiene-styrene (ABS). It is also used in the manufacture of resins, polyesters, and insulators, and in drug manufacture.
Air Limit:	100 ppm.
Water Limit:	No adverse level in drinking water has been established.

One of the early industrial applications of styrene was in the production of synthetic rubber during World War II. In the 1950s, its use in the manufacture of glass-reinforced plastics started, and the production of styrene has increased steadily since that time. Approximately 89% of styrene is used in the manufacture of reinforced plastics, including fiberglass. Workers most heavily exposed are those in polyester plastic industries, particularly the manufacture of small boats.

§ 7-5(i)(1). Exposure Limits.

The United States standard for styrene for an 8-hour TWA is 100 ppm. The acceptable ceiling concentration is 200 ppm, with an acceptable maximum peak of 600 ppm, for a maximum duration of 5 minutes in any 3 hours. The ACIGH has recommenced a TWA of 50 ppm.

§ 7-5(i)(2). Neurotoxic Effects.

The acute toxic effects of styrene have been evaluated in controlled exposure studies. In an exposure chamber study of 9 healthy males, no symptoms were observed at 52 and 117 ppm except for the unpleasant smell of styrene. Apparent adaptation to the smell was seen after 5 minutes of exposure. At exposure of 216 ppm for 20 minutes, the subjects began to complain of nasal irritation. Neurologic symptoms were not observed until exposure at 376 ppm for 25 minutes. Impairment in the Romberg test and a decrease in manual dexterity were observed. Also reported were headache, nausea, and a feeling of intoxication. In another test, set up to simulate a typical work day with exposures at 99 ppm for 7 hours with a 30-minute break at midday, eye and throat irritation were noted. Neurologic symptoms were limited to difficulty in the Romberg test.

In another exposure chamber study, 12 male subjects were exposed to styrene at levels increasing every 30 minutes from 0 to 50, 150, 250, and 350 ppm. At each 30-minute exposure, blood styrene levels increased (Gamberale, 1974). Alveolar concentrations increased during the first few minutes and then remained constant. While the subjects reported some feelings of impairment, they did not assess their work performance as adversely affected after exposure. Insignificant impairment of reaction time was noted up to 350 ppm. Perceptual speed and manual dexterity were not affected. Because of the observed increase in blood level throughout the 30-minute exposure intervals, the authors felt that the neurotoxic effects might have been more severe if the exposure times had been increased.

Gamberale and colleagues carried out a study of styrene exposure in workers employed in the manufacture of fiberglass boats at four different plants (Gamberale, 1975). The average duration of exposure was 2.7 years (in a range of 0.1 to 11.0 years). Reaction times in the exposed workers were prolonged and unstable. As the work day progressed, these effects became somewhat more pronounced. There was a direct correlation between the duration of employment and increases in reaction time. All test performances at all test periods were poorer in the exposed group than in controls.

Guillemin and Bauer examined workers at four separate plants for styrene concentration. The workers were employed in the manufacture of products fabricated from fiberglass-reinforced polyester plastics. They ranged in age from 21 to 57 years (with a mean of 28.0 years), and exposure times ranged from a few days to 12 years. Determination of symptoms, reaction times, and urine levels of the styrene metabolites mandelic and phenylglyoxcylic acids, as well as a neurologic examination, were carried out on a workday in the middle of the week. The exposed workers' most frequently noted complaints were irritation of the eyes and upper respiratory tract. No other specific symptoms were found in either the exposed workers or the control group. Workers exposed to more than 150 ppm had reaction times equally prolonged in the morning and afternoon, while workers exposed to less than 150 ppm had reaction times similar to those of the control workers. Only two exposed workers who were unsteady in the Romberg test in the morning but not at the end of the day demonstrated neurological findings. The data were insufficient to determine if the effects were subacute or chronic.

§ 7-5(i)(3). Chronic Effects.

The chronic effects of exposure to styrene have been extensively studied. Some studies noted a pattern of improvement in various neurologic parameters in some exposed workers after removal from exposure to styrene, but the improvement did not bring the exposed workers up to the level of those not exposed to styrene. Mutti, for example, investigated 50 exposed workers in 1975, and carried out follow-up examinations 6 years later on 15 of these workers (Mutti, 1984). The styrene concentration in the workers' environment had decreased from levels above 50 ppm in the original study to 20 to 25 ppm at follow-up. Urinary creatinine had decreased from a mean of about 400 mg/g to 200 mg/g. Results of simple reaction time (SRT) and block design tests had improved in the exposed workers, while performance in these tests and in logic memory and verbal memory had gone down in the control group of workers. However, performance in the exposed workers was still inferior to that of the controls. In a study of 21 workers exposed to styrene for a mean of 11.6 years (from a range of 6 to 21 years). At the initial examination, the workers complained of memory impairment, headache, fatigue, forgetfulness, and irritability.

Blood levels of styrene and urinary concentration of styrene metabolites have been found to correlate with results of neurologic tests. Cherry investigated workers in the English fiberglass boat industry

(Cherry, 1980). Styrene concentration was measured in the breathing zone and in the blood. Urinary excretion of mandelic acid was also evaluated. Neurologic testing included visual reaction times over ten minutes, vigilance task, digit symbol substitution, and forward and backward digit span. The subjects were tested in the morning and afternoon on Mondays. Exposure to styrene was highest in the morning, with a mean of 117 ppm, and afternoon concentrations were 52 ppm, yielding an average daily exposure of 92 ppm. Blood styrene concentration was 6.9 μmol/l. Mean mandelic acid excretion was 581 μmol/mmol creatinine. In patients with high blood styrene, backward digit span was performed less well than in controls, and morning and afternoon reaction times were almost identical. In subjects with low blood styrene levels, however, reaction times were similar to those of the control group. Also associated with high blood styrene were mood changes and excessive fatigue, particularly at the end of the week, suggesting a cumulative effect. In a later study, Cherry found that mandelic acid levels in the morning correlated with morning reaction time (Cherry, 1981). Some workers who had very slow excretion of mandelic acid also demonstrated slow reaction times. Reaction times improved in a group of workers who had been previously tested at high styrene levels and were re-tested at low levels.

Correlation between neurologic test performances and styrene metabolite excretion were also found in a study of 50 workers employed in the building of glass silos (Mutti, 1984). The mean duration of exposure was 8.6 years. The exposure level varied from 10 to 300 ppm. Fifty unexposed workers were matched pairwise in age, sex, educational level and general intelligence to form a control group. Testing was carried out when the patients had been removed from exposure for at least 15 hours. The test battery included vocabulary, visual choice reaction times, block design, memory, verbal memory (including recall after 30 minutes), digit symbols and imbedded figures. In several tests, particularly block design and reaction time, impaired performance was found. Exposure was expressed by urinary metabolite excretion for the duration of the experiment. The exposed workers had poorer performances than controls in all tests except digit symbol. Verbal learning was significantly impaired in workers whose urinary excretion of metabolites exceeded 150 mmol/mol creatinine, which corresponds to an air concentration of styrene of about 25 ppm. Impaired logical memory and visumotor and visuconstructive ability were seen in workers exposed to concentrations of greater than 50 ppm.

In some studies, a correlation between metabolite excretion and neurotoxic symptoms has not been found. Harkönen investigated 98 workers exposed to styrene (Harkönen, 1977). Mean duration of exposure was 2.5 years. The patients reported their symptoms on questionnaires, including general as well as acute symptoms experienced during exposure. General symptoms, such as dizziness, headache, and irritation of the mucous membranes, were reported much more frequently by the exposed workers than by the unexposed controls. Symptoms noted in the course of a workday included prenarcotic syndrome (nausea, dizziness, feeling of inebriation) and irritation of the eyes, throat, and skin. However, no correlation was found between mandelic acid excretion and any particular symptom. Eighty of the 96 workers were exposed to styrene at levels ranging from 5 to 25 ppm. Workers exposed to less than 25 ppm performed poorly on several tests, including simple reaction time, finger tapping, and a vocabulary subset from Wechsler's adult intelligence scale. Serum prolactin level correlated with increasing exposure before and after testing, while adrenocorticotropic hormone increased only after exposure.

Neurophysiologic effects have also been associated with exposure to styrene. A study of 33 exposed workers indicated significantly more neuropathy in exposed workers, even after adjustments for age (Rosén, 1978). Motor neuronography to determine maximal conduction velocity (MCV) was carried out on several nerves, including the median, ulnar, fibular, and posterior tibial. Sensory neuronography measurements were done on the median and ulnar nerves. While no change in MCV was shown, the duration of sensory action potentials was longer and the amplitude was lower than in the control group. The mean age of workers with neuropathy was higher than in those without the condition. However, when the data were adjusted for age, the exposed workers still demonstrated more signs of neuropathy than did the unexposed controls. In 27% of exposed patients, electroencephalography showed an increase in fast activity in the central and frontocentral areas. An increment in slow activity over both hemispheres was also noted. EEG abnormalities were more common in patients with chronic solvent intoxication, but the changes were not solvent-specific.

In a study of 96 workers exposed to styrene, EEGs and electromyograms (EMGs) were carried out on the 40 patients with the greatest number of complaints (Harkönen, 1977). Normal data from a neurophysiological laboratory served as a control. EEG abnormalities were observed in many of the exposed workers. The abnormalities, seen in 24%, were most often in the form of localized slow activity, diffuse theta activity, or bilateral spike and wave discharges above the expected 10%. EEG changes were seen in 33% of patients with the highest exposure to styrene (mandelic acid greater than 700 mg/dm^3) as compared with 10% in those with mandelic acid less than 700 mg/dm^3. Conduction velocities did not vary significantly from normal data. In another study of workers exposed to styrene in the fiberglass boat industry, workers with an average exposure of 1 year were compared to workers exposed for an average of 10 years (Dolmierski, 1976). EEG abnormalities were seen in 72% of the workers with short-term exposure. These abnormalities were primarily sharp-wave discharge and temporal high-voltage slow waves, which were accentuated during hyperventilation. The high rate of EEG abnormalities in the short-term exposure group may be indicative of an acute effect. Many in this group demonstrated abnormal tendon reflexes, nystagmus, and hand tremor. In the long-term exposure group, 22% had EEG abnormalities, mostly low- and medium-voltage theta waves. Increased frequency of fatigue and weakness were seen in workers with EEG changes. Because of health problems, about 50% of the workers quit their jobs within one to two years of starting their employment.

Adverse effects on hearing and equilibrium associated with styrene exposure have been reported. Five volunteers, with a mean age of 27 years, were exposed to 300 ppm for 1 hour in an exposure chamber (Ödqvist, 1982). They demonstrated eye movement disturbances, suggesting effects on the cerebellum or cerebellar-brainstem connections. Other tests, however, revealed no spontaneous positional or fixation nystagmus. In a similar study by the same investigator, 10 volunteers aged 20 to 30 years (with a mean of 23.9 years) were exposed to styrene at levels of 87 to 139 ppm while carrying out light work (Ödqvist, 1982). The subjects had not consumed alcohol for at least 24 hours before the investigation. Total uptake of styrene was 64% of the amount inspired (406 mg), and mean capillary blood concentration after 50 minutes of exposure was 2.7 ppm. Visual suppression test showed there was no change at a maximum amplitude of 60.. At 112., 8 of 10 exposed subjects had increased gain during exposure. In the saccade test, the maximum speed of saccade was enhanced.

Table 7.3
Chronic Effects of Styrene

Industry	n	Symptoms	Findings	Concentration	Reference
Fiberglass boats					
	106	—	RT.	10-310	Gamberale, 1975
	43	neuropsychiatric	abnormal EEG	periods>0.3 mg/l	Dolmierski, 1976
	98	neuropsychiatric	Psychomotor and visumotor performance.	30-35ppm	Lindstrom, 1976; Harkönen, 1979
	33	neuropsychiatric	MCV, SCV (dd). EEG changes	50-125 ppm	Wolff, 1978
	7	fatigue (nonsignificant)	RT. (transient)	37 mg/m^3	Kjelberg, 1979

Industry	n	Symptoms	Findings	Concentration	Reference
	6	neuropsychiatric	cerebral atrophy	—	Melgaard, 1979
	27	Exposure-related fatigue	Backward digit span. RT. in AM	90 ppm	Cherry, 1980, 1981
	11	Neuropsychiatric	MCV, SCV ulnar and median.	100 ppm	Triebig, 1985
	59	—	High frequency	60-140 mg/m^3	Muijser, 1988
	21	Neuropsychiatric	Encephalopathy	50 mg/m^3	Flodin, 1989
	105	—	Digit symbol.	30 ppm	Letz, 1989
	18	Neuropsychiatric fatigue	Vestibular	25-100 mg/m	Motter, 1990
Plastics					
	17	Neuropsychiatric	Abnormal EEG 71%	20-130 ppm	Klimka-Deutschova, 1962
	17	Irritation of mucous	RT.	>150 ppm	Gotell, 1972
	96	Neuropsychiatric	Abnormal EEG 24%	30-55 ppm	Sappolainen, 1976
	494	Prenarcotic symptoms	Neuropathy 16-19%	5-20 ppm	Lilis, 1978; Lorimer, 1978
	46	Neuropsychiatric	Vigilance and motor speed	>400 mg/m^3	Seeber, 1980
	59	—	High frequency hearing loss	60-140 mg/m^3	Muijser, 1988
	36	None	None	18 ppm	Triebig, 1989

§ 7-5(i)(4). Pharmacokinetics and Metabolism.

The concentration of styrene in the blood increases quickly during the first minutes after inhalation. Even in a steady-state concentration of alveolar air, the blood concentration continues to rise for more than 30 minutes, but starts to level off after 6 hours (Gamberale, 1974;

Ramsey, 1978; Ramsey, 1984). Exercise speeds up the increase in blood levels (Åstrand, 1974). The retention of inhaled styrene has generally been reported at about 65% (Bardojej, 1979; Åstrand, 1974; Kjellbërg, 1979; Wigaeus, 1984). At a time-weighted average (TWA) between 3 and 300 ppm, Sollenberg calculated the total uptake during a 5-day work week of 8-hour workdays to be 12.7 ppm (Sollenberg, 1988). In a study by Ödqvist, 5 young volunteers were exposed to 300 ppm styrene for 1 hour at light exercise (Ödqvist, 1982). The resulting alveolar concentration was 180 to 200 mg/m^3, and the capillary concentration was 8.5 to 8.9 mg/kg blood. The uptake was calculated to be 65%, which is equivalent to 1020 mg of styrene.

Absorption of styrene through the skin is about 9 to 15 mg/cm^2. Percutaneous absorption of styrene is of minor importance.

An affinity of styrene for nervous and adipose tissues has been demonstrated in animal studies. In a study by Bergman, autoradiography at low temperature showed that a 10-minute inhalation of styrene by mice resulted in high concentrations in these tissues (Bergman, 1979). While styrene was cleared from nervous tissue in about 1 hour, it was still detectable in adipose tissue more than 24 hours after exposure. In another animal study, exposure of rats to 45 ppm styrene for 1 to 8 hours resulted in a brain concentration corresponding to 70% of that in blood (Carlsson, 1981). After 8 hours of exposure, a major redistribution to subcutaneous fat was seen, with concentrations in that tissue of more than 4 times the blood concentration. After 4 hours of exposure at 240 ppm, the concentration of styrene in adipose tissue was 40 times that of the blood. At that exposure, concentrations of styrene metabolites were also higher in adipose tissue than in the blood. Withey, however, showed that after intravenous administration in rats of 13.37 mg/kg, styrene was evenly distributed in the heart, lungs, liver, spleen, kidneys, and brain (Withey, 1977). After 8 minutes, the concentration in the brain exceeded that in the blood.

In a study of human subcutaneous tissue, biopsies were taken 30 and 90 minutes after exposure to 293 mg/m^3 (Wigaeus, 1984). Concentrations of 62 and 53 µmol/kg with wide interindividual variations were seen. In another study, biopsies of subcutaneous fat were taken at the end of a work day (Kjellbërg, 1979). Concentration of styrene in the breathing zone averaged 37 mg/m^3, with a range of 11 to 59 mg/m^3. Styrene concentrations in adipose tissue ranged from 3.1 to 13.6 mg/kg. Retention of styrene in adipose tissue was estimated to average 92 mg, with a range of 5 to 229 mg. In a study by Engström, male volunteers were exposed to styrene at 210 mg/m^3 (50 ppm) for 30-minute work periods, at low, moderate, and heavy work intensities, each followed by a 30-minute rest period (Engström, 1978). Subcutaneous fat concentrations were found to be about 3.6 mg/kg at 2, 4 and 21 hours after exposure. The half-life ($T_{1/2}$) in fat was calculated to be 2.2 to 4.0 days. Detectable amounts of styrene remained in subcutaneous fat for 13 days.

Styrene is metabolized primarily in the liver. Small amounts are metabolized in extrahepatic tissues. The first metabolic step, the formation of styrene-7,8-oxide (SO), is catalyzed by the microsomal cytochrome P-450 system. SO is hydrated to styrene glycol (SG), catalyzed by epoxide hydratase. SG is transformed to either mandelic and phenylglyoxylic acids or hippuric acid. The transformation to hippuric acid is via benzoic acid. Some investigators have found that 85% to 90% of absorbed styrene is eliminated as mandelic acid and some 10% as phenylglyoxylic acid (Ramsey, 1978). Elimination has also been reported as 57% mandelic acid and 33% phenylglyoxylic acid (Guillemin, 1979).

Accumulation of styrene does not seem to occur at low doses. Wieczorek found that upon termination of exposure, the $T_{1/2}$ of elimination from subcutaneous adipose tissue ranged from 2 to 4 days (Wieczorek, 1988). Sollenberg has proposed that the excretion rate of mandelic acid plus phenylglyoxylic acid can be used as a reliable biological exposure index (Sollenberg, 1988). He has also proposed that the excretion rate of mandelic acid plus phenylglyoxylic acid in a urine sample obtained at the end of the work week provides a useful estimate of the styrene dose. These proposals were made on the basis of data obtained in a study of the excretion of mandelic and phenylglyoxylic acids during a work week of 5 8-hour days in workers with a mean absorption of styrene of 12.7 mmol. Mandelic and phenylglyoxylic acids were detected in the first urine samples and reached a peak after removal of the workers from exposure. Excretion did not return to baseline between work days. Mean half-times of excretion were 4.3 and 7.3 hours for mandelic and phenylglyoxylic acid, respectively.

Ohtsuji and Ikeda found that the urinary excretion of phenylglyoxylic acid and mandelic acid was a more sensitive indicator of exposure to styrene than mandelic acid (Ohtsuji, 1970). Löf found that the blood concentration of styrene glycol correlated linearly with the preceding uptake of styrene in workers exposed to styrene levels of about 100 mg/m^3, while styrene-7,8-oxide was at the detection limit (Löf, 1986). Bartolucci found a close correlation between TWA exposure shown by passive dosimeters and metabolites excreted in the urine (Bartolucci, 1986). Physical activity has a significant effect on the uptake of styrene and the level of excreted metabolites.

§ 7-5(j). Carbon Disulfide.

Carbon disulfide has been used in industry for more than 100 years. It was used in the felting process of hat manufacturing, which placed hat workers at risk of daily exposure. The resulting behavioral disorders may have contributed to the expression "mad as a hatter." Carbon disulfide can be used both as a solvent and as a raw product for synthesis. Today, carbon disulfide is used in the rayon industry and in the manufacture of carbon tetrachloride and cellophane (Timmerman, 1978). It is also used as a solvent for rubber paints and for lacquers.

In its pure state, carbon disulfide is a clear, volatile liquid with a slight, unobtrusive odor. Because of sulfur compound impurities, however, the commercial grades of carbon disulfide commonly used in industry have an unpleasant odor generally described as "foul" or "vile."

In the United States, there were few cases of occupational exposure until the introduction of the viscose rayon industry in the 1930s. Today, workers in the rayon industry run the greatest risk of exposure to carbon disulfide, particularly those in spinning operations and those working in the repair of equipment used in processes where carbon disulfide concentration is high.

The lungs are the major route of entry for carbon disulfide, but it can also be absorbed through the skin and the gastrointestinal tract. In persons not previously exposed, about 80% of inhaled carbon disulfide vapor is absorbed during the first 15 minutes. After 45 minutes, the rate of absorption drops to about 45% and stays there for quite some time. In people previously exposed, the rate of absorption is about 55% during the first 15 minutes.

§ 7-5(j)(1). Chronic Exposure.

Chronic exposure to carbon disulfide can affect all parts of the central and peripheral nervous systems. A Parkinson-like syndrome can occur, manifested by a wide range of symptoms and signs, including tremor, muscle spasm, speech disturbances, loss of memory and severe mental depression. Peripheral nerve involvement can result in a syndrome similar to polyneuritis. There may also be ocular disturbances.

Symptoms of a presenile type of cerebral arteriosclerosis in association with chronic exposure have been observed at the relatively early age of 40 to 55 years (Holmberg, 1994).

Mental disturbances have been associated with carbon disulfide exposure. In one study, a higher rate of suicide than in the general population was found among 4,899 workers in the rayon industry, aged 40 to 55 years (Mancuso, 1977). The investigators proposed that the biologic effects of abnormal mental and social behavior may be delayed and may occur later in response to environmental and social stresses.

Microscopic aneurysms have been seen in the retinas of exposed workers. In one study, these aneurysms were seen in 29% of Japanese workers exposed to carbon disulfide (Goto, 1971). The pathogenesis may be similar to that of diabetes; carbon disulfide may have a slight diabetogenic effect (Hotta, 1971). These investigators also found that carbon disulfide had a toxic effect on the optic nerve, resulting in decreased adaptability to darkness and difficulty in discerning colors.

Psychomotor effects and changes in nerve conduction have been seen in workers exposed to carbon disulfide. Less than 20 ppm has caused blurred vision, hand trembling, dizziness, and changes in nerve conduction velocities.

References.

Abbate, C., Giorgianni, C., Munao, F., Brecciaroli, R., *Neurotoxicity Induced by Exposure to Toluene.* Int. Arch. Occup. Environ. Health 1993; 64:389-92.

Abbritti, G., Siracusa, A., Cianchetti, C., et al., *Shoemakers' Polyneuropathy in Italy: the Etiological Problem.* Br. J. Ind. Med. 1976; 33:92-99.

ACGIH, *Threshold Limit Values for Chemical Substances and Physical Agents in the Work Environment.* Presented at the 1984 Annual Meeting of the American Conference of Governmental Industrial Hygienists, 1984.

Ad Hoc Subcommittee of the American Academy of Neurology AIDS Task Force, *Research Criteria for Diagnosis of Chronic Inflammatory Demyelinating Polyneuropathy (CIDP).* Neurology 1991; 41:617-18.

Allister, C., Lush, M., Oliver, J.S., Watson, J.M., *Status Epilepticus Caused by Solvent Abuse.* Br. Med. J. 1981; 283:1156.

Altenkirch, H., Mager, J., Soltenburg, G., Helmbrecht, J., *Toxic Polyneuropathies After Sniffing a Glue Thinner.* J. Neurol. 1977; 214:137-152.

Andersen, I., Lundqvist, G.R., Mølhave, L., et al., *Human Response to Controlled Levels of Toluene in Six-Hour Exposures.* Scand. J. Work Environ. Health 1983; 9:405-418.

Arlien-Søborg, P., Solvent Neurotoxicity. Boca Raton: CRC Press, 1992: 1-10.

Arlien-Søborg. P., Bruhn, P., Gyldensted, C., Melgaard, B., *Chronic Painter's Syndrome in House Painters: Chronic Toxic Encephalopathy in House Painters.* Acta Neurol. Scandinav. 1979; 60:149-156.

Åstrand, I., Ehrner-Samuel, H., Kilbom, H., Övrum, P., *Toluene Exposure. I. Concentration in Alveolar Air and Blood at Rest and During Exercise.* Work Environ. Health 1972; 9:119.

Åstrand, I., Engström, J., Övrum, P., *Exposure to Xylene and Ethylbenzene.* Scand. J. Work Environ. Health 1978; 4:185.

Åstrand, I., Kilbom, Övrum, P., *Exposure to Styrene. I. Concentration in Alveolar Air and Blood During Exercise and Metabolism.* Work Environ. Health 1974; 11:69-85.

Åstrand, I., Övrum, P., *Exposure to Trichloroethylene I. Uptake and Distribution in Man.* Scand. J. Work Environ. Health 1976; 4:199-211.

Åstrand, I., *Uptake of Solvents in the Blood and Tissue of Man.* Scand. J. Work Environ. Health 1975; 1:199-210.

Axelson, O., Hane, N., Hogstedt, C., *Current Aspects of Solvent-Related Disorders.* In: C. Zenz (ed.), Developments in Occupational Medicine. Chicago: Yearbook Medical Publishers, 1980: 237-248.

Bælum, J., Attwell, R., Skerfving, S., Örbäk, P., et al., *Toluene Metabolism During Exposure to Varying Concentrations Combined with Exercise.* Int. Arch. Occup. Environ. Health 1987; 59:281-294.

Baker, E.L., *A Review of Recent Research on Health Effects of Human Occupational Exposure to Organic Solvents.* J. Occup. Med. 1994; 36:1079-1092.

Baker, E.L., Letz, R.E., Eisen, E.A., et al., *Neurobehavioral Effects of Solvents in Construction Painters.* J. Occup. Med. 1988; 30:116-123.

Baker, E.L., Smith, T.J., *Evaluation of Exposure to Organic Solvents.* In: J.M. Harrington (ed.), Recent Advances in Occupational Health. Edinburgh: Churchill Livingstone, 1984: 89-105.

Baker, T.S., Rickert, D.E., *Dose-Dependent Uptake, Distribution, and Elimination of Inhaled n-Hexane in the Fischer-344 Rat.* Toxicol. Appl. Phramacol. 1981; 61:414-422.

Bakke, O.M., Scheline, R.R., *Hydroxylation of Aromatic Hydrocarbons in the Rat.* Toxicol. Appl. Pharmacol. 1970; 16:691-700.

Ballantyne, B., Marrs, T., Turner, P. (eds.), General and Applied Toxicology. NY: Stockton Press, 1993; 4:89-100.

Balso, A., Aksoy, M., *Neurologic Abnormalities in Chronic Benzene Poisoning.* Environ. Res. 1982; 27:457-465.

Bardojej, Z., Bardodejova, E., *Biotransformation of Ethyl Benzene, Styrene, and Methylstyrene in Man.* Am. Ind. Hyg. Assoc. J. 1979; 31:206-209.

Barnes, G.E., *Solvent Abuse; A Review.* Int. J. Addict. 1979; 14:1-26.

Barrett, L., Garrel, S., Danel, V., Bebru, J.L., *Chronic Trichloroethylene Intoxication: A New Approach by Trigeminal Evoked Potentials?* Arch. Environ, Health 1987; 42:297-302.

Bartolucci, G.B., Perbellini, L., Gori, G.P., *Occupational Exposure to Solvents: Field Comparison of Active and Passive Samplers and Biological Monitoring of Exposed Workers.* Ann. Occup. Hyg. 1986; 30:295-306.

Bartonicek, V., *Metabolism and Excretion of Trichloroethylene After Inhalation by Human Subjects.* Br. J. Ind. Med. 1962; 19:134.

Bass, M., *Sudden Sniffing Death.* JAMA 1970; 212:2075-2079.

Bergman, K., *Whole-Body Autoradiography and Allied Tracer Techniques in Distribution and Elimination Studies of Some Organic Solvents.* Scand. J. Work. Environ. Health 1979; 5 (Supp. 1):263.

Bernad, P.G., et al., *Neurotoxicity and Behavior Abnormalities in Cohort Chronically Exposed to Trichloroethyene.* Vet. & Human Toxicology, December, 1987; 29(6):475.

Bird, M.G., *Industrial Solvents: Some Factors Affecting Their Passage Into and Through the Skin.* Ann. Occup. Hyg. 1981; 24:235-244.

Bleecker, M.L., Bolla, K.I., Agnew, J, et al., *Dose-Related Subclinical Neurobehavioral Effects of Chronic Exposure to Low Levels of Organic Solvents.* Am. J. Indust. Med. 1991; 19:715-728.

Bolla, K.I., Schwartz, B.S., Agnew, J., *Subclinical Neuropsychiatric Effects of Chronic Low-Level Solvent Exposure in US Paint Manufacturers.* J. Occup. Med. 1990; 32:671-677.

Bove, F.J., Letz, R., Baker, E.L., *Sensory Thresholds Among Construction Trade Painters: A Cross-Sectional Study Using New Methods for Measuring Temperature and Vibration Sensitivity.* J. Occup. Med. 1989; 31:320-325.

Brooks, S.M., et al., Environmental Medicine. St. Louis: Mosby, 1995;17:201-214.

Brugnone, F., Perbellini, L., Grigolini, L., Apostoli, P., *Solvent Exposure in a Shoe Upper Factory.* Int. Arch. Occup. Environ. Health 1978; 42:51-62.

Buiatti, E., Cecchini, S., Ronchi, O., et al., *Subclinical Neuropathic Disorders and Precautionary Measures in the Shoe Industry.* Br. J. Ind. Med. 1978; 35:168-173.

Carlsson, A., *Distribution and Elimination of ^{14} C-Styrene in Rat.* Scand. J. Work Environ. Health 1981; 7:45-50.

Carlsson, A., Ljungquist, E., *Exposure to Toluene.* Scand. J. Work Environ. Health 1982; 8:56-62.

Carpenter, C., Kinkead, E.R., Geary, D.L., et al., *Petroleum Hydrocarbon Toxicity Studies. V. Animal and Human Response to Vapors of Mixed Xylenes.* Toxicol. Appl. Pharmacol. 1975; 33:543-558.

Channer, K.S., Stanley, S., *Persistent Visual Hallucinations Secondary to Chronic Solvent Encephalopathy: Case Report and Review of the Literature.* J. Neurol. Neurosurg. Psychiatr. 1983; 46:83-86.

Cherry, N., Hutchins, H., Pace, T., Waldron, H.A., *Neurobehavioral Effects of Repeated Occupational Exposure to Toluene and Paint Solvents.* Br. J. Ind. Med. 1985; 42:291-300.

Cherry, N., Johnston, J.D., Venables, H., et al., *The Effects of Toluene and Alcohol on Psychomotor Performance.* Ergonomics 1983; 26:1081-1087.

Cherry, N., Rogers, B., Venables, H., et al., *Acute Behavioural Effects of Styrene Exposure: A Further Analysis*. Br. J. Ind. Med. 1981; 38:346-350.

Cherry, N., Waldron, H.A., Wsells, G.G., *An Investigation of the Acute Behavioral Effects of Styrene on Factory Workers*. Br. J. Ind. Med. 1980; 37:232-240.

Cornblath D.R., *Electrophysiology in Guillain-Barre Syndrome*. Neurology 1990; 27 (Supp.):517-520

Cronk, S.L., Barkley, D.E.H, Farrell, M.F., *Respiratory Arrest After Solvent Abuse* Br. Med. J. 1985; 290:897-898.

Demers, R.Y., Markell, B.L., Wabeke, R., *Peripheral Vibratory Sense Deficits in Solvent-Exposed Painters.* J. Occup. Med. 1991; 33:1051-1054.

Dick, R.B., Setzer, J.V., Wait, R., et al., *Effects of Acute Exposure of Toluene and Methyl Ethyl Ketone on Psychomotor Performance.* Int. Arch. Occup. Environ. Health 1984; 54:91.

DiVincenzo, V.G., Hamilton, M.L., Kaplan, C.J., et al., *Studies on the Respiratory Uptake and Excretion and the Skin Absorption of Methyl-n-Butyl Ketone in Humans and Dogs*. Toxicol. Appl. Pharmacol. 1978; 44:593-604.

Dolmierski, F., Kwiatkowski, S.R., Nitka, J., *Clinical and Experimental Research into the Pathogenesis of Toxic Effect of Styrene. VII. Appraisal of the Nervous System in Workers Exposed to Styrene.* Bull. Inst. Marit. Trop. Med. Gdynia. 1976; 27:193-196.

Echeverria, D., Fine, L., Langolf, G., et al., *Acute Neurobehavioral Effects of Toluene*. Br. J. Ind. Med. 1989; 46:483-495.

Ehyai, A., Freemon, F.R., *Progressive Optic Neuropathy and Sensorineural Hearing Loss Due to Chronic Glue Sniffing.* J. Neurol Neurosurg. Psychiatr. 1983; 46:349-351.

Ekberg, K., Barregård, Hagberg, S., Sällsten, G., *Chronic and Acute Effect of Solvents on Central Nervous System Functions in Floorlayers*. Br. J. Ind. Med. 1986; 43:101-106.

Elofsson, S.A., Gamberale, F., Hinmarsh, T, et al., *Exposure to Organic Solvents. A Cross-Sectional Epidemiologic Investigation on*

Occupationally Exposed Car and Industrial Spray Painters with Special Reference to the Nervous System. Scand. J. Work Environ. Health 1980; 6:239-273.

Engström, J., Bjurström, R., *Exposure to Xylene and Ethylbenzene.* Scand J Work Environ. Health 1978; 4:195-203.

Engström, J., Husman, K., Pfaffi, P.,Riihimäki, V., *Evaluation of Occupational Exposure to Xylene by Blood, Exhaled Air, and Urine Analysis.* Scand J Work Environ. Health 1978; 4:114-121.

Engström, J., *Styrene in Subcutaneous Adipose Tissue After Experimental and Industrial* Exposure. Scand J Work Environ. Health 1978; 4 (Supp. 2):119-120.

Fabre, R., Truhaut, R., Laham, S., *Recherches Toxicologiques Sur les Solvants de Remplacement Dubenzene. IV. Etude des Xylenes.* Arch. Mal. Prof. 1960; 21:20.

Feldman, R.G., *Trichloroethylene.* In: P.J. Vinken, G.W. Bruyn (eds.), Handbook of the Nervous System. Amsterdam: North-Holland Publishing Co., 1979: 457-464.

Ferguson, R.K., Vernon, R.J., *Trichloroethylene in Combination with CNS Drugs.* Arch. Environ. Health 1970; 20:462-467.

Fernandez, J.G., Droz, P.O., Humbert, B.E., Caperos, J.R., *Trichloroethylene Exposure in Simulation of Uptake, Excretion, and Metabolism, Using a Mathematical Model.* Br. J. Ind. Med. 1977; 34:43-55.

Fernandez, J.G., Humbert, B.E., Droz, P.O., Caperos, J.R., *Exposition au Trichloroéthyléne. Bilan de l'Absorption de l'excrétion du Métabolisme sur des Subjets Humains.* Arch. Mal. Prof. 1975; 36:397.

Fiserova-Bergerova, V., *Toxicokinetics of Organic Solvents.* Scand. J. Work Environ. Health 1985; 11 (Supp. 1):7-21.

Fiserova-Bergerova, V., Vlach, V., Cassady, J.C., *Predictable "Individual Differences" in Uptake and Excretion of Gases and Lipid Soluble Vapors Simulation Study.* Br. J. Ind. Med. 1980; 37:42-49.

Fornazzari, L., Wilkinson, D.A., Kapur, B.M., et al., *Cerebellar, Cortical, and Functional Impairment in Toluene Abusers.* Acta. Neurol. Scand. 1983; 67:319-329.

Franchini, I., Mutti, A., Arfini, G., *Styrene-Induced Brain Dysfunction. A Longitudinal Study.* Presented at the 2d Meeting of the International Neurotoxicology Association (INA), Sitges, Spain, 1989, 250.

Gade, A., Mortensen, L., Bruhn, P., *"Chronic Painter's Syndrome." A Reanalysis of Psychological Test Data in a Group of Diagnosed Cases Based on Comparisons with Matched Controls.* Acta. Neurol. Scand. 1988; 77:293-306.

Gamberale, F., Annwall, G., Hultengren, M., *Exposure to Xylene and Ethylbenzene. III. Effects on Central Nervous System Functions.* Scand J. Work Environ. Health 1978; 4:204-211.

Gamberale, F., Hultengren, M., *Exposure to Styrene* II. *Psychological Functions.* Work Environ. Health 1974; 11:86-93.

Gamberale, F., Hultengren, M., *Toluene Exposure. II. Psychophysiological Functions.* Work Environ. Health 1972; 9:131.

Goetz, C.G., Neurotoxins in Clinical Practice. New York: Spectrum Publications, 1985: 645-690.

Goldie, I., *Can Xylene (Xylol) Provoke Convulsive Seizures*? Ind. Med. Surg. 1960; 29:33.

Gonzales, E.G., Downey, J.A., *Polyneuropathy in a Glue Sniffer.* Arch. Phys. Med. Rehabil. 1972; 53-63.

Goto, D.S., et al., *Studies on Chronic Carbon Disulfide Poisoning — Pathogenesis of Retinal Microaneurysm Due to Carbon Disulfide, with Special Reference to a Subclinical Defect of Carbohydrate Metabolism.* Int. Arch. Arbeitsned. 1971; 28:115-126.

Governa, M., Calisti, R., Coppa, G., Tagliavento, G., *Urinary Excretion of 2,5-Hexanedione and Peripheral Polyneuropathies in Workers Exposed to Hexane.* J. Toxicol. Environ. Health 1987; 20:219-228.

Grabski, D.A., *Toluene Sniffing Producing Cerebellar Degeneration.* Am. J. Psychiatr. 1961; 3:271.

Grandjean, E., Münchinger, R., Turrian, V., et al., *Investigations into the Effects of Exposure to Trichloroethylene in Mechanical Engineering.* Br. J. Ind. Med. 1955; 12:131-145.

Guillemin, M.P., Bauer, D., *Human Exposure to Styrene,* Int. Arch. Occup. Environ. Health 1979; 44:249-263.

Hane, M., Axelson, O., Blume, J., et al., *Psychological Function Changes Among House Painters*. Scand. J. Work Environ. Health 1977; 3:91-99.

Hänninen, H, Aniti-Poika, M., Juntunen, J., et al., *Exposure to Organic Solvents and Neuropsychological Dysfunction: A Study on Monozygotic Twins.* Br. J. Ind. Med. 1991; 48:18-25.

Hänninen, H., *Psychological Picture of Manifest and Latent Carbon Disulfide Poisoning.* Br. J. Ind. Med. 1971; 28:374-381.

Harkönen, H., *Relationship of Symptoms to Occupational Styrene Exposure and to the Findings of Electroencephalographic and Psychological Examinations*. Int. Arch. Occup. Environ. Health 1977; 40:231-239.

Herskowitz, A., Ishii, N., Schaumberg, H., *n-Hexane Neuropathy. A Syndrome Occurring as a Result of Industrial Exposure.* N. Engl. J. Med. 1971; 285:82-85.

Holmberg, B., Zenz, C., Dodson, V.N., *The Polymer Industry. Sulfide.* In: C. Zenz, O.B. Dickerson, E.P. Horvath (eds.), Occupational Medicine, 3d Ed. St. Louis: Mosby, 1994: 719-753.

Hormes, J.T., Filley, C.M., Rosenberg, N.L., *Neurologic Sequelae of Chronic Solvent Vapor Abuse.* Neurology 1986; 36:698-702.

Hotta, R., Savic, S., *Fluorescin Angiography in Ophthalmodynamometric Study on Carbon Disulfide Exposure.* Presented at International Symposium on Toxicology of Carbon Disulfide. Banya Koviljaca, Yugoslavia: May 1971.

Huang C., Chu, N., Chang, S., Shin, T., *Biphasic Recovery in n-Hexane Polyneuropathy*. Acta. Neurol. Scand. 1989; 80:610-615.

Hydén, D., Larsby, B., Andersson, H, et al., *Impairment of Visuo-Vestibular Interaction in Humans Exposed to Toluene*. Otolaryngology. 1983; 45:262-269.

Imbriani, M., Ghittori, S., Pezzagno, G., Capodaglio, E., *n-Hexane Urine Elimination and Weighted Exposure Concentrations.* Arch. Occup. Environ. Health 1984; 55:33-41.

Inoue, O., Seiji, K., Watanabe,T., et al., *Possible Ethnic Differences in Toluene Metabolism: A Comparison Study of Chinese, Turkish, and Japanese Solvent Workers.* Toxicol. Lett. 1986; 34:167-174.

Iregren, A., Åkerstedt, T., Olson, B.A., Gamberale, F., *Experimental Exposure to Toluene in Combination with Ethanol Intake.* Scand. J. Work Environ. Health 1986; 12:128-136.

Iregren, A., *Effects on Psychological Test Performance of Workers Exposed to a Single Solvent (Toluene): A Comparison with Effects of Exposure to a Mixture of Organic Solvents.* Neurobehav. Toxicol. Teratol. 1982; 4:695-701.

Kadyrov, G.K., Muzyka, V., *Chronic Effect of Benzene Vapour upon the GABA System in Rat Brain.* Work Environ. Health 1970; 10:140-143.

Katz, G.V., O'Donoghue, J.L., DiVincenzo, G.D., Terhaar, C.J., *Comparative Neurotoxicity and Metabolism of Ethyl n-Butyl Ketone and Methyl n-Butyl Ketone in Rats.* Toxicol. Appl. Pharmacol. 1980; 52:153-158.

Keane, J.R., *Toluene Optic Neuropathy.* Ann. Neurol. 1978; 3:390.

Kilburn, K.H., Seidman, B.C., Warshaw, R., *Neurobehavioral and Respiratory Symptoms of Formaldehyde and Xylene Exposure in Histology Technicians.* Arch. Environ. Health 1985 40:229-233.

Kilburn, K.H., Warshaw, R., Thornton, J.C., Husmark, I., *An Examination of Factors That Could Affect Choice Reaction Time in Histology Technicians.* Am. J. Ind. Med. 1989; 15:679-686.

King, M.D., Day, R.E., Oliver, J.S., et al., *Solvent Encephalopathy.* Br. Med. J. 1981; 283:663-665.

Kjellbërg, A., Wigaeus, E., Engström, J., et al., *Lågtidseffekter av Styrenex-Position Vid en Plastbåtsindustri.* Arbeite och Hälsa. 1979; 18:5.

Klaucke, D.N., Johansen, M., Vogt, R.L., *An Outbreak of Xylene Intoxication in a Hospital.* Am. J. Ind. Med. 1982; 3:173-178.

Knave, B., Kolmodin-Hedman, B., Persson, H.E., Goldberg, J.M., *Chronic Exposure to Carbon Disulfide: Effects on Occupationally*

Exposed with Special Reference to the Nervous System. Work Environ. Health 1974; 11:49-58.

Knox, J.W., Nelson, J.R., *Permanent Encephalopathy from Toluene Inhalation*. N. Engl. J. Med. 1966; 275:1494.

Korobkin, R., Asbury, A.K., Sumner, A.J., Nielsen, S.L., *Glue-Sniffing Neuropathy*. Arch. Neurol. 1975; 32-158-162.

Landrigan, P.J., Stein, G.F., Kominsky, J.R., et al., *Common-Source Community and Industrial Exposure to Trichloroethylene*. Arch, Environ. Health 1987; 42:327-332.

Larsen, F., Leira, H.L., *Organic Brain Syndrome and Long-Term Exposure to Toluene; A Clinical Psychiatric Study of Vocationally Active Printing Workers*. J. Occup. Med. 1988; 30:875-878.

Lawrence, W.H., Partyka, E.K., *Chronic Dysphasia and Trigeminal Anesthesia After Trichloroethylene Exposure*. Ann. Intern. Med. 1981; 95:710.

Lindström, K., Härkönen, H., Hernberg, S., *Disturbances in Psychological Functions of Workers Occupationally Exposed to Styrene*. Scand. J. Work Environ. Heath 1976:3:129-139.

Lodén M., *The In Vitro Permeability of Human Skin to Benzene, Ethylene Glycol, Formaldehyde, and n-Hexane*. Acta Pharmacol. Toxicol. 1986; 58:382.

Löf, A., Lundgren, E., Nydahl, E.M., Nordqvist, M.B., *Biological Monitoring of Styrene Metabolites in Blood*. Scand. J. Work. Environ. Health 1986; 12:70.

Mahmood, Z., *Cognitive Function of Solvent Abusers*. Scott. Med. J. 1983; 269:1340.

Maizlish, N.A., Fine, L.J., Walbers, J., et al., *A Neurological Evaluation of Workers Exposed to Mixtures of Organic Solvents*. Br. J. Ind. Med. 1987; 44:14-25.

Mancuso, T.F., Locke, B.Z., *Carbon Disulfide as a Cause of Suicide: Epidemiological Study of Viscose Rayon Workers*. J. Occup. Med. 1977; 14:595-606.

Massengale, O.N., Glaser, H.H., LeLievre, R.E., *Physical and Psychologic Factors in Glue Sniffing.* N. Engl. J. Med. 1963; 269:1340.

Matsumura, M., Inoue, N., Ohnishi, A., et al., *Toxic Polyneuropathy due to Glue-Sniffing.* J. Neurol. Sci. 1974; 21:101.

Matushita, T., Arimatsu, Y., Ueda, A., et al., *Hematological and Neuromuscular Response of Workers Exposed to Low Concentration of Toluene Vapor.* 1975; 13:115.

Means, E.D., Prockop, L.D., Hooper, G.S., *Pathology of Lacquer Thinner Induced Neuropathy.* Ann. Clin. Lab. Sci. 1976; 6:240.

Mendell, J.R., Sahenk, Z., Saida, K., et al., *Alterations of Fast Axonal Transport in Experimental Methyl-n-Butyl-Ketone Neuropathy.* Brain Res. 1977; 133:107-118.

Metrick, S.A., Brenner, R.P., *Abnormal Brainstem Auditory Evoked Potentials in Chronic Paint Sniffers.* Ann. Neurol. 1982; 12:553-556.

Mikkelson, S., *A Cohort Study of Disability Pension and Death Among Painters with Special Regard to Disabling Senile Dementia as an Occupational Disease.* Scand. J. Soc. Med. Supp. 1980; 16:34-43.

Molhave, L., *Volatile Organic Compounds and the Sick Building Syndrome,* In: Lippmann, M. (ed), Environmental Toxicants, NY: VanNostrand Reinhold, 1992.

Morley, R., Eccleston, D.W., Douglas, C.P., et al., *Xylene-Poisoning: A Report on One Fatal Case and Two Cases of Recovery After Prolonged Unconsciousness.* Br. Med. J. 1970; 3:442.

Müller, G., Spassovski, M., Henschler, D., *Metabolism of Trichloroethylene in Man.* Arch. Toxicol 1974; 32:283-295.

Mutti, A., Falzoi, M., Lucertini, S., et al., *N-hexane Metabolism in Occupationally Exposed Workers.* Br. J. Ind. Med. 1984; 41:533-538.

Mutti, A., Mazzuchi, A., Rustichelli, P., et al., *Exposure-Effect and Exposure-Response Relationships Between Occupational Exposure to Styrene and Neurophysiological Functions.* Am. J. Ind. Med. 1984; 5:275-286.

Nomiyama, K., Nomiyama, H., *Respiratory Elimination of Organic Solvents in Man.* Int. Arch. Arbeitsmed. 1974; 32:85.

Ödqvist, L.M., Larsby, B., Tham, R., et al., *Vestibulo-Oculomotor Disturbances in Humans Exposed to Styrene.* Acta Otolaryngol. 1982; 94:487.

Ogata, M., Tomokuni, K., Takatsuka, Y., *Urinary Excretion of Hippuric Acid and m- or p-Methylhippuric Acid in the Urine of People Exposed to Vapours of Toluene and m-or p-Xylene in a Test of Exposure.* Br. J. Ind. Med. 1970; 27:43-50.

Oge, A., Yazici J., Boyaciyan, A., et al., *Peripheral and Central Conduction in n-Hexane Polyneuropathy.* Muscle and Nerve 1994; 17:1416-1430.

Ohtsuji, H., Ikeda, M., *A Rapid Colorimetric Method for the Determination of Phenylglyoxylic and Mandelic Acids.* Br. J. Ind. Med. 1970; 27:150.

Ørbæk, P., Nise, G., *Neurasthenic Complaints and Psychometric Function of Toluene-Exposed Rotogravure Printers* 1989; 16:67-77.

Ørbæk, P., Rosen, I., Svensson, K., *Electroneurographic Findings in Patients with Solvent-Induced Central Nervous System Dysfunction.* Br. J. Ind. Med. 1988; 45:409-414.

Passero, S., Battistini, N., Cioni, R., et al., *Toxic Polyneuropathy of Shoe Workers in Italy. A Clinical, Neurophysiological and Follow-up Study.* Ital. J. Neurol. Sci. 1983; 4:463-472.

Prockop, L.D., Alt, M., Tison, J., *Huffer's Neuropathy.* JAMA 1974; 229:1083-1084.

Pyykkö, K., Tähti, H., Vapaatalo, H., *Toluene Concentrations in Various Tissues of Rats After Inhalation and Oral Administration.* Arch. Toxicol. 1977; 38:169-176.

Ramsey, J., Andersen, M.E., *A Physiologically Based Description of the Inhalation Pharmacokinetics of Styrene in Rats and Humans.* Toxicol. Appl. Pharmacol. 1984; 73:159-175.

Ramsey, J., Anderson, H.R., Bloor, K., Flanagan, R.J., *An Introduction to the Practice, Prevalence, and Chemical Toxicology of Volatile Substance Abuse*. Human Toxicol. 1989; 8:261-269.

Ramsey, J., Young, J.D., *Pharmacokinetics of Inhaled Styrene in Rats and Humans*. Scand. J. Work Environ. Health 1978; 4 (Supp. 2):84-91.

RCA, A., Bozievic, D., Karacic, V., *Visual Evoked Potentials in Individuals Exposed to Long-Term Low Concentrations of Toluene*. Arch. Toxicol. 1995; 69:337-40.

Riihimäki, V., *Conjugation and Urinary Excretion of Toluene and m-Xylene Metabolites in Man*. Scand. J. Work Environ. Health 1979; 5:135-142.

Riihimäki, V., Pfäffli, P., *Percutaneous Absorption of Solvent Vapours in Man*. Scand. J. Work Environ. Health 1978; 4:73-85.

Riihimäki, V., Savolainen, K., *Human Exposure to m-Xylene and Acute Effects on the Central Nervous System*. Ann. Occup. Hyg. 1980; 23:411-422.

Roe, O., *Past, Present, and Future Fights Against Methanol Blindness and Death*. Tans. Ophthalmol. Soc. U.K. 1969; 89:235-242.

Rosén, I., Haeger-Aronsen, B., Rehnström, S., Welinder, H., *Neuropsychological Observations After Chronic Styrene Exposure*. Scand. J. Work Environ. Health 1978; 4 (Supp. 2):184-194.

Rosenberg, N.L., Spitz, M.C., Filley, C.M., et al., *Central Nervous System Effects of Chronic Toluene Abuse — Clinical Brainstem Evoked Response and Magnetic Resonance Imaging Studies*. Neurotoxicol. Teratol. 1988; 10:489-495.

Rosenblath, T., *Neurasthenie Hervorgerufen Durch Einathmung von Xylol-Dämpfen*. Sachverständigen Ztg. 1902; 8:197.

Ruff, R.L., Petito, C.K., Acheson, L.S., *Neuropathy Associated with Chronic Low Level Exposure to n-Hexane*. Clin. Toxicol. 1981; 515-519.

Salvini, M., Binaschi, S., Riva, M., *Evaluation of the Psychophysiological Functions in Human Subjects Exposed to Trichloroethylene*. Br. J. Ind. Med. 1971; 28:293-295.

Sandmark, B., Broms, I., Löfgren, L., Carl-Göran, O., *Olfactory Function in Painters Exposed to Organic Solvents.* Scand. J. Environ. Health 1989; 15:60-63.

Santesson, C.G., *Chronic Poisoning with Coal Tar Benzene: Four Deaths*. Arch. Hyg. (Munich) 1897; 31:336.

Sasa, M., Igarashi, S., Miyazaki, T., et al., *Equilibrium Disorders with Diffuse Brain Atrophy in Long-Term Toluene Sniffing.* Arch. Otol. Rhinol. Laryngol. 1978; 221:163-169.

Sato, A., Nakajima, T., *Differences Following Skin or Inhalation Exposure in the Absorption and Excretion Kinetics of Trichloroethylene and Toluene.* Br. J. Ind. Med. 1978; 35:43-49.

Sato, A., Nakajima, T., Fujiwara, Y., Hirosawa, K., *A Pharmacokinetic Model to Study the Excretion of Trichloroethylene and Its Metabolites After an Inhalation Exposure.*Br. J. Ind. Med. 1977; 34:56-63.

Savolainen, K, Riihimäki, V., Lane, A., Kekoni, J., *Short-Term Exposure of Human Subjects to m-Xylene and 1,1,1-Trichloroethane.* Int. Arch. Occup. Environ. Health 1981; 49:89-98.

Savolainen, K, Riihimäki, V., Muona, O, et al., *Conversely Exposure-Related Effects Between Atmospheric M-Xylene Concentrations and Human Body Sense of Balance.* Acta Pharmacol. Toxicol. 1985; 57:67-76.

Savolainen, K. Linnavuo, M., *Effects of m-Xylene on Human Equilibrium Measured with a Quantitative Method.* Acta Pharmacol. Toxicol. 1979; 44:315-318.

Savolainen, K., *Combined Effects of Xylene and Alcohol on the Central Nervous System.* Acta Pharmacol. Toxicol. 1980; 46:366-372.

Savolainen, K., Pfäffli, P., Tengén, M., et al., *Trichloroethylene and 1,1,1-Trichloroethane: Effects on Brain and Liver After Five Days Intermittent Inhalation.* Arch. Toxicol. 1977; 38:229-237.

Scelsi, R., Poggi, P., Fera, L. Gonella, G., *Toxic Polyneuropathy Due to n-Hexane.* J. Neurol. Sci. 1980; 47:7-19.

Sedivec, V., Flek, J., *The Absorption, Metabolism, and Excretion of Xylene in Man.* Int. Arch. Occup. Environ. Health 1976; 37:205-217.

Selling, L., *Benzol as a Leukotoxin; Studies on Degeneration Regeneration of Blood and Hematopoietic Organs.* John's Hopkins Hospital Rep. 1917; 17:83.

Senczuk, w., Orlowski, J., *Absorption of m-Xylene Vapours Through the Respiratory Tract and Excretion of m-Methylhippuric Acid in Urine.* Br. J. Ind. Med. 1978; 35:50-55.

Seppäläinen, A.M., Savolainen, K., Kovala, T., *Changes Induced by Xylene and Alcohol in Human Evoked Potentials.* Electroencephalogr. Clin. Neurophysiol. 1981; 5:148-155.

Seppäläinen, A.M., Tolonen, M., *Neurotoxicity of Long-Term Exposure to Carbon Disulfide in the Viscose Rayon Industry. A Neurophysiological Study.* Work Environ. Health 1974; 11:145.

Shirabe, T., Tsuda, T., Erao, A., Akari, S., *Toxic Poluneuropathy Due to Glue Sniffing:* J. Neurol. Sci. 1974; 21:101-113.

Sollenberg, J., Bjurström, R., Wrangskog, K., Vesterberg, O., *Biological Exposure Limits Estimated from Relations Between Occupational Styrene Exposure During a Work-Week and Excretion of Mandelic and Phenylglyoxylic Acid in Urine.* Int. J. Arch. Occup. Environ. Health 1988; 60:365-370.

Spencer, P.S., Couri, D., Scahaumber, H.H., *n-Hexane and Methyl n-Butyl Ketone.* In: P.S. Spencer, H.H. Schaumberg (eds.), Neurotoxicology. Baltimore: William and Wilkins, 1980: 456-475.

Spencer, P.S., Schaumberg, H.H., Sabri, M.I., Veronesi, B., *The Enlarging View of Hexacarbon Neurotoxicity.* CRC Crit. Rev. Toxicol. 1980; 279-356.

Spurgeon, A., Gray, C.N., Sims, J., et al., *Neurobehavioral Effects of Long-Term Occupational Exposure to Organic Solvents — Two Comparable Studies.* Am. J. Ind. Med. 1992; 22:325-335.

Stewart R., Dodd, H.C., Gay, H.H., Erley, D.S., *Experimental Human Exposure to Trichloroethylene.* Arch. Environ. Health 1970; 20:64-71.

Stewart, R.D., Dodd, H.C., *Absorption of Carbon Tetrachloride, Trichloroethylene, and Tetrachloroethylene, Methylene Chloride, and 1,1,1-Trichloroethane Through the Human Skin.* Am. Ind. Hyg. Assoc. J. 1964; 25:439-446.

Stewart, R.D., Hake, C.L., Lebrun, A.J., et al., *Effects of Trichloroethylene on Behavioral Performance Capabilities.* In: C. Xintaras, B. Johnson, I. Groot, Behavioral Toxicology. Washington, D.C.: U.S. Dep't of Health, Education, and Welfare, 1974.

Takeichi, S., Yamada, T., Shikata, I., *Acute Toluene Poisoning During Painting.* Forensic Sci. Int. 1986; 32-109-115.

Takeuchi, Y., Hisanaga, N., *Cerebellar Dysfunction Caused by Sniffing of Toluene-Containing Thinner.* Ind. Health 1981; 19:163-169.

Tarsh, M.J., *Schizophreniform Psychosis Caused by Sniffing Toluene.* J. Soc. Occup. Med. 1979; 29:131-133.

Timmerman, R.W., *Carbon Disulfide.* In: G.J. Bushey, I. Campbell, A. Klingsberg, L. van Nes (eds.), Kirk-Othmer Encyclopedia of Chemical Technology, 4th Ed. New York: John Wiley-Interscience, 1978: 742.

Towfighi, J., Gonatas, N.K., Pleasure, D., et al., *Glue Sniffer's Neuropathy.* Neurology 1976; 238-243.

Triebig, G., Schaller, K.H., Valentin, H., *Investigations on Neurotoxicity of Chemical Substances at the Workplace.* Int. Arch. Occup. Environ. Health 1985; 56:239-247.

Triebig, G., Trautner, P., Weltle, D., et al., *Untersuchungen zur Neurotoxizität von Arbeitsstoffen.* Int. Arch. Occup, Environ. Health 1982; 51:25-34.

Van Vliet, C., Swaen, G.M.H., Meijers, J.M.M., *Prenarcotic and Neuraesthenic Symptoms Among Dutch Workers Exposed to Organic Solvents.* Br. J. Industr. Med. 1989; 46:586-590.

Veulemans, H., Van Viem, E., Jannssens, H., et al., *Experimental Human Exposure to n-Hexane.* Int. Arch. Occup. Environ. Health 1982; 49:251-263.

Wallén, M., *Toxicokinetics of Toluene in Occupationally Exposed Volunteers.* Scand. J. Work Environ. Health 1986; 12:588-593.

Wieczorek, H., Piotrowski, J.K., *Kinetic Interpretation of the Exposure Test for Styrene.* Int. Arch. Occup. Environ. Health 1988; 61:107-113.

Wigaeus, E., Löf, A., Nordqvist, M., *Uptake, Distribution, Metabolism, and Elimination of Styrene in Man. A Comparison Between Single Exposure and Co-Exposure with Acetone.* Br. J. Ind. Med. 1984; 41:539-546.

Wilczok, T., Bienick, G., *Urinary Hippuric Acid Concentration After Occupational Exposure to Toluene.* Br. J. Ind. Med. 1978; 35:330-334.

Winchester, R.V., Madjar, V.M., *Solvent Effects on Workers in the Paint, Adhesive, and Printing Industries.* Ann. Occup. Hyg. 1986; 30:307-317.

Windemuller, F.J.B., Etteman, J.H., *Effects of Combined Exposure to Trichloroethylene and Alcohol on Mental Capacity.* Int. Arch. Occup. Environ. Health 1978; 41:77-85.

Winck, C.L., Wecht, C.H., Collom, W.D., *Toluene Fatality from Glue Sniffing.* Penn. Med. 1968; 71:81-86.

Withey, J.R., Collins, P.G., *Pharmacokinetics and Distribution of Styrene Monomer in Rats After Intravenous Administration.* J. Toxicol. Environ. Health 1977; 3:1011-1020.

World Health Organization, *Chronic Effects of Organic Solvents on the Central Nervous System. Environmental Health 5.* Copenhagen, WHO, 1985.

World Health Organization, *Organic Solvents and the Central Nervous System.* Environ. Health. 1990.

World Health Organization, *Recommended Health-Based Limits in Occupational Exposure to Selected Organic Solvents.* Technical Report Series No. 664, Copenhagen, 1981.

Chapter 8

METALS

One of the liveliest topics in occupational health and safety practice is the recognition of effects on the nervous system arising out of exposure at work to a growing list of commonly encountered chemicals. The severe neurotoxic impact of overexposure to certain agents, such as mercury, manganese, lead (both the metal and certain organic compounds), carbon disulfide, carbon monoxide, dinitro-o-cresol, and several insecticides, has long been recognized. Over the past several decades, there have been dramatic episodes of clinical neuropathies traced to exposures to acrylamide, methyl-n-butyl ketone (MBK), and butylazo-hydroxy-methylhexane (BHMH). Meanwhile, a lengthening tally of solvents and other chemical agents have been demonstrated or suspected to cause neurological damage. The effects of neurotoxic agents on the nervous system can be diverse and, although either peripheral or central effects may predominate from exposure to any single neurotoxin, the involvement of both peripheral and central nervous systems is common.

—*Proctor and Hughes' Chemical Hazards of the Workplace*, 3d Ed. (1991).

§ 8-1. In General.

Many metals are essential for life in small or trace amounts. Metals are involved in the synthesis and function of neurotransmitters (chemicals required for transmitting nerve impulses). Some metals, including iron, zinc, selenium, manganese, copper, aluminum, chromium, and molybdenum, are referred to as trace elements or trace nutrients, and are required as cofactors for vital enzymes. Disease can result from a dietary deficiency of trace metals. However, many of these same metals are toxic in large quantities. Other heavy metals are not essential. (See Table 8.1.)

Table 8.1
Essential and Nonessential Metals and Minerals

Essential:
Calcium
Chromium
Cobalt

Copper
Iron
Magnesium
Manganese
Molybdenum
Selenium
Zinc

Nonessential:
Aluminum
Arsenic
Lead
Mercury
Thallium

Much is unknown about the toxic mechanisms of heavy metals. In general, they are thought to exert adverse neurotoxic effects by interfering with the transmission of nerve impulses. Among the possible mechanisms are damage to the cell membranes of nerve cells, interference with neurotransmitters, and interaction with other metals.

§ 8-2. Lead.

Lead was one of the first metals to be used by man. It was abundant, cheap, and easily worked and shaped. Its compounds were found to be attractively colored and were used in paints, cosmetics, jewelry, pottery glazes, and other artistic applications. Lead toxicity has been with us since the beginning of recorded history, and it is still with us. The ruling class of Rome may have been poisoned by drinking wine from lead-lined vessels and water delivered by lead pipes (Gilfillan, 1966). Ancient physicians were probably familiar with the symptoms of lead toxicity. The use of lead increased during the Middle Ages and again during the Industrial Revolution. By the mid-nineteenth century, "painter's colic" had become well-known. Until the middle of the present century, most paint pigments were compounds of lead and other heavy metals. “White lead” was the most widely used paint color until about the middle of the present century.

The use of lead increased sharply with the advent of the automobile, as did levels of lead contamination in the environment. Lead storage batteries, organic lead salts as additives for gasoline, and rubber manufacturing processes accounted for these increases. Lead is no longer widely used in paints or gasoline, or in many other consumer products which formerly contained it. The level of contamination, however, is still quite high, although considerably lower than it was 25 years ago.

Data from the Third National Health and Nutrition Examination Surveys (NHANES III) show that from 1976 to 1991 the mean blood lead levels in persons aged 1 to 74 years dropped from 12.8 μg/dL to 2.8 μg/dL (Pirkle, 1994). In non-Hispanic white children under the age of 6 years, mean blood levels decreased from 13.7 μg/dL to 3.2 μg/dL. In non-Hispanic black children under 6 years of age, mean blood levels decreased from 20.2 μg/dL to 5.6 μg/dL. Over the same time period, the prevalence of blood levels of 10 μg/dL or greater decreased from 85% to 5.5% in non-Hispanic white children under 6 years of age, and from 97.7% to 20.6% in non-Hispanic black children under 6 years of age. Nevertheless, it has been estimated that in the period from 1988 to 1991, approximately 1.7 children in the United States under the age of 6 years had blood lead levels of 10 μg/dL or higher (Brody, 1994).

Lead/acid batteries are still the most widely used type of automotive battery. Lead from these batteries, battery oxides, and lead alkyds are the major sources of lead exposure in the United States today. Epidemics of lead poisoning have occurred in areas where low-income populations have been exposed to lead battery casings.

Lead is a heavy, soft metal, bluish to gray in color. Its relatively low melting point of 327.4. C (621.3. F) contributed to its early use. At 500. C to 600. C (932. F to 1112. F), lead gives off fumes in measurable amounts that can be harmful if inhaled. As the temperature rises, the rate of evaporation increases. In nature, lead occurs in several inorganic compounds or ores. Lead sulfide (galena) is the most common source of commercial lead. Other commercially important lead compounds included lead carbonate (cerusite), lead sulfate (aglesite), and lead chromate (crocoisite). Lead also occurs in organic compounds. Among the more important of these are tetraethyl and tetramethyl lead. When these "antiknock" additives were used in gasoline, they became a major source of environmental lead contamination. Because of the natural abundance of lead, the environment has never been lead-free. There has always been a "background" exposure from air, food and water. This level of exposure is probably much higher than it was before the Industrial Revolution (Saryan, 1994).

Leaded paint has long been a major source of toxic exposure to lead compounds. Basic lead carbonate (white lead), basic lead sulfate, lead silicate, and leaded zinc oxide are among the pigments used for outdoor paints. Chromates of lead make brightly colored paints, including yellows, greens, and reds. An oxide of lead, generally referred to as red lead, is used widely as a primer or rust retardant coating for metals. In the United States, leaded paint was used routinely for both indoor and outdoor painting until the 1970s. In 1977 and 1978, the U.S. Product Safety Commission banned the indoor use of paint with lead content greater than .06% by weight. The ingestion by children of peeling lead paint chips has been a problem in older buildings, particularly in inner city settings where buildings have not been properly maintained. Lead concentrations in paint chips can be as high as 40%. In a report of the Department of Health and Human Services, it was estimated that as many as 12 million children in the United States lived in housing containing lead paint, and that many suffered from lead exposure (U.S. Dep't of HHS, 1988, 1991; U.S. Dep't of HUD, 1990).

Leaded gasoline has also been a significant source of toxic exposure to lead, particularly in urban areas. When leaded gasoline was used, young children living in the city were exposed to air/lead concentrations about 10 times greater than those in most rural areas (Christian, 1964).

Lead has no known function in the human body. At any serum level, therefore, lead is a contaminant. Lead poisoning has always been more of a problem in young children than in adults. In the same environmental setting, children, particularly those under age five years, will have higher mean blood levels than adults (EPA, 1977). Children below the age of 3 are at maximal susceptibility to lead toxicity (Graef, 1979). Children absorb lead at a higher rate and are more likely to ingest nonfood items that may contain lead. In adults, about 10% of ingested lead is absorbed from the intestine, while in children the rate of absorption ranges from 40% to 50% (Krigman, 1980).

The National Health and Nutrition Examination Survey (NHANES II) demonstrated a very close association between the declining use of leaded gasoline and declining mean blood levels between 1976 and 1980 (U.S. Dep't of HHS, 1991). The NHANES III data discussed earlier, which covered the period from 1988 to 1991, demonstrated a further decline in overall mean blood levels. The geometric mean blood level found in NHANES II was 0.62 μmol/L (12.8 μg/dL); NHANES III data indicated that the mean had dropped to 0.14μmol/L (2.8 μg/dL) (Brody, 1994). These figures represent a major reduction in overall lead exposure, corresponding to further reduction in the use of leaded gasoline. There are still, however, some areas for concern. Lead blood levels are much higher in children than in adults, in blacks than in whites, and in city residents than in rural residents. It was estimated that 1.7 million children between the ages of 1 and 5 years have levels of 0.48 μmol/L (10 μg/dL) or greater. According to guidelines set in 1991 by the Centers for Disease Control and Prevention, these levels are high enough to be of concern (CDC, 1991). Also of concern is that leaded gasoline is still used in Europe and other parts of the world. There have been instances of lead encephalopathy from sniffing gasoline containing tetraethyl lead (Chisolm, 1992).

Industrial exposure occurs mainly in jobs where workers are exposed to lead fumes or lead powders. High-risk occupations include bookbinding, demolition of ships, papermaking, plumbing, production of brass and bronze, and the manufacture of lead storage batteries. The storage battery industry uses the largest amounts of lead, accounting for almost two-thirds of total consumption in the United States. Almost 80% of lead from discarded batteries is recycled, making old batteries the major source of lead for the secondary lead smelting and refining industry (Saryan, 1994).

§ 8-2(a). Biochemistry and Metabolism.

In addition to ingestion, lead can enter the body by inspiration of metal vapors or powders, and by absorption through the skin. About one-third of the lead taken into the body of an adult is absorbed through the lungs from atmospheric lead or its vapor (Cohen, 1977). The rate of lead absorption can be influenced by diet. It is increased by a high-fat, low-mineral diet, and decreased by a diet with high mineral content (Barltop, 1975). In rats fed a subtoxic dose of lead, studies have shown that an iron-deficient diet resulted in increased organ levels of lead (Six, 1978). Once lead is absorbed, it is carried by red blood corpuscles. In humans, lead can be detected in blood, soft tissue, and bone. The half-life in bone can be 10 years or more, while the half-life in blood can be as short as two weeks.

Lead diminishes the supply of glucose to the brain. It retards the activities of several key enzymes involved in the energy-releasing reactions of glycolysis and the tricarboxylic acid cycle (Goetz, 1985). Lead also interferes with the enzymes required for the synthesis of hemoglobin. One such enzyme is ferrochelatase, required for the synthesis of heme, a precursor of hemoglobin (Bernad, 1990).

§ 8-2(b). Clinical Effects.

The major adverse effects of lead are hematologic, neurologic, renal, gastrointestinal, and cardiovascular. Neurologic adverse effects can involve the central, peripheral and autonomic nervous systems. The association between low blood lead levels and low IQ is a controversial topic and has been studied for decades (Needleman, 1979; Needleman, 1980; Palca, 1991).

§ 8-2(b)(1). Central Nervous System.

Encephalopathy associated with lead can be acute, subacute, or chronic, and can stem from exposure to organic and inorganic forms of lead. It is generally agreed that the developing brain is more susceptible to lead toxicity. Thus, children are likely to be more severely affected. Lead-induced encephalopathy is considered to be a separate disease in young children and adults.

Acute lead encephalopathy from industrial exposure is rare today. High blood lead concentrations in excess of 100 µg/dL are generally needed to induce this disease. When it does occur, the prognosis is poor. Severe delirium is a frequent early manifestation, often accompanied by seizures and combative, irrational behavior (Goetz, 1985). Swelling of the brain, often accompanied by petechial hemorrhages, is seen frequently in acute lead encephalopathy. The swelling is believed to be a manifestation of vascular injury. The most extensive neuronal damage is usually seen in the cortex of the cerebellum. However, changes also occur in the cerebral cortex (Saryan, 1994). The clinical course varies with the age and condition of the patient, and with complicating factors such as alcoholism. As the disease progresses, symptoms reflecting the brain edema develop, such as forceful vomiting, apathy leading to somnolence, intractable seizures, and, in severe cases, death from cardiac arrest. In some cases, seizures and coma may occur without the warning signs of somnolence and apathy.

Before the availability of chelation therapy, about two-thirds of children with acute lead encephalopathy died. The mortality rate today is about 5%. However, approximately 25% of the survivors have permanent brain damage (Smith, 1989). Severe sequelae may occur, including mental retardation, blindness, and epilepsy with cortical atrophy. Sequelae may also include less obvious problems, such as lack of sensory perception, poor learning ability, aggressiveness, destructive behavior and hostility (Finkle, 1983). Subacute lead encephalopathy has been described in children, and may be more common in adults than previously thought. The existence of subacute lead encephalopathy was suspected when industrial lead toxicity was common. Lead workers were seen to develop subtle, generalized symptoms, such as sleep disturbances, memory dysfunction, and a tendency to be easily distracted.

Chronic lead encephalopathy in adults is characterized by psychomotor disturbances and dementia. These symptoms are probably due to the primary effects of chronic lead exposure on brain cells. They may also be due to lead-induced cirrhosis of the liver, nephropathy, and hypertension (Graef, 1979). Other possible manifestations include optic atrophy, mild facial or ocular nerve paresis, and laryngeal paralysis resulting in speech difficulties.

Symptoms and signs of lead encephalopathy usually develop slowly in children. Early manifestations, such as ataxia, clumsiness, listlessness and drowsiness, may be overlooked in a small child. In many instances, medical help is not sought until the occurrence of convulsions, coma, or respiratory arrest. This sudden deterioration is probably due to rapid increases in intracranial pressure. The worst prognosis is seen in children with significant increases in intracranial pressure accompanied by papilledema and brainstem compression, possibly leading to respiratory compromise (Goetz, 1985). The sequelae of lead encephalopathy, which can be quite severe, include permanent brain damage with mental retardation, seizures, and optic atrophy (Chisholm, 1979).

Children chronically exposed to lead can be affected for the rest of their lives. If, as is usually the case, there are no obvious symptoms and signs such as convulsions and coma, chronic lead exposure in children is often undiagnosed. It has been long known that children exposed to lead as infants tend not to do as well as those who are not exposed. Psychomotor testing has demonstrated significant differences between exposed and unexposed children (de la Burde, 1975). It has also been demonstrated that adverse effects on intelligence can occur in children if their mothers are exposed to low levels of lead during pregnancy (Baghurst, 1992; Bellinger, 1987). It was demonstrated that fetuses could be adversely affected at blood lead concentrations below

25 μg/dL, which is well below the highest acceptable level for young children as defined in 1987 by the Centers for Disease Control.

§ 8-2(b)(2). Peripheral Neuropathy.

Involvement of peripheral nerves is often seen in chronic lead intoxication occurring in adults. Lead intoxication is associated with several specific mononeuropathies. Both sensory and peripheral nerves are affected, although the effect on motor nerves is often more pronounced. Sensory complaints are most often paresthesias and spontaneous pain. Motor manifestations include local weakness, atrophy and fasiculations. A characteristic feature is that the paralysis usually occurs in extensor muscles, and the effect is often unilateral. The most used muscles are often the ones affected. Wrist drop, for example, has been seen in painters using lead compounds as pigments and tends to occur in the right hands of the painters. Other muscles may also be affected, including extensors of the legs, muscles of the upper body, and muscles that move the eyes. Weakness, lowered tone, and, in some cases, atrophy of extensors, have also been observed. As is the case with encephalopathy, industrial peripheral nerve paralysis in association with exposure to lead is now relatively rare (U.S. Dep't of Labor, 1990).

§ 8-3. Mercury.

Mercury is one of only a few metals that are liquid at room temperature. It exists as the metal, as inorganic mercurous (monovalent) and mercuric (divalent) salts, and as organic (covalent) compounds. Inorganic mercury can be transformed to methyl mercury, a highly toxic compound. Mercury and its compounds have been used in human activities since prehistoric times. Cinnabar, the red ore of mercury (mercury sulfide), was used by prehistoric men to add color to paintings on cave walls. Commonly referred to as quicksilver, mercury was being mined during the time of ancient Rome. The toxic effects were well known by then, and only slaves and convicts worked in the mercury mines. The term "mad as a hatter" refers to the practice of using mercuric nitrate in the felting process. The chronic exposure resulting from this work was associated with a syndrome of neurologic disorders including marked personality changes.

Mercury is used widely in industry in the manufacture of electrical equipment, paints, measurement and control systems, detonators (fulminate of mercury), and catalysts. Mercury is used in dentistry in the "silver" amalgam used for filling cavities. Mercury compounds are also used in agriculture, primarily as a fungicide. The use of mercury to separate gold and silver from ores is a major source of environmental pollution in areas where protective measures are not observed. Waterways around the gold mines in the Brazilian state of Para have been heavily polluted. In this method, an amalgam of liquid mercury and ore is made, and the mercury is driven off as a vapor by heating the amalgam.

Runoff from agricultural use of mercury compounds also contaminates waterways. Some of this mercury is converted to methyl mercury, the most dangerous form of the metal, by the action of certain microorganisms that flourish in aquatic environments. The methyl mercury is passed along in the food chain from plankton to predatory fish, many of which are food sources for humans. In passing from plankton to fish, the concentration of methyl mercury increases several thousandfold. The eating of fish containing methyl mercury was the cause of the mercury poisoning epidemic in Minamata, Japan, in 1952. Many of the victims suffered irreversible damage to the cerebral cortex and cerebellum (Takeuchi, 1989). The effects of methylmercury on fetuses, including microencephaly, cerebral palsy, and mental retardation, are similarly devastating.

§ 8-3(a). Factors Affecting Toxicity.

The toxicity of mercury depends on its chemical form and method of entry into the body. The ingestion of metallic mercury poses little risk of toxicity. Mercuric sulfide, which is more toxic than metallic mercury, forms on the surface of the metal. Thus the more surface exposure, the more toxic metallic mercury is likely to be. Because of the poor absorption of mercury, oral doses of 100 to 500 grams have been given with little effect other than diarrhea (National Research Council, 1977). Inhalation of mercury vapor is the major industrial source of mercury poisoning. Elemental mercury is quite volatile and vaporizes at room temperature. Once the vapor is inhaled, it is absorbed rapidly through the lungs. Animal studies have shown that 10 times more mercury accumulates in the brain following a single exposure to mercury vapor than after intravenous injection of a similar quantity of mercuric mercury (Berlin, 1969). Absorption of mercury through the skin is insignificant. However, skin contact can result in dermatitis in susceptible individuals. Mucus membranes can also be so affected (Meddler, 1968; Friberg, 1986).

There is considerable controversy over the existence of a toxic effect of the mercury in dental amalgams. The present official position of the American Dental Association is that there is little risk (Council on Dental Materials, 1989). Data from some studies have shown a relationship between the surface area of amalgams and urinary and plasma mercury levels (Molin, 1989; Molin, 1990). As yet, however, there is no conclusive evidence of any adverse effects, other than allergic reactions, from exposure to dental amalgams (Velen, 1990).

§ 8-3(b). Acute and Chronic Mercury Poisoning.

Mercury poisoning can be acute or chronic. Acute poisoning has been associated with inhaling high concentrations of mercury vapor or dust. Inhaling vapors has been associated with bronchitis, bronchiolitis, and interstitial pneumonia (Dreisbach, 1983). Signs and symptoms of exposure to high levels of mercury vapor include tightness and pain in the chest, difficult breathing, and coughing. These may be followed by nausea, vomiting, metallic taste, headache, abdominal pain, diarrhea, and, in some instances, albumin in the urine. Three to four days after the onset of symptoms, the salivary glands swell, gingivitis occurs, there may be a dark line of mercury sulfide on inflamed gums, teeth may loosen, and ulcers may appear on the lips and cheeks. As the disease progresses, symptoms of nephritis and gastroenteritis may appear. In severe cases, death may occur at any time after the exposure. In milder cases, recovery may occur in two weeks. Cases of acute mercury poisoning have occurred at concentrations ranging from 1.2 to 8.5 mg/m^3. Survivors may develop psychopathologic symptoms and muscle tremors which could become chronic (Patty, 1982).

Some compounds of mercury are corrosive, and ingesting them causes immediate burning pain and a feeling of constriction. Within a few minutes of ingestion there is acute epigastric pain, followed by diffuse abdominal pain and continuous vomiting of bloody, mucoid material. There may also be liquid, bloody feces and painful defecation. In severe cases, the patient may go into shock and die. In milder cases, the gastroenteritis subsides with local treatment. Mercurial stomatitis, which consists of glossitis and ulcerative gingivitis accompanied by heavy salivation, may appear a day or two after the ingestion. If untreated, there may be necrosis of the jaw, infection, and loosening of the teeth. Other possible complications include ulcerative colitis, liver necrosis, and kidney problems which could result in death from azotemia (Aposhian, 1959).

Chronic mercury poisoning is most often associated with industrial exposure. In recent years, however, with the adoption of safety procedures, the incidence of industrial mercury exposure has declined in most industrialized countries. A variety of symptoms and signs have been reported in association with chronic mercury poisoning. (See Table 8.2.)

Table 8.2
Signs and Symptoms of Chronic Mercury Poisoning

Mouth

General inflammation
Gingivitis
Tender and discolored gums
Loose teeth

Alveolar destruction of teeth (x-ray diagnosis)
Swollen salivary glands
Increased salivation or mouth dryness
Excretion of mercury in the saliva
Tongue inflammation

Neurologic

Tremor
Neuralgia
Ataxia
Paresthesia
Exaggerated knee jerks
Altered plantar reflexes
Vasomotor disturbances (blushing, excessive perspiration)
Disturbances of muscles that move the eyes
Decreased peripheral vision/blindness
Personality changes

(Gilman, 1990; Grant, 1986; Levine, 1982; Wood, 1973)

The tremor of chronic mercury poisoning is observed most frequently in the fingers, and later in the arms and legs. Tremor in the eyelids has also been reported (Grant, 1986). A change in handwriting is often the first indication of chronic mercury poisoning. Personality changes, such as the "mad hatter" syndrome, are among the most common findings. In mild cases, they may occur in the absence of other symptoms. Observed symptoms have included erethism, irritability, irascibility, excitability, fearfulness, depression, shyness, timidity, moroseness, fatigue, drowsiness, and weakness. Excessive criticizing has also been observed. Erethism and tremor are sometimes reversible (Gilman, 1990).

§ 8-3(c). Inorganic Mercury Salts.

Mercury in inorganic salts or compounds is not well absorbed in the intestine. Skin absorption has not been shown to be significant. Inorganic mercury readily crosses the blood-brain barrier, but to a lesser extent than mercury vapor. Inorganic mercury salts occur in two main groups: monovalent (mercurous), and divalent (mercuric). In the past, the mercurous compound calomel was widely used as a medication. It is thought that George Washington's death may have been hastened by the liberal use of calomel during his final illness. In the early twentieth century, calomel was used as a teething powder in infants. It was sometimes associated with a syndrome called "pink disease," characterized by a body rash and pain in the extremities (acrodynia), thought to be related to an affect on the sympathetic nervous system. Other symptoms included chills, irritability, photophobia, anorexia, insomnia and excessive perspiration (Warkany, 1953). Fatal poisoning in adults from an accidental overdose of a laxative containing mercurous chloride has been reported (Davis, 1974). Autopsy revealed cerebral atrophy and loss of cells in the cerebellum.

Chronic exposure to mercuric mercury is almost always associated with some occupational activity which puts the worker at risk of inhaling dust of mercury compounds such as mercuric nitrate. The "mad hatter" syndrome is the best known of the neurologic syndromes associated with this exposure. The symptoms are similar to those seen in poisoning from mercury vapor and include erethism, incoordination, tremor, and neuropsychological changes. Acute exposure is usually associated with adverse effects on the renal and gastrointestinal systems, rather than on the nervous system. The effects can be quite severe. They may include abdominal pain and bloody diarrhea, which can progress to circulatory collapse and death. Survivors may experience kidney failure.

§ 8-3(d). Organic Mercury Compounds.

Organic mercury compounds are used as fungicides for treating seeds and for preventing mold growth on turf, and also in paper mills to prevent the formation of "slime." They have been a major source of environmental pollution. Organic mercury compounds can be classified into two major groups: 1) arylmercury and alkoxyalkylmercury, and 2) alkylmercuric compounds. The former are unstable in mammals, while the latter are short-chain compounds which are stable in mammals.

Phenyl mercury and methoxymethylmercury are examples of the arylmercury and alkoxyalkylmercury group. They are rapidly absorbed, both in the gastrointestinal tract and by inhalation. Once absorbed, they are decomposed into inorganic mercuric ions. Phenyl mercury and methoxymethylmercury cross the blood-brain barrier to about the same extent as inorganic mercury. There have been reports of an association between phenylmercury and a degeneration of spinal motor neurons similar to that seen in amyotrophic lateral sclerosis (Kantarjian, 1964; Adams, 1983). However, other studies have failed to show significant mercury accumulation, or any specific neuronal changes in the central nervous system, in association with the exposure to the mercury compound (Currier, 1968). The issue remains controversial, however, with the recent demonstration of the accumulation of mercuric mercury in the spinal cord and brainstem following the injection of inorganic mercury (Arvidson, 1992).

Alkyl mercury compounds include methylmercury, considered to be the most dangerous of the mercury compounds, and ethylmercury. Methylmercury is by far the most toxic of the mercury compounds. After ingestion, it is readily distributed from the blood to body tissues. The highest initial concentrations are in the liver (Clarkson, 1972). It readily enters the brain, but at rates slower than in other tissues and via mechanisms that are not fully understood. Several days are required for peak concentrations to accumulate in the brain (Sakai, 1974; Magos, 1976).

The toxic potential of methylmercury was dramatically brought to the world's attention by the massive outbreak of mercury poisoning in Minamata, Japan, in 1956 and 1965 (Takeuchi, 1968). The syndrome, generally referred to as "Minamata disease," occurred among people who had consumed fish and shellfish contaminated by methylmercury. Distinguished from methylmercury poisoning resulting from direct exposure to the compound, Minamata disease develops over an extended period of time, while the syndrome associated with direct exposure is manifested after a relatively short period of time.

The outbreak of Minamata disease was one of the worst environmental disasters of modern times. Industrial discharge of mercury into Minamata Bay and adjacent waters started in 1932. The peak levels of contamination occurred in 1956. Discharge was completely stopped in 1968, but the waters remained contaminated for quite some time. Levels of mercury exceeding 100 ppm were found in mud samples taken from Minamata Bay in 1974. Similar, but smaller, outbreaks that occurred in Iraq were associated with contaminated grain.

Gold mining in areas upstream of the Amazon river in Brazil has resulted in a severe mercury pollution problem. Mercury is used in a gold extraction process in which 2 to 10 grams of mercury are required to extract 1 gram of gold. In 1989, the Brazilian government began to enforce a law banning the mercury process. However, several measures of mercury pollution — including mercury content in human hair, river bed mud, and fish and shellfish — continue to increase in areas downstream from the gold mining areas (Harada, 1997). Natural methylation of inorganic mercury has raised concern in Canada and Brazil.

§ 8-3(d)(1). Symptoms of Methylmercury Poisoning (Minamata Disease).

The nervous system is the major target of methylmercury poisoning. The disease can be acute or chronic, and the symptoms vary widely with each patient, but some manifestations occur more frequently than others. Typically, a patient with acute methylmercury poisoning develops symptoms referred to collectively as the Hunter-Russell syndrome. The syndrome includes ataxia, dysarthria, auditory disturbance, sensory impairment, and constriction of the visual field (Minamata Disease Research Group, 1968). Patients with mild cases may have a variety of vague, subjective complaints, including headache, muscle and joint pains, memory disturbances, vertigo and dizziness, trembling, fatigue, and increased susceptibility to cold. Fainting and convulsions have also been reported (Tsubaki, 1977; Fujino, 1994). Some patients develop muscular dystrophy hemilateral and spinal symptoms (Tsubaki, 1977; Harada, 1982).

The sensory deficits are generally believed to result from damage to the peripheral nervous system. Sensory fibers have been observed to be selectively damaged in association with methylmercury poisoning (Takeuchi, 1985). Sensory disturbances are often evident around the mouth and in the extremities, and taste and smell may be impaired. The central nervous system may also be involved. Narrowing of the visual field occurs in the later stages of the disease, and is considered to be almost pathognomonic by some authorities (Minamata Disease Research Group, 1968; Harada, 1995).

The symptoms of chronic methylmercury poisoning are essentially the same as those seen in the acute disease. However, the symptoms come on slowly, usually over a period of 5 to 10 years. Which symptoms appear, the degree of severity, and the time required for development of the disease vary widely. Terms such as "gradually progressive type," "delayed onset type," and "escalatingly progressive type" have been used in attempts to classify different types or forms of the disease. A patient may continue to develop new symptoms even after exposure to methylmercury is reduced or ceased. Committees formed in Japan for the purpose of identifying victims established sensory disturbances and either cerebellar ataxia or constriction of visual fields as the criteria for diagnosis (Harada, 1997).

§ 8-3(d)(2). Pathologic Findings.

Acute disease has been associated with damage to the central nervous system, particularly the cerebral and cerebellar cortex. Damage has also been seen in the visual center of the brain (which is on the occipital lobe in the back of the brain), in the sensory and motor areas, and in the temporal cortex where the auditory center is located (Takeuchi, 1977; Takeuchi, 1985). Chronic disease is associated with lesions in the cerebellar and cerebral cortex and peripheral nerves. The severity of the lesions varies (Takeuchi, 1985).

§ 8-3(d)(3). Congenital Methylmercury Disease.

Organic mercury passes readily through the placenta and can seriously damage the brain of the fetus (Minamata Disease Research Group, 1968). It was observed that many children in the Minamata area who had not eaten contaminated fish developed symptoms and signs of infantile cerebral palsy. The rate of cerebral palsy in the affected areas was about 9.0%, compared to about 0.02% in the general population of Japan (Minamata Disease Research Group, 1968; Harada, 1986).

Symptoms and signs of congenital methylmercury disease include mental retardation, strabismus, primitive reflexes, cerebellar ataxia, dysarthria, hypersalivation, seizures, deformed limbs, and growth retardation. Pathologic findings include general atrophy and hypoplasia of the cerebral cortex, various abnormalities in brain cells, and hypoplasia of the corpus callosum. Abnormalities in the cerebellum include hypoplasia of the granular cell layer and other cells layers, and degeneration of granular cells, which is characteristic of Minamata disease (Takeuchi, 1979, Harada, 1986).

Data obtained on the intake of methylmercury from the events in Japan and Iraq led to the establishment of a total body load of 25 mg of methylmercury as necessary to induce minimal symptoms of sensory disturbance and 100 mg for typical symptoms (Amin-Zaki, 1974).

§ 8-3(d)(4). Long-Term Studies of Methylmercury Poisoning.

In a 30-year follow-up study, the brain weights of persons exposed to methylmercury in the Minamata area were compared with those of a control group who had died suddenly or from an accident. The brain weights in the Minamata cases had decreased by 80 to 200 mg compared to the controls (Takeuchi, 1996).

In a review article, Gilbert pointed out the long-term risk of low levels of methylmercury exposure to the developing fetus (Gilbert, 1995). The fetus is particularly susceptible to methylmercury exposure. Adverse effects on the fetus occur at levels of exposure that produce few if any symptoms and signs of illness in the mother. Gilbert recommends that women of childbearing age limit their exposure to potential sources of methylmercury. On the basis of results from human and animal studies, he recommends further that the accepted reference dose of methylmercury by reduced from 0.06 to 0.025 micrograms per kilogram of body weight a day.

In the United States, a family who consumed pork containing methylmercury provided an opportunity for long-term studies on Minamata-type mercury poisoning (Davis, 1994). In August 1969, a family in New Mexico inadvertently fed their hogs grain that had been treated with a fungicide containing methylmercury. A hog was killed a month later, and the family, which included a pregnant mother, ate the pork over the next 3 months. Three of the children, aged 20, 13, and 8 years, and the neonate developed severe neurological signs. The mother, father, and two children aged 9 and 16 years were asymptomatic. For reasons unknown, it is believed these 2 children seldom ate in the household. Neurologic symptoms and signs included confusion, ataxia, constricted visual fields, seizures, somnolence, cortical blindness, dementia, hemiparesis, loss of proprioception, and choreoathetosis (abnormal movements). When the baby was born, it had a weak cry and was lethargic, mentally retarded, blind, spastic, and exhibited myoclonic jerks.

Follow-up studies of the affected individuals, including neuropsychological testing, were carried out 22 years later. A female who was 42 years old at follow-up, had a verbal IQ of 86 (low), mild attentional deficit, poor coordination, poor word retrieval, and no peripheral vision. MRI revealed loss of tissues in various parts of the cerebrum and cerebellum. The mercury level in her hair was 2,436 ppm, which is extremely high. A male who was 35 years old at follow-up had a verbal IQ of 99, and demonstrated some of the same deficits as the female. In addition, he had a moderate learning deficit, dysfluent speech and hyperactive reflexes. His MRI findings were similar to those of the 42-year-old female. A female who was 8 years old at the time of exposure died at 29 years of age. Before her death, she was mute and blind, and had dementia, quadriparesis, and seizures. Autopsy showed extensive abnormalities. All three major parts of the brain — cerebrum, cerebellum, and brainstem — were greatly reduced in size, weighing only 440 gm. Atrophy was seen in almost all lobes of the brain. The individual who was a fetus at the time of exposure died at age 21. His symptoms and signs were similar to those of the female who died at age 29. The father and mother, who were 72 and 70 years of age respectively at the time of follow-up, were essentially asymptomatic. The father had spatial deficits and poor tandem gait. His MRI was normal, but the mother's showed mild atrophy in some parts of the cerebellum.

The experience of this family graphically illustrates that the younger the patient, the more severe the effects of mercury poisoning on the nervous system. The child exposed in utero suffered the worst neurological damage. Neither parent was severely affected. Similar patterns of effects were seen in the Minamata and Iraqi epidemics.

§ 8-4. Arsenic.

Arsenic is utilized in the manufacture of insecticides, herbicides, wood preservatives, microelectronics, and some pharmaceuticals, particularly veterinary products. Workers in these industries may be at risk of exposure, as may be workers in some mining and smelting operations, particularly copper, lead and zinc (La Dou, 1986; Farmer, 1990; Lagerkvist, 1994). In the smelting of these metals, arsenic is removed as an impurity. People living near smelters and other industries emitting arsenic are subject to environmental exposure from inhalation of dust and contamination of soil and water (Milham, 1974; Baker, 1977; Franzblau, 1989; Engel, 1994).

Arsenic exists in three valence states: metalloid (0 oxidation state), arsenite (trivalent state), and arsenate (pentavalent state). It also exists in organic and inorganic forms. The toxicity of arsenic varies with the valence state, the organic or inorganic form, and with physical factors such as physical state (gas, liquid, powder), particle size, solubility, and rates of absorption and elimination. In general, the toxicity of inorganic arsenic is greater than that of organic arsenic. The toxicity of the trivalent form is greater than that of pentavalent arsenic. The most toxic form of arsenic, however, is arsine gas, which is used in the microelectronics industry. The clinical syndrome it produces is quite different from that produced by other arsenic compounds (HHS, 1990).

The use of arsenic in industry has declined since the 1960s. In the late 1980s, almost three-quarters of the arsenic used in the United States was for wood preservation; less than 1% was used in electronics. However, with the growth of the microelectronics industry associated with computers and other applications, the use of arsenic is increasing. Gallium arsenide is used in microwave generators, lasers, photoelectric chemical cells, and semiconductors. Arsine gas is also used in the manufacture of semiconductors. Exposure to arsine may occur during accidental releases of gas in the manufacturing process, during transport, or when arsine unexpectedly forms chemically after the addition of an acid to substances containing low levels of arsenic.

Among the general population, the main route of arsenic exposure is ingestion of food and water containing arsenic. Groundwater can be contaminated from natural sources, such as arsenic in bedrock, or from pollution, such as runoff from pesticides containing arsenic. Areas in the United States with the highest natural groundwater concentrations of arsenic are those near geothermal activity, including the

Southwest, Northwest, and Alaska. Epidemics of arsenic toxicity associated with contaminated well water have been reported in the United States, Argentina, Chile, Germany, Taiwan, and the United Kingdom.

The sources of about 80% of the natural dietary intake of arsenic are meat, fish, and poultry. The highest concentrations are seen in fish and other seafood — especially bivalves (oysters, clams) and certain cold-water and bottom-feeding fish — and in algae. This arsenic is in the form of arsenobetaine and arsenocholine. Often referred to as "fish arsenic," these substances have low toxicity to humans and are rapidly excreted in the urine (Maher, 1985; Lau, 1987). Smokers may inhale small amounts of arsenic residue from tobacco leaves sprayed with insecticide. Larger amounts of arsenic may be ingested in the form of wine made from grapes sprayed with insecticides containing arsenic.

Table 8.3
Sources of Arsenic

Natural Sources

Mineral ores
Groundwater
Seafood
Kelp

Products

Anti-fouling and other paints
Cattle and sheep dips
Fungicides
Herbicides
Insecticides
Wood preservatives

Industrial Processes

Burning fossil fuels
Burning wood impregnated with arsenic preservatives

Clarifying glass
Electronics manufacturing
Hardening metal alloys
Preserving animal hides

Exposure to arsenic can be acute or chronic. Acute exposure is usually associated with accidental or intentional ingestion. However, industrial exposure has also resulted in acute poisoning (Renwick, 1981). Chronic poisoning has been associated with industrial exposure and long-term use of contaminated water and foods.

The effects of acute arsenic poisoning are multi-systemic. Arsenic can interfere with biochemical pathways involving lipoic acids, resulting in a condition similar to thiamine deficiency and neurologic effects such as peripheral neuropathy (Dreisbach, 1983). Acute poisoning is usually manifested by severe inflammation of the gastrointestinal tract, often accompanied by hemorrhage. Cardiogenic shock may also occur (Landrigan, 1992). Symptoms and signs include difficult swallowing, abdominal cramps, diarrhea, dehydration, weak pulse, and low blood pressure. If not treated, or if the poisoning is too massive to treat, the patient will suffer stupor, coma, convulsions and death. The seizures are probably a manifestation of encephalopathy. The liver and kidneys may also be affected. Survivors may develop chronic encephalopathy (Fincher, 1987). Intense short-term exposure is often associated with peripheral neuropathy developing two-to-three weeks later (Heyman, 1956).

The effects of chronic arsenic poisoning are also multi-systemic. The major neurologic manifestation of arsenic poisoning is peripheral neuropathy. Other affected systems and organs include skin, the liver, the cardiovascular system, and the respiratory system. The formation of new blood cells may also be impaired (Woods, 1977). The skin manifestations can be quite severe, and include the risk of cancer. Chronic exposure has been associated with eczematous and follicular dermatitis, warts, hyperkeratosis of the palms and soles, and hyper pigmentation, particularly around the eyes, neck, nipples, and armpits.

The presence of concurrent skin manifestations and neuropathy increases the suspicion of arsenic exposure. Skin cancer associated with arsenic is dose-related. In addition to industrial and natural exposure, skin cancer has been associated with medications containing arsenic (Fitzpatrick, 1993). Cancers in other parts of the body have also been associated with chronic exposure to arsenic. Changes in cutaneous bleeding time have been noted in association with arsenic ingested in seafood (Meltzer, 1994).

The peripheral neuropathy associated with arsenic poisoning is symmetric and manifests nitially as mild paresthesias in the feet. Patients may complain of pain and swelling in the hands and feet. As the disease progresses, the vibratory and position senses may be affected, leading to ataxia and impaired coordination (Heyman, 1956). EMG studies may show slowing of nerve conduction velocities. A patient who ingested arsenic in the opium to which he was addicted experienced respiratory difficulties because of slowed conduction in the phrenic nerve, which controls the movement of the diaphragm. He presented with watery diarrhea and vomiting characteristic of arsenic poisoning (Bansal, 1991).

Patients often exhibit a symmetric decrease in pin, touch, and temperature sensations. The decrease in these senses usually starts in the feet. In severe disease, there may be symmetric muscle weakness which is usually more pronounced distally. In some instances, the neuropathy may be at least partially reversible (Franzblau, 1989). Encephalopathy is rare in patients who survive, and is usually associated with high levels of exposure.

The amount of arsenic in the body can be assessed by measuring total arsenic concentrations in hair, blood, and urine. Of these, urine testing appears to be the most useful indicator of recent arsenic exposure (Landrigan, 1992). Concentration in hair is a useful indicator of past arsenic exposure. However, it does not distinguish between absorbed and deposited arsenic. The arsenic hair content could appear to be increased after swimming in water contaminated by arsenic (Yamauchi, 1989). In a study of workers in a semiconductor fabrication facility, it was found that nonoccupational sources of arsenic contributed more to arsenic levels in the hair of workers than did occupational exposure in plants where safe work practices were followed (dePeyester, 1995). Blood level determinations are of little practical value (Mealey, 1959).

The timing of the collection of urine for testing is important. In cases of suspected industrial exposure, urine collected at the end of the work week should provide the most accurate information (Roy, 1983). Urine collected in the morning, or in random spot checks, is useful for determination of the absorption of arsenic (Baker, 1977). If the subject has eaten seafood 48 to 72 hours before the test, the results can be complicated or invalidated. However, the arsenic in seafood is excreted as arsenobetaine. Separation of the concentration of this metabolite from the other quantifications can produce valid results (Yamauchi, 1989).

§ 8-5. Thallium.

Thallium is one of the most toxic of metals affecting the nervous system. The neurotoxic effects can result from acute and chronic exposure. Both the peripheral and central nervous systems can be affected. As is the case with lead, thallium has no known function in the body and is not required as a trace element, although it occurs in small amounts in almost all living things. It is a natural constituent of the earth's crust and can be obtained from dust residues in zinc and lead smelters because of its existence as an impurity in the ores of these metals. Thallium forms compounds in monovalent and trivalent states. The trivalent compounds are water soluble and are found in both fresh water and sea water.

Thallium has a number of commercial uses, including thallium sulfate, a lethal poison used for rat and ant control. Thallium is used in the manufacture of optical glass, photoelectric cells, imitation gemstones, dyes, pigments, fireworks, high-quality metal alloys, and cements. Thallium compounds are used in devices that detect infrared radiation and in military communication devices. A liquid alloy with mercury is used in electric switches, thermometers, and relays.

Environmental thallium pollution results from cement plants, iron alloy production, mining operations, and burning coal. Of these, coal-burning, mostly from power plants, appears to be the major source. Ambient air levels of thallium near power plants have been determined to contribute amounts much greater than might be expected in nature.

Thallium is efficiently absorbed in the intestine at a rate approaching 100%. It is rapidly distributed throughout the body and enters cells of all organs, including those of the nervous system. In blood, it tends to be in the red blood cells rather than the plasma. Most excretion is via the kidneys and intestine. However, a small but detectable amount is excreted in hair, providing a test for assessment of exposure (Kazantzis, 1986). Thallium compounds can also be absorbed through the skin. Toxicity through the percutaneous route was a frequent side effect of topical medications containing thallium salts (Rick, 1979).

Once thallium enters the body, it is excreted slowly. In studies of experimental ingestion in humans, it was found that 45% of the dose was still in the body 24 days after ingestion (Moeschlin, 1980). In cases of acute poisoning, thallium could still be detected in urine, feces, and hair five months after ingestion (Sabbioni, 1980). In addition to hair, some thallium is excreted in sweat, tears, and milk. Thallium crosses the placenta and has been in the urine, feces, and meconium of infants whose mothers had experienced thallium poisoning during pregnancy (Sabbioni, 1980).

Cases of thallium poisoning have declined in recent years. Thallium compounds are no longer used for treating syphilis, gonorrhea, tuberculosis, gout, or scalp fungus (Moeschlin, 1980). The use of thallium sulfate for rodent control is now regulated, and its use for that purpose had declined (Saddique, 1983). Industrial exposure has also declined, but thallium poisoning still occurs. Cement plants appear to present the greatest exposure hazard today (Schaller, 1980).

§ 8-5(a). Neurologic Effects.

Thallium is taken up by cerebral tissue much more slowly than by other tissues. However, thallium levels decline more slowly in the brain than in other organs (Sabbioni, 1980; Eden-Rad, 1982). Thallium appears to accumulate in the nervous system only after repetitive ingestion, and in an uneven pattern (Davis, 1981).

§ 8-6. Manganese.

Manganese is the fourth most widely used metal in the world, after iron, aluminum, and copper. It is used in the manufacture of steel alloys, dry batteries, paints, enamels, and chlorine gas. Manganese compounds are used as fungicides, pesticides, and bactericides. The compound mehtylcyclopentadienyl (MMT) is an antiknock additive in lead-free gasoline. Workers exposed to manganese dust and vapor can be at risk of adverse neurotoxic effects.

Parkinson-like symptoms in workers employed in grinding manganese ores were described in the 1830s (Couper, 1837). These observations came only 20 years after the classic paper of James Parkinson. The effects of chronic manganese intoxication are still generally referred to as manganese Parkinsonism. Symptoms include asthenia, hypokinesia, rigidity (sometimes accompanied by dystonia), impotence, and insomnia. The symptoms progress as long as exposure continues and may continue to progress after the patient is removed from exposure. Recovery is rare (Cotzias, 1968; Huang, 1989).

Acute manganese intoxication, often referred to as locura manganica, is usually mild and transient. It is seen most often in manganese miners, and seldom in manganese industry workers. The syndrome includes memory impairment, disorientation, emotional instability, hallucinations, and behavioral disturbances such as involuntary laughter.

Manganese is a vital trace element. It is required for growth, for the formation of bone and connective tissue, and for the metabolism. Manganese deficiency during pregnancy can result in abnormal development of the inner ear and reproductive systems (Schramm, 1986). Manganese is required for the function of a number of important enzymes, including glutamine synthease, pyruvate carboxylase, and galactosyl transferase. A possible association between manganese deficiency and a reduction in the threshold for epileptic seizures has been proposed. However, while low manganese levels have been found in association with seizures, some investigators have proposed that the low manganese levels are secondary to the genetic mechanisms responsible for the epilepsy (Hurley, 1963; Carl, 1986; Carl, 1993).

Some pathological changes in the brain have been associated with manganese neurotoxicity. In normal conditions, manganese is distributed fairly uniformly throughout the brain. About 80% of brain manganese is in the enzyme glutamine synthease (Wedler, 1984). After toxic exposure, manganese tends to accumulate in a part of the brain called the basal ganglia. Autopsies and chronic studies in humans and animals have shown neuropathological changes in the basal ganglia in association with manganese intoxication (Yamada, 1986; Eriksson, 1987; Bird, 1984). The basal ganglia are involved in the control and regulation of motor activity, such as the movement of muscles, and complex behavioral activity (Alexander, 1990; Groenwegen, 1993). Typical autopsy findings include atrophy of the basal ganglia, characterized by loss of neurons and gliosis. Neurochemical studies in monkeys have shown that manganese had the greatest toxic effect on dopaminergic neurons.

§ 8-6(a). Differentiating Between Manganese and True Parkinsonism.

Levodopa is a widely used drug in the treatment of Parkinson's disease. However, in recent studies of miners with chronic manganism, the drug has not been particularly successful in the treatment of manganese Parkinsonism (Lu, 1994; Huang, 1993). The results of this study were contrary to those of an earlier investigation in which levodopa was found to be more beneficial in the treatment of manganese

Parkinsonism than to patients with Parkinson's disease (Cotzias, 1971).

Positron emission tomography (PET) in miners exposed to manganese showed a decline in cortical and subcortical glucose consumption. No change in the utilization of 6-fluorodopa was seen. High blood manganese levels, not accompanied by high urinary levels, are generally found in association with exposure to the metal (Mergler, 1994).

§ 8-7. Zinc.

Zinc is an essential trace element. Dietary zinc deficiency can result in central nervous system disorders and peripheral neuropathy (Browning, 1994). Zinc is abundant in the earth's crust and is used extensively in a variety of industrial applications. Zinc ore deposits may contain varying amounts of cadmium, arsenic and manganese. Zinc smelting operations, therefore, may expose workers to the adverse effects of those metals. Refined zinc is used in the manufacture of brass and various noncorrosive alloys. Compounds of zinc are used in the ceramic, chemical, pharmaceutical, agricultural, and paint industries.

Until recent years, most nutrition research has focused on the effects of zinc deficiency. It has become apparent, however, that in addition to industrial exposure, overdosing of zinc supplements may also have a variety of adverse effects. "Metal fume fever," a reaction to inhalation of zinc oxide fumes and fumes of other metal oxides, is well-known to metal workers (Bertholf, 1988). The first symptoms are usually respiratory, and the patient often complains of having a "cold in the chest." The patient generally looks and feels distressed, may have a fever, and the pulse rate may be quite elevated (100 to 120 beats a minute). If the symptoms are due to zinc, the disease is self-limiting and the patient usually recovers in a few days

Most reports of acute zinc toxicity have been associated with food poisoning. Some cases have been attributed to the storage of food in galvanized containers (Brown, 1964; Fosmire, 1990). In these incidents, it was not possible to quantify the amount of zinc ingested. Typically, the foods were somewhat acidic and were stored long enough for zinc to leach out of the galvanized coating. Symptoms included nausea, vomiting, epigastric pain, abdominal pain, and diarrhea. Neurologic manifestations were seen in a 16-year-old boy who ingested 12 grams of elemental zinc over a 2-day period. His symptoms included lethargy, light-headedness, slight staggering gait, and difficulty in writing (Murphy, 1970).

Excessive use of supplements and dosages of zinc prescribed for various therapeutic purposes have been associated with severe copper deficiency (Porter, 1977; Prasad, 1978). The zinc dosages in these instances were between 100 and 300 mg a day. Symptoms included anemia, leukopenia, and neutropenia. The serum copper levels returned to normal when the zinc therapy was discontinued. Even moderate intake of zinc has been associated with copper imbalance. Typically, zinc supplementation is around 100 mg a day (The RDA is 15 mg a day). However, this adverse effect is not seen in all individuals using that level of zinc supplementation (Festa, 1985; Greber, 1978; Burke, 1981).

Heavy metal exposure may have negative effects on the autonomic nervous system (ANS), peripheral nervous system (PNS), as well as the central nervous system (CNS). The usual techniques to evaluate ANS function may be used (EKG, R2R variability, tilt table techniques). In a study of gunmetal workers, the R-R interval (a characteristic of the electrocardiogram (ECG)) was found to be significantly reduced from the norm. This variation reflects changes in both the sympathetic and parasympathetic divisions of the autonomic nervous system. Peripheral nerve conduction velocity was also reduced in these workers. Gunmetal is composed of lead, zinc and copper. The mean blood lead levels in the workers was 34 μg/dL, a level associated with subclinical lead toxicity. Nonsignificant reductions in an ECG measure called the Mayer wave-related sinus arrhythmia ($C\text{-}CV_{MWSA}$) were observed, but were significantly correlated with the plasma zinc concentration.

Some investigators have suggested a possible link between zinc and Alzheimer's disease (Constantinidis, 1997). One hypothesis is that in Alzheimer's disease, the deposit of extracellular β-amyloid in the cortex is activated by free zinc. This results in the disturbance of the blood-brain barrier, allowing the entrance of toxic metals into the brain. These metals displace the zinc in vital enzymes, which then cannot function properly. The possibility of a role for zinc in the etiology of Alzheimer's disease is very controversial.

§ 8-8. Cadmium.

The major source of exposure to cadmium is the nickel-cadmium battery industry. Cadmium most often affects the respiratory and urinary systems. The neurologic effects of cadmium are thought be secondary to its effects on the lungs and kidneys. Manifestations of neurologic effects include headache, vertigo, tremor, and increased knee-jerk reflex. Also observed are anorexia, anosmia, and disturbances in sensory and motor function. Brain atrophy has been seen on CAT scan (Babitch, 1988; Bar-Sela, 1992).

Adverse effects on the sense of smell were observed in workers exposed to cadmium fumes in refrigerator coil manufacturing plant (Rose, 1992). The subjects were 55 workers with chronic exposure to cadmium fumes during brazing operations. About 44% of the workers were mildly hyposmic, and some 13% were moderately to severely hyposmic. The affected workers also had high urinary cadmium levels. Disturbances of urinary function are a major adverse effect of long-term exposure to cadmium (Cárdenas, 1992). A study of workers in a nickel-cadmium battery factory showed 34 with headache, 16 with vertigo, and 32 with general or muscle weakness. CAT scan showed brain atrophy in 6 workers.

Elevated levels of cadmium in children have been associated with adverse effects on their neurologic development. Prolongation of the auditory evoked potential components was seen in association with high levels of cadmium and lead in hair (Thatcher, 1985). Lead and cadmium were found to affect different aspects of cognitive functioning. Lead had a greater affect on performance IQ, while cadmium's major effect was on verbal IQ. This difference may be due to the fact that lead affects dopamine levels, while cadmium affects levels of norepinephrine, acetylcholine, and serotonin levels.

A few studies have attempted to determine an association between cadmium and Alzheimer's disease. As is the case with aluminum and zinc, the results of some studies suggest the possibility of such a relationship, but none to date has provided definitive data. There have also been attempts to find elevated levels of several heavy metals (aluminum, calcium, lead, manganese, mercury) in the spinal cord, brain, cerebrospinal fluid, and blood of patients with amyotrophic lateral sclerosis (ALS). A 1990 study found evidence of such an association (Khare, 1990), while a 1992 study did not (Sillevis Smitt, 1992).

§ 8-9. Aluminum.

Aluminum is a relatively light, ductile metal that is a good conductor of heat and electricity. When the metal is exposed to air, a thin coating of aluminum oxide forms on the surface and acts as a barrier to corrosion. Aluminum is used in alloys with copper, zinc, magnesium and other metals.

Aluminum and its compounds are used widely in industry. Aluminum is used in the construction of aircraft, automobiles, kitchen utensils, containers, wrapping and packing materials, and building panels. Its compounds are used in paints, abrasives, insulating materials, cosmetics, pesticides, and medical products. Aluminum hydroxide is the active ingredient in several brands of antacid. Aluminum chloride hexahydrate is used in antiperspirants.

Aluminum phosphide is used to fumigate stored grain bins against insects and rodents. The substance is quite toxic if ingested. The compound can give off a gas called phosphine, which can be fatal if inhaled (Mistra, 1988; Wilson, 1980). Most deaths involving phosphine in the United States are suicidal, but accidental deaths have occurred. Aluminum phosphide and phosphine are a major problem in India where several hundred cases of poisoning are known to have occurred.

§ 8-9(a). Toxic Effects.

Toxic effects of aluminum and its compounds have been observed in the respiratory and central nervous systems, and in bone and blood-forming organs. The respiratory effects are the most frequent, and can be classified into two major categories: restrictive pulmonary disease, and obstructive pulmonary disease. Both are most often associated with industrial exposure (Sjögren, 1994).

Encephalopathy associated with aluminum was first observed in patients with renal failure on dialysis (Alfrey, 1980). The patients began to develop a dysfunction of the brain, ranging from fluctuating to permanent. The major symptoms were tremor, speech and language disorders, myoclonus, and epilepsy. Personality changes and intellectual deterioration were also observed. Recovery was the exception, and most patients died within a year of the onset of symptoms (Bugiani, 1990). The problem was found to be related to the presence of aluminum in the dialysis fluids and to the use of drugs containing aluminum to lower phosphate levels (Flendrig, 1976). The condition is rare today, and generally limited to subclinical intoxication. The dialysis fluid is monitored and the aluminum level is kept below 0.4 μmol/L. Patients with the encephalopathy had aluminum levels ranging from 7 μmol/L to 30 μmol/L (Sjögren, 1994). Aluminum-free phosphate binders are used today.

§ 8-9(b). Aluminum and Alzheimer's Disease.

Alzheimer's disease is characterized by deterioration of the mental functions involved with memory, judgment, and abstract thinking, and by changes in personality and behavior. While there is much data suggesting an association between aluminum and Alzheimer's disease, there is as yet no definitive proof. On autopsy, the brains of Alzheimer's victims are characterized by senile plaque, amyloid, and degeneration of neurofibrils. Aluminum has been found in amyloid and senile plaque (Flendrig, 1976).

Epidemiologic studies have shown a possible association between aluminum in drinking water and Alzheimer's disease (Flaten, 1990; Martyn, 1989; Neri, 1991). Studies in Norway demonstrated that in areas where the aluminum concentration in water was greater than 4.1 μmol/L, the risk of Alzheimer's was 1.5 times greater than in areas where the aluminum concentration was less than 4.1 μmol/L (Flaten, 1990). Similar results were obtained in a Canadian study (Neri, 1991). In this study, the risk was 1.5 times higher in areas where the aluminum content in water was greater than 7.4 μmol/L, compared to areas where the concentration was 0.4 μmol/L. An English study showed a risk 1.5 times greater in districts where the aluminum content in water was greater than 4.1 μmol/L compared to districts where the concentration was less than 0.4 μmol/L (Martyn, 1989).

Other studies have not yielded data showing an association. Antacids containing aluminum are a major source of ingested aluminum, accounting for far more aluminum intake in a single recommended dose than years of drinking water with a concentration of about 4.0 μmol/L. However, no association between intake of antacids and Alzheimer's disease has yet been found (Graves, 1990). The epidemiologic studies are by no means conclusive. Diagnostic criteria may not be the same in different areas, and the aluminum content in drinking water is a fraction of total intake. It is possible that drinking water may contain unknown complexes of aluminum that are more easily absorbed and pass through the blood-brain barrier. Also, it has been found that the lesions in the brains of patients who have died of dialysis encephalopathy are quite different from those seen in the brains of Alzheimer's patients (Bugiani, 1990).

§ 8-10. Selenium.

Selenium is an essential trace element in humans, but it is also toxic at concentrations that occur in the environment. In nature, it is often found in association with sulfur, and to a lesser extent with gold, silver, antimony, and mercury. Selenium compounds occur in some soils, where they may accumulate in plants and cause poisoning in livestock.

Selenium has a variety of applications in industry. It is incorporated into alloys to enhance hardness. It is used to increase resistance to abrasion in rubber hoses and cables. Selenium increases electrical conductivity and is used in the manufacture of photoelectric cells and diodes. Selenium is also used in the glass and ceramics industry, in cosmetics, and in antidandruff shampoo.

The major occupational problem associated with selenium is dermatitis. Liver damage is a risk at high concentrations. Selenium toxicity has occurred in copper refinery workers. Symptoms included fatigue, nose and eye irritation, indigestion and stomach pain (Holness, 1989).

§ 8-11. Gallium.

Gallium, which was not identified as an element until 1875, was not used for industrial purposes until the 1970s. It is one of the few metals that are liquid at or near room temperature. Gallium does not exist in its free state in nature, and no specific gallium ores are known. It is found in small quantities in association with ores of zinc, aluminum, iron, and other metals. Its compounds are used by the electronics industry in transistors, rectifiers, and diodes.

Theoretically, gallium can have devastating effects on the neuromuscular system, as well as on other organ systems. As far as is known, there are no biodetoxification mechanisms for gallium in humans. However, almost all that is known about gallium toxicity has come from animal studies (Dudley, 1950; Dudley, 1949). Toxicity from occupational exposure is rare. A 43-year-old woman exposed to gallium fluoride fumes experienced neurologic symptoms a few days after exposure, and a rash as well. Muscular weakness and pain persisted for 3 months (Ferm, 1970).

Gallium arsenide is a gas, which is increasingly being used in the microelectronics industry. It may have toxic effects if inhaled.

Gallium is not well absorbed from the gastrointestinal tract. If gallium citrate is injected subcutaneously or intravenously, some 30% to 48% will be stored in bone. When the gallium is released from the bone about 3 months later, a variety of toxic effects may occur, including hyperexcitability, blindness, and terminal paralysis. Other adverse effects include anorexia, kidney damage, nausea, edema, and dermatitis (Dickerson, 1994).

References.

Adams, C.R., Ziegler, D.K., Lint, J.T., *Mercury Intoxication Simulating Amyotrophic Lateral Sclerosis*. JAMA 1983; 250:642-643.

Alexander, G.E., Crutcher, M.D., *Functional Architecture of Basal Ganglia Circuits: Neural Substrates of Parallel Processing.* TINS 1990; 13:266-271.

Alfrey, A.C., *Aluminum Metabolism in Uremia.* Neurotoxicology. 1980; 1:43-53.

Amin-Zaki, L., Elhassani, S., Majeed, M.A., Clarkson, T.W., Doherty, R.A., Greenwood, M., *Introuterine Methylmercury Poisoning in Iraq*. Pediatrics 1974; 54:587.

Aposhian, H.V., et al., *N-acetyl-dl-penicillamine, a New Oral Protective Agent Against the Lethal Effects of Mercuric Chloride.* J. Pharmacol. Toxicol. 1959; 126:131.

Arvidson, B., *Inorganic Mercury Is Transported from Muscular Nerve Terminals to Spinal and Brainstem Motor Neurons.* Muscle Nerve 1992; 125:1089-1094.

Babitch, J.A., *Cadmium Neurotoxicity.* In: J.C. Bondy, K.N. Prasad (eds.), Metal Neurotoxicity. Boca Raton, FL: CRC Press, 1988: 141-166.

Baghurst, P.A., McMichael, A.G., Wigg, N.R., et al., *Environmental Exposure to Lead and Children's Intelligence at the Age of 7 Years — the Port Pirie-Cohort Study*. N. Engl. J. Med. 1992; 327:1279-84.

Baker, E.L. Jr., Hayes, C.G., Landrigan, P.J., et al., *A Nationwide Survey of Heavy Metal Absorption in Children Living Near Primary Copper, Lead, and Zinc Smelters.* Am. J. Epidemiol. 1977; 106:261-273.

Bansal, S.K., Haldar, N., Dhand, U.K., Chopra, J.S., *Phrenic Neuropathy in Arsenic Poisoning.* Chest 1991; 100:878-880.

Barltop, D., Khoo, H.E., *The Influence of Nutritional Factors on Lead Absorption.* Postgrad. Med. 1975; 51:795-800.

Bar-Sela, M., Levy, M., Westin, J.B., *Medical Findings in Nickel-Cadmium Battery Workers.* Isr. J. Med. Sci. 1992; 28:578-583.

Bellinger, D., Leviton, A., Waternaux, C., Needleman, H., Rabinowitz, M., *Longitudinal Analyses of Prenatal and Postnatal Lead Exposure and Early Cognitive Development.* N. Engl. J. Med. 1987; 316:1037-43.

Berlin, M., Nordberg, G., Serenius, F., *On the Site and Mechanism of Mercury Vapor Resorption in the Lung.* Arch. Environ. Health 1969; 18:42-50.

Bernad, P.G., *Clinical and Laboratory Evaluation of Patients Exposed to Neurotoxins.* Clinical Toxicology I. 10(2). June, 1990: 387-402.

Bertholf, R.L., *Zinc.* In: H. Seiler, H. Sigel, A.M. Sigel (eds.), Handbook on Toxicity of Inorganic Compounds. New York: Marcel Dekker, 1988: 788-800.

Bird, E.D., Anton, A.H., Bullock, B., *The Effect of Manganese Inhalation on Basal Ganglia Dopamine Concentrations in Rhesus Monkey.* Neurotoxicology 1984; 5:59-65.

Brody, D.J., Pirkle, J.L., Kramer, R.A., et al., *Blood Levels in the U.S. Population: Phase I of the Third National Health and Nutrition Examination Survey. (NHANES III, 1988 To 1991).* JAMA 1994; 272:277-283.

Brown, M.A., Thom, J.V., Orth, G.L., et al., *Food Poisoning Involving Zinc Contamination.* Arch. Environ. Health 1964; 8:637-640.

Browning, J.D., O'Dell, B.L., *Low Zinc Status in Guinea Pigs Impairs Calcium Uptake by Brain Synaptosomes.* J. Nutr. 1994; 436-443.

Bugiani, O., Ghetti, B., *Aluminum Encephalopathy: Experimental v Human.* In: M. De Broe, J.W. Coburn (eds.), Aluminum and Renal Failure, Developments in Nephrology, Vol. 26. Dordrecht: Kluwer, 1990.

de la Burde, B., Choate, M.S., *Early Asymptomatic Lead Exposure and Development at School Age.* J. Pediatr. 1975; 87:638.

Burke, D.M., Demico, F.J., Taper, I.J., Ritchey, S.J., *Copper and Zinc Utilization in Elderly Adults.* J. Gerontol. 1981; 35:558-563.

Cárdenas, A., Ramis, I., Hotter, G., et al., *Human and Experimental Studies on Renal Eicosanoid Response to Long-Term Cadmium Exposure.* Toxicol. Appl. Pharmacol. 1992; 116:155-160.

Carl, G.F., Keen, C.L., Gallagher, B.B., et al., *Association of Low Blood Manganese Concentrations with Epilepsy.* Neurology 1986; 36:1584-1587.

Carl, G.F., Blackwell, F.K., Barnett, F.C., et al., *Manganese and Epilepsy: Brain Glutamine Synthease and Liver Arginase Activities in Genetically Epilepsy Prone and Chronically Seizured Rats.* Epilepsia 1993; 34:441-446.

Chisolm, J.J., Jr., Barltrop, D., *Recognition & Management of Children with Increased Lead Absorption.* Arch. Dis. Child. 1979; 54:249-262.

Chisolm, J.J., Jr., *Increased Lead Absorption and Lead Poisoning (Plumbism).* In: Behrman, R.E. (ed.), Nelson Textbook of Pediatrics, 14th Ed. Philadelphia: W.B. Saunders, 1992; 1788-91.

Christian, J.R., Celewyz, B.S., Andelman, S.L., *A Three-Year Study of Lead Poisoning in Chicago: II. Case Findings in Asymptomatic Children Using Urinary Coprophyrin as a Screening Test.* Am. J Pub. Health 1964; 54:1245.

Clarkson, T.W., *The Pharmacology of Mercury Compounds.* Annu. Rev. Pharmacol. 1972; 12:375.

Cohen, M.M., *Biochemical Aspects of Lead Neurotoxicity.* In: P.J. Vinken, G.W. Bruyn (eds.), Handbook of Clinical Neurology. Amsterdam: North-Holland Publishing Co., 1977: 65-72.

Constantinidis, J., *Zinc-Toxicity in Alzheimer's Disease: An Emerging Hypothesis*. In: M. Yasui, M.J. Strong, K. Ota, M.A. Verity (eds.), Mineral and Metal Toxicity. Boca Raton, FL: CRC Press, 1997: 147-156.

Cotzias, C.G., Horiuchi, K., Fuenzalida, S., Mena, I., *Chronic Manganese Poisoning — Clearance of Tissue Manganese Concentration with Persistence of the Neurological Picture.* Neurology 1968; 18:376-382.

Cotzias, C.G., Papavasiliou, P.S., Ginos, J., et al., *Metabolic Modification of Parkinson's Disease and of Chronic Manganese Poisoning*. Rev. Med. 1971; 22:305-326.

Council on Dental Materials, *Instruments and Equipment: Council on Dental Therapeutics. Safety of Dental Amalgam, an Update.* JAMA 1989; 119:204-205.

Couper, J., *On the Effects of Black Oxide of Manganese when Inhaled into the Lungs*. Br. Ann. Med. Pharmacol. 1837; 1:41-42.

Currier, R.D., Haerer, A.F., *Amyotrophic Lateral Sclerosis and Metallic Toxins.* Arch. Environ. Health 1968; 17:712-719.

Davis, L.E., Kornfeld, M., Mooney, H.S., et al., *Methylmercury Poisoning: Long-Term Clinical, Radiological, Toxicological, and Pathological Studies of an Affected Family*. Ann. Neurol. 1994; 35:680-688.

Davis, L.E., Wands, J.R., Weiss, S.A., *Central Nervous System Intoxication from Mercurous Chloride Laxatives.* Arch. Neurol. 1974; 30:428-431.

Davis, L.E., Standefer, J.C., Kornfeld, M., et al., *Acute Thallium Poisoning. Toxicological and Morphological Studies of the Nervous System*. Ann. Neurol. 1981; 10:38.

Department of Health and Human Services, *Case Studies in Environmental Medicine*. Washington: Public Health Service, 1990.

Dickerson, O.B., Smith, T.H.F., *Gallium, Germanium, and Indium.* In: C. Zenz, O.B. Dickerson, E.P. Horvath (eds.), Occupational Medicine, 3d. Ed. St. Louis: Mosby, 1994: 501-505.

Dreisbach, R.H., Handbook of Poisoning, 11th Ed. Los Altos, CA: Lange Medical Publications, 1983; 264.

Dudley, H.C., Levine, M.D., *Gallium Toxicity*. J. Pharmacol. 1949; 95:487-493.

Dudley, H.C., Henry, K.E., Lindsley, B.F., *Studies on the Toxic Action of Gallium (I)*. J. Pharmacol. 1950; 98:409-417.

Eden-Rad, J., Marafante, E., Sabbioni, E., et al., *Placental Transfer and Retention of 201Tl-Thallium in the Rat.* Toxicol. Lett. 1982; 11:275.

Engel, R.R., Smith, A.H., *Arsenic in Drinking Water and Mortality from Vascular Disease: An Ecologic Analysis in 30 Counties in the United States*. Arch. Environ. Health 1994; 49:418-427.

Eriksson, H., Mägiste, K., Plantin, L.O., et al., *Effects of Manganese Oxide on Monkeys as Revealed by a Combined Neurochemical, Histological, and Neurophysiological Evaluation.* Arch. Toxicol. 1987; 61:46-52.

Expert Group of National Institute of Public Health, *Methylmercury in Fish. A Toxicologic-Epidemiologic Evaluation of Risks*. Stockholm: Uno S. Andersons Tryckeri, 1971.

Farmer, J.G., Johnson, L.R., *Assessment of Occupational Exposure to Arsenic.* 1990; 47:3442-3448.

Ferm, V.H., Carpenter, S.J., *Teratogenic and Embryopathic Effects of Indium, Gallium, and Germanium.* Toxicol. Appl. Pharmacol. 1970; 16:166-170.

Festa, M.D., Anderson, H.L., Dowdy, R.P., Ellerieck, M.R., *Effect of Zinc Intake on Copper Excretion and Retention in Men.* Am. J. Clin. Nutr. 1985; 41:285-292.

Fincher, R.E., Koerker, R.M., *Long-Term Survival in Acute Arsenic Encephalopathy.* Am. J. Med. 1987; 82:549-552.

Finkel, A.J., Hamilton & Hardy's Industrial Toxicology, 4th Ed. Boston: John Wright-PSG, 1983.

Fitzpatrick, T.B., et al., *Dermatology*. In: General Medicine, 4th Ed., New York: McGraw-Hill, 1993; 1776-77.

Flaten, T.P., *Geographical Associations Between Aluminum in Drinking Water and Death Rates with Dementia (Including Alzheimer's Disease), Parkinson's Disease and Amyotrophic Lateral Sclerosis in Norway.* Environ. Geochem. Health 1990; 121:152-167.

Flendrig, J.A., Kruis, H., Das, H.A., *Aluminum and Dialysis Dementia.* Lancet 1976; ii235.

Fosmire, G.J., *Zinc Toxicity.* Am. J. Clin. Nutr. 1990; 51:225-227.

Franzblau, A., Lillis, R., *Acute Arsenic Intoxication from Environmental Arsenic Exposure.* Arch. Environ, Health 1989; 44:385-390.

Friberg, L., Nordberg, C.F., Vouk, V.B. (eds), Handbook of Toxicology of Metals. Amsterdam: Elsevier, 1986.

Fujino, T., *Clinical and Epidemiological Studies on Chronic Minamata Disease, Part 1. Study on Katsurajima Island.* Kumamoto Med. J. 1994; 44:139-155.

Gage, J.C., Swain, A.A.B., *The Toxicity of Alkyl and Alkyl Mercury Salts.* Biochem. Pharmacol. 1961; 8:77 (Abstract 250).

Gilfillan, S.C., *Lead Poisoning and the Fall of Rome.* J. Occup. Med. 1966; 7:53.

Giblet, J.A., *An Outbreak of Lead Poisoning (in the Canklow District of Rotterdam*). Public Health 1955; 1118.

Gilbert, S.G., Grant-Webster, K.S., *Neurobehavioral Effects of Developmental Methylmercury Exposure.* Environ. Health Perspect. 1995; 103 (Supp. 6):135-142.

Goetz, C.G., New Toxins in Clinical Practice. New York: SP Medical & Scientific Books, 1985; 1:3-16.

Gilman, A.G., et al., Pharmacological Basis of Therapeutics, 8th Ed. Elmsford, NY: Pergamon Press, 1990.

Graef, J.W., *Clinical Aspects of Lead Poisoning.* In: P.J. Vinken, G.W. Bruyn (eds.), Handbook of Clinical Neurology. Amsterdam: North-Holland Publishing Co., 1979.

Grant, W.M., Toxicology of the Eye, 3d Ed. Springfield, IL: Thomas, 1986.

Graves, A., White, E., Koepsell, T.D., *The Association Between Aluminum-Containing Products and Alzheimer's Disease.* J. Clin. Epidemiol. 1990; 43:35-44.

Greber, J.L., Zaikis, S.C., Abernathy, R.P., et al., *Zinc, Nitrogen, Copper, Iron, and Manganese Balance in Adolescent Females Fed Two Levels of Zinc.* J. Nutr. 1978; 108:1449-1456.

Groenwegen, H.J., Roeling, T.A.P., Voorn, P., Berendse, H.W., *The Parallel Arrangement of Basal Ganglia-Thalamocortical Circuits: A Neuronal Substrate for the Role of Dopamine in Motor and Cognitive Functions?* In: E.C. Wolterm, P. Scheltens (eds.), Mental Dysfunction of Parkinson's Disease. Dordrecht: ICG Printing, 1993: 3-18.

Harada, M., *Congenital Minamata Disease. Intrauterine Methyl-Mercury Poisoning.* In: J.L. Sever, Teratogen Update, Environmental Birth Defects Risks. New York: Alan R. Liss, 1986: 123-126.

Harada, M., *Minamata Disease: Methylmercury Poisoning in Japan Caused by Environmental Pollution.* Crit. Rev. Toxicol. 1995; 25:1-24.

Harada, M., *Minamata Disease: Organic Mercury Poisoning Caused by Ingestion of Contaminated Fish.* In: E.F. Jellife, D.B. Jellife (eds.), Adverse Effects of Food. New York: Plenum Press, 1982: 135-148.

Harada, M., *Neurotoxicity of Methylmercury: Minamata and the Amazon.* In: M. Yasui, M.J. String, K. Ota, M.A. Verity (eds.). Mineral and Metal Neurotoxicology. Boca Raton, FL: CRC Press, 1997: 177-188.

Heyman, A., Pfeiffer, J.B., Willett, R.W., et al., *Peripheral Neuropathy caused by Arsenical Intoxication.* 1956; 254:401-409.

Holness, Tarashuk, I., *Health Status of Copper Refinery Workers with Specific Reference to Selenium Exposure.* Arch. Environ. Health 1989; 44:291-297.

Huang, C.C., Chu, N.S., Lu, C.S., et al., *Chronic Manganese Intoxication.* Arch. Neurol. 1989; 46:1104-1106.

Huang, C.C., Lu, C.S., Chu, N.S., *Progression After Chronic Manganese Exposure.* Neurology 1993; 43:1479-1483.

Hurley, L.S., Woolley, D.E., Rosenthal, F., et al., *Influence of Manganese on Susceptibility of Rats to Convulsions.* Am. J. Physiol. 1963; 204:493-496.

Kantarjian, A.A., *A syndrome Clinically Resembling Amyotrophic Lateral Sclerosis Following Chronic Mercurialism.* Neurology 1964; 639-644.

Kazantzis, G., *Thallium.* In: L. Friberg, G.F. Nordberg, V. Vouk (eds.), Handbook on the Toxicology of Metals, 2d Ed. Amsterdam: Elsevier Science Publishers, 1986.

Khare, S.S., Ehmann, W.D., Kasarskis, E.J., Markesbery, W.R., *Trace Element Imbalances in Amyotrophic Lateral Sclerosis.* Neurotoxicology. 1990; 11:521-532.

Krigman, M.R., Bouldin, T.W., Mushak, P., *Lead.* In: P.S. Spencer, H.H. Schaumberg (eds.), Experimental and Clinical Neurotoxicology. Baltimore: Williams and Wilkins, 1980: 490-507.

La Dou, J., *Health Issues in the Microelectronics Industry.* Occup. Med. 1968; 1:1-11.

Lagerkvist V.J., Zetterlund, B., *Assessment of Exposure to Arsenic Among Smelter Workers; A Five-Year Follow-up.* Am. J. Ind. Med. 1994; 25:477-488.

Landrigan, P.J., *Arsenic.* In: W.N. Rom (ed.), Environmental and Occupational Medicine. Boston: Little, Brown and Co., 1992: 773-779.

Lau, B.P., Michalik,P., Porter, C.J., Krolik, S., *Identification and Confirmation of Arsenobetaine and Arsenocholine in Fish, Lobster, and Shrimp by a Combination of Fast Atom Bombardment and Tandem Mass Spectrometry.* Biomed. Environ. Mass. Spectrum. 1987; 14:723-732.

Levine, S.P., et al., *Elemental Mercury Exposure: Peripheral Neurotoxicity.* Br. J. Ind. Med. 1982; 39:136.

Lu, C.S., Huang, C.S., Calne, D.B., *Levodopa Failure in Chronic Manganism.* Neurology 1994; 44:1600-1602.

Magos, L., Butler, W.H., *The Kinetics of Methyl Mercury Administered Repeatedly to Rats.* Arch. Toxicol. 1976:35:25.

Maher, W.A., *The Presence of Arsenobetaine in Marine Animals.* Comp. Biochem. Physiol. C. 1985; 80:199-201.

Martyn, C.N., Barker, D.J.P., Osmknd, C., et al., *Geographical Relation Between Alzheimer's Disease and Aluminum in Drinking Water.* Lancet 1989; 1(8629):59-62.

Mealey, J., Jr., Brownell. G.L., Sweet, W.H., *Radioarsenic in Plasma, Urine, Normal Tissues, and Intracranial Neoplasms.* Arch. Neurol. Psychiatr. 1969; 81:310-319.

Meltzer, H.M., Mundal, H.H., Alexander, J., et al., *Does Dietary Arsenic and Mercury Affect Cutaneous Bleeding Time and Blood Lipids in Humans?* Biol. Trace Elem. Res. 1994; 46:135-153.

Mergler, D., Huel, G., Bowler, R., et al., *Nervous System Dysfunction Among Workers with Long-Term Exposure to Manganese.* Environ. Res. 1994; 64:151-180.

Milham, S., Jr., Strong, T., *Human Arsenic Exposure in Relation to a Copper Smelter.* Environ. Res. 1974; 7:176-182.

Minamata Disease Research Group, Minamata Disease. Kumamoto, Japan: Medical School of Kumamoto University, 1968.

Mistra, U.K., Tripathi, A,K., Pandey, R., Bhargwa, B., *Acute Phosphine Poisoning Following Ingestion of Aluminum Phosphide.* Human Toxicol. 1988; 7:343-345.

Moeschlin, S., *Thallium Poisoning.* Clin. Toxicol. 1980; 17:133.

Meddler, J., Forbears, J.D., *Allergic Contact Dermatitis Due to Metallic Mercury.* Arch. Environ. Health 1968; 17:960.

Molin, M., *Mercury, Selenium, and Glutathione Peroxidase, in Dental Personnel.* Acta. Odontologica Scandinavica 1989; 47:383-390.

Molin, M., *Mercury, Selenium, and Glutathione Peroxidase Before and After Amalgam Removal in Man.* Acta. Odontologica Scandinavica 1990; 48:189-202.

Murphy, J.V., *Intoxication Following Ingestion of Elemental Zinc.* JAMA 1970; 212:2119-2120.

National Research Council, *Drinking Water and Health.* 1977.

Needleman, H.L., Low Level Lead Exposure: The Clinical Implications of Current Research. New York: Raven Press, 1980.

Needleman, H.L., Gunnoe C., Leviton A., et al., *Deficits in Psychologic and Classroom Performance of Children with Elevated Dentine Lead Levels*. N. Engl. J. Med. 1979; 300:689-95.

Neri, L.C., Hewitt, D., *Aluminum, Alzheimer's Disease and Drinking Water*. Lancet 1991; 338:390.

Palca, J., *Get-the-Lead-Out Guru Challenged*. Science 1991; 253:842-44.

Patty, Patty's Industrial Hygiene and Toxicology. 3d Ed., Vols. 2A, 2B, 2C. New York: John Wiley and Sons, 1981-82.

de Peyster, A., Silvers, J.A., *Arsenic Levels in Hair of Workers in a Semiconductor Fabrication Facility*. A. Ind. H.G. Assoc. J. 1995; 56:377-383.

Pirkle, J.L., Brody, D.J., Gunter, E.W., *The Decline in Blood Lead Levels in the United States: the National Health and Nutrition Examination Surveys (NHANES)*. JAMA 1994; 272:284-291.

Porter, K.G., McMaster, D., Elmes, M.E., Love, A.H., *Anaemia and Low Serum Copper During Zinc Therapy*. Lancet 1977; 2:774.

Prasad, A.S., Brewer, G.J., Schoomaker, E.B., Rabbani, P., *Hypocupremia Induced by Zinc Therapy in Adults*. JAMA 1978; 240:2166-2168.

Rick, J.J.G.M., *Thallium Poisoning*. In: P.J. Vinken, G.W. Bruyn (eds.), Handbook of Clinical Neurology. Amsterdam: North-Holland, 1979; 239.

Renwick, J.H., Harrington, J.M., Waldron, JA, et al., *Long-Term Effects of Acute Arsenical Poisoning*. J. Soc. Occup. Med. 1981; 31:144-147.

Rose, C.S., Heywood, P.G., Costanzo, R.M., *Olfactory Impairment After Chronic Occupational Cadmium Exposure*. J. Occup. Med 1992; 34:600-605.

Roy, M., *Arsenic and Medical Surveillance*. Occup. Health Ontario 1983; 3:17-29.

Saddique, A., Peterson, C.D., *Thallium Poisoning, a Review*. Vet. Hum. Toxicol. 1983; 25:16.

Sakai, K., *Time-Dependent Distribution of ^{203}Hg-methylymercuric Chloride in Tissues and Cells of Rats*. Jpn. J. Exp. Med. 1974; 45:63.

Saryan, L.A., Zen, C., *Lead and Its Compounds*. In: C. Zenz, O.B. Dickerson, E.P. Horvath (eds.), Occupational Medicine, 3d Ed. St. Louis: Mosby, 1994: 506-541.

Schaller, K.H., Manke, G., Raithel, H.J., et al., *Investigations of Thallium-Exposed Workers in Cement Factories*. Int. Arch. Occup. Environ. Health 1980; 47:223.

Schramm, V.L., Wedler, F.C. (eds.), Manganese in Metabolism and Enzyme Function. New York: Academic Press, 1986.

Sillevis Smitt, P.A.E., van Beek, H., Baars, A.-J., et al., *Increased Metallothionein in the Liver and Kidney of Patients with Amyotrophic Lateral Sclerosis*. Arch. Neurol. 1992; 49:721-724.

Sjögren, B., Elinder, C., *Aluminum and Its Compounds*. In: C. Zenz, O.B. Dickerson, E.P. Horvath (eds.), Occupational Medicine, 3d Ed. St. Louis: Mosby, 1994: 458-465.

Six, K.M., Goyer, R.A., *The Influence of Iron Deficiency on Tissue Content and Toxicity of Ingested Lead in the Rat*. J. Lab. Clin. Med. 1978; 79:128-136.

Smith, M.A., Grant, L.D., Sors, A.I. (eds.), Lead Exposure and Child Development: An International Assessment. Dorcrecht, the Netherlands: Kluwer Academic Publishers, 1989.

Takeuchi, T., *Pathology of Minamata Disease*. In: M. Kutsuma (ed.), Minamata Disease. Study Group of Minamata Disease, Kumamoto University, Japan, 1968: 141-288.

Takeuchi, T., *Pathology of Fetal Minamata Disease. The Effect of Methylmercury on Intrauterine Life of Human Being*. Pediatrician 1977; 6:69-87.

Takeuchi, T., Eto, K., Eto, N., *Neuropathology of Childhood Cases of Methylmercury with Prolonged Symptoms, with Particular Refer-*

ence to the Decortication Syndrome. Neurotoxicology 1979; 1:1-20.

Takeuchi, T., *Human Effects of Methylmercury as an Environmental Neurotoxicant.* In: K. Blum, L. Manzo (eds.), Neurotoxicology. New York: Marcel Dekker, 1985: 345-367.

Takeuchi, T., Eto, K., Tokunaga, H., *Mercury Level and Histochemical Distribution in a Human Brain with Minamata Disease Following a Long-Term Clinical Course of 26 Years.* Neurotoxicology 1989; 10:651-658.

Takeuchi, T., Eto, K., Kino, Y., Tokunaga, H., *Human Brain Disturbance by Methylmercury Poisoning, Focusing on the Long-Term Effect on Brain Weight.* Neurotoxicology 1996; 17:187-190.

Thatcher, R.W., Lester, M.L., *Nutrition, Environmental Toxins and Computerized EEG: A Mini-max Approach to Learning Disabilities*. J. Learn. Disabil. 1985; 18:287-297.

Tsubaki, T., Irukayama, K., Minamata Disease: Methylmercury Poisoning in Minamata and Niigata, Japan. Amsterdam: Elsevier, 1977.

United States Environmental Protection Agency, *Air Quality Criteria for Lead.* Office of Research and Development, Washington, D.C.: EPA-600/8-77-107, 1977.

U.S. Department of Health and Human Services, Agency for Toxic Substances and Disease Registry. *The Nature and Extent of Lead Poisoning in Children in the United States: A Report to Congress.* 1988.

U.S. Department of Health and Human Services, Centers for Disease Control. *Environmental Lead Poisoning in Young Children.* 1991.

U.S. Department of Health and Human Services, Centers for Disease Control. *Strategic Plan for the Elimination of Childhood Lead Poisoning,* 1991a.

U.S. Department of Health and Human Services, Centers for Disease Control, Housing and Urban Development, Office of Policy Development and Research. *Comprehensive and Workable Plan for the*

Abatement of Lead-Based Paint in Privately Owned Housing: Report to Congress.
U.S. Department of Labor, Occupational Safety and Health Administration. *Lead Standard.* 20CFR1919.1025 (revised July 1, 1990). Washington, D.C.: U.S. Government Printing Office, 1990.
Velen, N.K., *Stomatitis and Systemic Dermatitis from Mercury in Amalgam Dental Restorations*. Dermatol. Clin. 1990; 8:157-160.
Warkany, J., Hubbard, D.M., *Acrodynia and Mercury.* J. Pediatr. 1953; 42:365-369.
Wedler, F.C. Denman, R.B., *Glutamine Synthease: The Major Mn (II) Enzyme in Mammalian Brain.* Curr. Top. Cell. Regul. 1984; 24:153-169.
Wilson, R., Lovejoy F.H., Jaeger, R.J., Landrigan, P.L., *Acute Phosphine Poisoning Aboard a Grain Freighter.* JAMA 1980; 244:148-150.
Wolters, E.C., Huang, C.C., Clark, C., *Positron Emission Tomography in Manganese Intoxication.* Ann. Neurol. 1976 14:339-352.
Wood, R.W., et al., *Hand Tremor Induced by Industrial Exposure to Inorganic Mercury.* Arch. Environ. Health, 1973; 26:249.
Woods, J.S., Fowler, B.A., *Effects of Chronic Arsenic Exposure on Hematopoietic Function in Adult Mammalian Liver.* Environ. Health Perspect. 1977; 19:209-213.
Yamada, M., Ohno, S., Okayasu, I., et al., *Chronic Manganese Poisoning: A Neuropathological Study with Determination of Manganese Distribution in the Brain.* Acta. Neuropathol. (Berl.) 1986; 70:273-278.
Yamauchi, H., Takahashi, K., Mashiko, M., Yanamaru, Y., *Biological Monitoring of Gallium Arsenide- and Inorganic Arsenic-Exposed Workers by Determination of Inorganic Arsenic and its Metabolites in Urine and Hair.* Am. Ind. H.G. Assoc. J. 1989; 50:606-612.

Chapter 9

ORGANOPHOSPHATE INSECTICIDES

As crude a weapon as the caveman's club, the chemical barrage has been hurled against the fabric of life.

—Rachel Carson, *Silent Spring* (1962).

§ 9-1. Overview.

A pesticide, by definition, is any agent intended for destroying, repelling or preventing a pest. Pesticides can be divided into three categories: insecticides, rodenticides and herbicides. Organophosphates were first synthesized by Lassaigne in the early 1800s, by reacting alcohol and phosphoric acid. In 1932, Lange noted the toxic effects of these derivatives and alerted German industrialists of their potential as insecticides. Between 1938 and 1944, Schrader developed 1-methylethyl methylphosphonofluoridate (Sarin), parathion and paraxon. The German Ministry of Defense recognized the value of these compounds as chemical warfare agents in WWII and produced large amounts of Tabun and Soman. Organophosphorus compounds are now one of the most frequently used groups of pesticides in the world. They are used in agriculture, forestry, public health, and by the general population as insecticides, fungicides, herbicides, and acaricides. See Table 9.1 for a list of commonly used organophosphorous compounds.

Table 9.1
Commonly Used Organophosphate Insecticides

Chlorpyrifos
Diazinon
Dichlorvos
Malathion
Parathion

Nearly all American families (97.8%) use pesticides at least once per year (Davis, 1992). The home is the most common setting for use of organophosphate insecticides, followed by use in the yard and on pets. There are now more than 250 organophosphate pesticide brand names registered in the United States, and this group of compounds accounts for as much as 80% of all pesticide-related hospital admissions (Bardin, 1994). Organophosphate poisoning with insecticides can be accidental, homicidal, or suicidal.

Other potent organophosphate agents that have been developed as nerve gas for chemical warfare include mustard gas and the more modern agent Sarin (used in the recent Tokyo subway terrorist action). Many organophosphates are neurotoxic. Some anticholinesterase agents may be therapeutic in certain disease states. Echothiophate eye drops are used to treat glaucoma, neostigmine is therapeutic in myasthenia gravis, and cyclophosphamide may be therapeutic in cancer.

Organophosphates can be absorbed via the respiratory tract, the gastrointestinal tract, or through the skin. Onset of toxicity varies from minutes to hours, depending on the agent and route of absorption. Organophosphorus compounds are very dangerous due to their high acute toxicity, but they have a low potential for accumulation. Ingestion usually results in gastrointestinal disturbances, dermal exposure results in muscle disturbances and fasciculations, and inhalation results in respiratory effects. Sufficient dosage inhibits both plasma and tissue cholinesterase, and results in a cholinergic crisis of prolonged duration.

The complexity of the nervous system is reflected in the wide variety of toxic actions that can be exerted upon it by hazardous chemicals and by the large number of symptoms and signs associated with these actions. Three main biochemical reactions are responsible for organophosphate effects: inhibition of cholinesterase activity; inhibition of neuropathy target esterase (NTE); and release of alkyl groups attached to the phosphorus atom, and the alkylation of macromolecules RNA and DNA.

Cholinesterase inhibition is the specific effect and principal mechanism of action of organophosphates. Accumulation of acetylcholine at the nerve ending produces muscarinc and nicotinic effects. In lower doses, over stimulation of the parasympathetic system occurs with muscarinic effects, whereas in higher doses stimulation of ganglionic fibers and myoneural junctions predominate with nicotinic effects. The central nervous system is affected as well, by direct impact on the choline receptors of the nerve cells. Acute intoxications with organophosphates are very serious health problems. The percentage of lethal cases is very high in accidental and intentional intoxication (Kaloynaov, 1991).

The clinical picture is dominated by cholinergic symptoms of a different grade. As illustrated in Table 9.2, the most common of them are salivation, lacrimation, urination, diarrhea, gastrointestinal cramps and emesis. Hence, the term "SLUDGE" syndrome. Other muscarinic effects include miosis, bradycardia, bronchorrhea and bronchoconstriction. Nicotinic effects involve the autonomic ganglia and skeletal muscles and may result in diaphoresis, mydriasis, tachycardia, hypertension, muscle weakness, paralysis, and possibly death.

Together with the symptomatic treatment, an adequate specific therapy with cholinolytics (atropine) and ChE reactivators is applied. Pralidoxime may also be an effective antidote. The intoxicated person may never recover completely. Rare cases of renal involvement and failure have been documented (Abend, 1994). Such disturbances of the cholinergic system during rapid development of the brain have been shown to lead to permanent changes in cholinergic and behavioral variables in neonatal mice as they become adults (Eriksson, 1991).

In addition to acute cholinergic poisoning, a few newer OP compounds with great lipid solubility may cause cyclical or delayed OP syndromes. These include intermediate syndrome and organophosphate-induced delayed neuropathy (OPIDN). The intermediate syndrome may follow treatment and resolution of the cholinergic signs of OP toxicity, but it may also occur without the acute poisoning. Although this syndrome is not well understood, there is some evidence that it is due to pejunctional dysfunction of the neuromuscular synapses. Any OP can cause this syndrome, and it is called "intermediate" because it occurs before the delayed neuropathy. Starting one to four days following the resolution of cholinergic findings, patients report proximal, truncal and neck flexor muscle weakness, decreased deep tendon reflexes, cranial nerve palsies and respiratory depression. There are no associated sensory deficits. However, EMG shows an abnormal pattern on repetitive nerve stimulation, implicating neuromuscular junction dysfunction. Nerve conduction studies are normal (Jamal, 1997).

OPIDN is a specific neurotoxic effect that occurs two to three weeks after exposure and that may be irreversible. It consists of a distal symmetrical sensory motor mixed peripheral neuropathy mainly affecting the lower limbs with burning and tingling sensations, and causing muscle weakness and ataxia. In severe cases it may develop into flaccid paralysis and result in death. The precise biochemical abnormality responsible for the development of the OPIDN is unknown, but it appears to occur partly through inhibition of neurotoxic esterase (NTE) (Jamal, 1997). See § 9-3 regarding delayed neurotoxicity.

Chronic intoxications are believed to be rather rare. A positive relationship has been found, however, between family pesticide use (no-pest strips in the home, pesticides to control termites, flea collars on pets, diazinon in the garden or yard, and herbicides to control weeds in the yard) and childhood brain cancer (Davis, 1993). This case-control study also identified significant positive associations for use of pesticide bombs in comparison to cancer controls. Because of small sample sizes, potential recall bias, multiple comparisons, and lack of detailed exposure verification, however, further research must be done to confirm these findings.

Treatment for OP intoxication should not be delayed for receipt of cholinesterase levels, but red blood cell cholinesterase (RBC) and plasma tests are helpful. RBC is a more difficult test to obtain than plasma. It has a large range of normal, which proves less helpful in acute toxicity, but comparison to baseline is useful in cases of workplace monitoring. RBC regenerates at 1% per day. 2-PAM treatment regenerates the enzyme, so levels must be obtained before treatment is started. Levels measured by plasma tests decline faster acutely and regenerate faster than RBC, and plasma tests are easier to obtain in most hospitals.

§ 9-2. Monitoring.

Erythrocytes from mammalian species contain acetylcholinesterase (AChE). This enzyme is also found in varying amounts in the plasma, where it occurs mixed in different proportions with butyrylcholinesterase. The function of AChE ion erythrocytes is unknown, and inhibition of the enzyme in either or both of these blood compartments does not appear in and of itself to have any adverse consequences. Although inhibition of AChE in the blood may or may not be well-correlated with inhibition of the enzyme in functional sites, blood cholinesterase activity is used as a specific test for exposure and is included as a principal means for biologic monitoring. Recently, NTE measurement in peripheral lymphocytes has been suggested as a biochemical test for delayed neuropathy caused by organophosphates. Alkylphosphates in urine provide good information regarding absorption and excretion of organophosphate pesticides.

Organophosphates lower the levels of cholinesterase by forming complexes. Because the reaction with organophosphates and esterases is irreversible, inhibition of these effects is dependent on the molecular synthesis of new peptides. An assessment of red blood cell cholinesterase levels can be informative in evaluating organophosphate exposure. Laboratory tests should reveal depression of plasma and red blood cell esterases for acute exposures.

The changes in neurophysiological parameters are often expressed more than the biochemical ones, such as cholinesterase inhibition after exposure to organophosphates. The same correlation between physiological and biochemical changes was seen in subchronic experiments when rats were treated with low doses (1/50 and 1/100 LD50) of organophosphates. This effect can be more serious with successive exposed generations.

§ 9-3. Delayed Neurotoxicity.

An insidious property of certain organophosphorus pesticides is their ability to produce delayed neurotoxicity, often referred to as OPIDN (organophosphate-induced delayed neuropathy), in humans. Experimental techniques have been developed to screen for this property by using domestic hens as the test species (Derelanki, 1995). The hen has been found to be one of the most sensitive species for detecting delayed neurotoxicity. The ability to produce delayed neurotoxicity resides in the pesticide's ability to inhibit the brain enzyme neurotoxic esterase (NTE). A minimum of 70% NTE inhibition after a single exposure and 45% after multiple exposures to organophosphorous compounds, and subsequent aging of NTE, are biochemical prerequisites for the development of delayed neurotoxicity (Husain, 1995). However, the NTE assay itself, when conducted in vitro, misses organophosphates that are activated into OPIDN-causing agents in the body (Chow, 1986). Also, pre-treatment with non-neuropathic NTE inhibitors, such as phenylmethanesulfonyl fluoride, protects from OPIDN (Moretto, 1992). However, when given after organophosphates, these compounds promote OPIDN.

Organophosphorus pesticides that have been known to produce delayed neurotoxicity in humans include chlorpyrifos, diazinon, Mipafox, EPN, Trichlornat, Leptophos, Methaminophos, and Trichlorphon. Distal paralysis usually occurs three weeks after the beginning of the intoxication. Electroneuromyography is used for diagnosis. Behavioral deviations and EEG changes are often related to central nervous system impairment due to organophosphates. It should be noted that there is a marked age-related dependency in sensitivity to OPIDN: the young of a given species are more resistant than the adults are (Richardson, 1995).

Exposures to organophosphorous compounds seldom involve only the organophosphorous compound of interest, but may also include other organophosphorous compounds, solvents, and drugs, particularly when the compound of interest is a pesticide. Therefore, the possibility exists for toxic chemical interactions that may be additive, antagonistic, synergistic, or potentiative with respect to the toxic endpoint being measured. A classic example of potentiation is the dramatic increase in the acute cholinergic toxicity of malathion produced by pretreatment with inhibitors of carboxylesterases, which mediate the detoxification of malathion.

In screening chemicals for neurotoxicity, the general approach has been to utilize both behavioral and neuropathological endpoints. The use of behavior and morphology in assessing neurotoxicity has been adopted because both endpoints are relevant indicators of nervous system damage. However, behavior and neuropathology often show differing sensitivities for detecting neurotoxicity, so this combination approach increases the probability of detecting neurotoxicity and provides a more comprehensive assessment of nervous system damage.

The mechanisms by which organophosphorus esters cause their psychopharmacologic and neurologic trauma have been studied at great length, though it would be fair to state that only the relationship between chemical structure and neurotoxicity has proven to be a fruitful field of investigation (Ecobichon, 1982). That most of the neurotoxic agents have been anticholinesterase agents led to the obvious hypothesis involving nervous tissue cholinesterases.

Behavioral toxicology holds that toxic effects may manifest themselves as subtle disturbances of behavior and function long before any classic symptoms of organophosphate poisoning become apparent (Ecobichon, 1982). This may be due to the fact that increasing levels of corticosterone and catecholamines follow organophosphate intoxication similar to those observed during stress, including elevation of adaptive enzymes such as tyrosine aminotransferase (Kassa 1994).

Table 9.2
Signs and Symptoms of Acute Organophosphate Intoxication

Site of Action	Signs and Symptoms
Eyes	Increased lacrimation, slight mycosis, blurred vision, eye pain when focusing, frontal headache, conjunctive hyperemia
Respiratory system	Rhinorrhea, hyperemia, tightness in chest, prolonged wheezing, bronchoconstriction, increased secretion, dyspnea, slight chest pain, cough, edema of the lung
Gastrointestinal system	Increased salivation, anorexia, vomiting, abdominal cramps, heartburn, diarrhea, tenesmus, involuntary defecation
Sweat glands	Increased secretion
Striated muscles	Easy fatigue, mild weakness, twitching, fasciculation, cramps, generalized weakness including respiratory muscles, dyspnea, cyanosis

Site of Action	Signs and Symptoms
Central nervous system	Giddiness, tension, anxiety, tremor, restlessness, excessive dreaming, insomnia, nightmares, headaches, apathy, withdrawal and depression, drowsiness, concentration difficulty, slow recall, confusion, slurred speech, ataxia, convulsions, cyanosis, fall in blood pressure
Circulatory system	Bradycardia, decreased cardiac output, cardiac arrest, vasomotor center paralysis

§ 9-4. Sensory Effects.

Relatively little attention appears to have been paid to purely sensory effects of organophosphorous compounds. For many of these substances, cholinergic effects on the autonomic and motor systems tend to dominate the clinical picture (Taylor, 1990). Nevertheless, current information suggests that sensory effects of organophosphorous compound exposures could be assigned at least tentatively to three categories according to reversibility and probable mechanism (Richardson, 1995). First, some reversible sensory perturbations such as visual disturbances resulting from acute or repeated exposures to organophosphorous compounds are likely to be direct manifestations of cholinergic toxicity, either on innervation within the eye or on subcortical mechanisms of visual integration. Second, some longer-term sensory changes might arise from alteration in central cholinergic receptor density or other accommodations to prolonged cholinesterase inhibition, but the effects of such changes on sensory functions do not appear to have been well-characterized. Third, slowly reversible or permanent sensory deficits may be associated with suprathreshold acute or repeated exposures to compounds capable of producing OPIDN.

Based on the many reports of TOCP neuropathy, sensory effects in OPIDN have been considered mild when compared with motor dysfunction. However, the degree of sensory involvement would naturally be expected to vary according to exposure severity. Factors that might be expected to affect the degree and pattern of sensory involvement include organophosphorous compound structure, species, age, presence of interacting chemicals, dose amount, and dose chronicity (Hayes, 1982). One must also consider that anxiety and/or depression may evolve secondarily to the patient's concerns about carcinogenicity or teratogenic health effects and this may also simulate additional symptoms.

§ 9-5. Individual Organophosphate Insecticides.

§ 9-5(a). Chlorpyrifos.

Chlorpyrifos (diethyl 3,5,6-trichloro-2-pyridyl phosphorothionate) is a broad spectrum organophosphate insecticide. Since its development in 1965, this compound has become widely used for a variety of agricultural and public health applications. Because chlorpyrifos is increasingly employed for new uses and as a replacement for chlorinated hydrocarbon insecticides, demand for this product is expected to continue to grow (Richardson, 1995). A natural consequence of more extensive use of chlorpyrifos is that more people and other non-target organisms will have the opportunity to become exposed. Increased exposure, in turn, would be expected to result in an increase in the frequency of reports of toxic sequelae attributed to this compound.

Chlorpyrifos is metabolically activated by oxidative desulfuration to chlorpyrifos oxon, which produces neurotoxicity following inhibition of target esterases in the peripheral and central nervous systems. The bulk of bioactivation occurs in the liver, and detoxification takes place largely in the liver and plasma. The moderate toxicity of chlorpyrifos in humans has been attributed to hydrolytic detoxification of the oxon by A-esterases such as paraoxonase, which is more active toward chlorpyrifos oxon than paraoxon (Richardson, 1995). As a result of this hydrolytic cleavage of chlorpyrifos oxon to products that are much more water-soluble than the starting material, this insecticide is eliminated relatively rapidly from fish, rats, and humans, and is considered to have a low potential to accumulate after repeated exposures to relatively low doses.

It has been established that acute inhibition of AChE results in an accumulation of acetylcholine in cholinergic synapses, which causes hyperexcitation of postsynaptic neurons or end organs mediated by the action of muscarinic or nicotinic acetylcholine receptors. This cholinergic hyperexcitation gives rise to the well-known signs and symptoms of acute organophosphate intoxication described in Table 9.2. Chlorpyrifos and its oxon also interact directly with muscarinic receptors in the rat striatum. Chlorpyrifos oxon alters the postreceptor signal transduction and may interfere with normal cellular signaling, thereby disturbing neurological function. This direct interaction of chlorpyrifos oxon with muscarinic receptors is a potential mechanism of neurotoxicity that is independent of AChE inhibition.

Subchronic or chronic intoxication by organophosphorous compounds such as chlorpyrifos may result in the development of tolerance to many of the effects seen after acute exposures (Hoskins, 1992). Tolerance has been attributed to down-regulation of muscarinic as well as nicotinic receptors as an adaptive response to elevated neurotransmitter levels, although other less well-characterized effects may contribute to the phenomenon. However, there appear to be sensitive sub-groups of the human population who are sensitive to organophosphates such as chlorpyrifos and who suffer sensory neuropathy after exposure (Kaplan, 1993). These patients were previously healthy individuals who experienced symptoms of peripheral sensory neuropathy, memory loss, and mental slowing after repeated respiratory and dermal exposure to chlorpyrifos in enclosed, commercially fumigated sites. Whether or not chlorpyrifos causes OPIDN symptoms continues to be a source of controversy in the literature and in the courtrooms (Richardson, 1993a, 1993b).

Since chlorpyrifos is lipophilic, it passes through the placenta of developing mammalian embryos/fetuses. Muto et al. showed that prenatal exposure to relatively low concentrations of chlorpyrifos may be associated with embryotoxicity, fetal lethality and behavioral neurotoxicity (Muto, 1992). Recent studies have shown, however, that chlorpyrifos exposure to dams during gestation produces more extensive neurotoxicological effects in the dam relative to the developing fetus (Chanda, 1995). In vivo inhibition of maternal and fetal brain AChE activity by chlorpyrifos oxon suggested that the prenatal brain AChE activity was somewhat more sensitive.

§ 9-5(b). Diazinon.

Diazinon is O,O-diethyl O-(2-isopropyl-6-methyl-4-pyrimidinyl) phosphorothionate. Percutaneous absorption of diazinon in humans ranges from 2.87% to 3.85% (Webster, 1993). The authors noted no difference between levels of absorption from different body sites (forearm or abdomen) or from different vehicles (acetone solution or lanolin wool grease). The percutaneous absorption in vitro through human skin was 14.1 ± 9.2% of the applied dose.

The excretion pattern of C14 following intravenous administration of [14C] diazinon to rhesus monkeys and following topical administration in humans suggests that some interesting pharmacokinetic parameters and/or metabolism may be occurring. Diazinon is also known to induce a dose-related inhibition of protein synthesis in HL-60 (human leukemia cell line) cells at 24 hours at 40 μg/ml medium (Marinovich, 1994).

Recent studies have found elevated risks for farmers who personally handled, mixed or applied pesticides such as diazinon (OR=1.5) (Cantor, 1992). These white male farmers were shown to be at increased risk for developing non-Hodgkin's lymphoma, especially when first use was prior to 1965 and when protective clothing was not worn.

Since home gardeners also use copious amounts of diazinon, and since some states now require grass clippings to be disposed of communally to be reused as mulch, there has been a controversy over how much diazinon actually remains in the mulch distributed to residents. A recent study, however, showed that, under natural degradation processes, composted grass clippings containing diazinon, chlorpyrifos, isofenphos, and pendimethalin during the summer should be free of pesticide residues by the time the compost is used in the following growing season (Lemmon, 1992).

Hypertonicity has been documented in an infant who resided in a home which received a diazinon misapplication (Wagner, 1994). Six months after investigation, the levels of diazinon in the house were close to an order of magnitude higher than is normally expected immediately after application. When the infant was removed from the home, muscle tone returned to normal.

Diethyl phosphate (DEP), an organophosphate metabolite of diazinon, was found in the urine of symptomatic persons who resided in a household that had been sprayed with diazinon 4.5 months earlier (Richter, 1992). Since DEP is usually fully excreted within 48-72 hours after exposure has ended, the DEP levels were proof of current exposure-absorption, and the verifying cholinesterase depressions were enzymatic evidence of a metabolic effect. Pre- and post-decontamination data with regard to symptoms, DEP, cholinesterase, and surface and air levels underscore the utility of alkyl phosphate metabolites for monitoring exposure to organophosphorous compounds such as diazinon.

§ 9-5(c). Dichlorvos.

Dichlorvos is O,O-dimethyl-O-2,2-dichlorovinylphosphate. As an insecticide, dichlorvos has the highest vapor pressure of any organophosphorus compound commonly in use (Hayes, 1982). This makes it practical to produce insecticidal concentrations of it in closed spaces. Dichlorvos is an effective broad-spectrum antihelminthic. The USEPA will soon revoke the food additive registration of this cholinesterase-inhibiting insecticide due to NTP test results showing unequivocal evidence of carcinogenicity in rats (Mennear, 1994).

Quail eggs treated with dichlorvos showed inhibition of both butyrlcholinesterase (which is in the yolk and subembryonic membrane) and acetylcholinesterase (in the embryo) (Kaltner, 1993). This enzyme inhibition leads to retardation of the development of the embryo, to reduced accumulation of glucose and amino acids in the subembryonic liquid, and finally to death of the embryo, suggesting that the developmental retardation is due to the restricted supply of glucose and amino acids.

Pathological lesions induced by dichlorvos are characterized by degeneration of axons and myelin (Julka, 1992), and most of the resulting conditions are associated with damage to the cellular and subcellular membranes, which contain a variety of polyunsaturated fatty acids (PUFA). Current theories of cell injury by environmental toxicants implicate peroxidation of PUFA, leading to the degradation of phospholipids in a variety of pathological states. Peroxidative damage has been proposed as an index of cellular deterioration. The brain is the most susceptible organ to peroxidative damage because of high oxygen tension, low mitotic rate, high lipid content, and low concentration of antioxidants.

Testing on the rat central nervous system has illustrated that dichlorvos exposure resulted in a marked inhibitory effect on AChE activity in serum and different regions of the CNS and produced significant increases in the activities of the antioxidant enzymes superoxide dismutase (SOD) and catalase (Julka, 1992). These were accompanied by a decrease in the values of lipid peroxidation, also indicating neurotoxicity. Studies such as this help physicians identify enzymes such as SOD and catalase, which may enhance the disposal of potentially toxic radicals.

Illness caused by dichlorvos is generally similar to that caused by other organophosphate insecticides, but is remarkable for the rapidity of onset and disappearance of symptoms. It is not irritating or sensitizing, but it has been reported to cause persistent asthma in a young male after inhalation of the chemical (Deschamps, 1994). Dichlorvos inhibits human plasma cholinesterase more rapidly than red cell cholinesterase.

§ 9-5(d). Malathion.

Malaoxon (O,O-dimethyl-S-1,2-bis-(ethoxycarbonyl) ethyl phosphorothioate) is an active oxygen analogue of the organophosphate malathion. Malaoxon causes cholinergic convulsions and neuronal injury in both young and old rats, but old rats are much more sensitive than the young ones to the neurotoxic effects of malaoxon.

§ 9-5(e). Parathion.

Parathion is an organophosphate insecticide with the chemical composition of O-O-diethyl O-4-nitrophenyl phosphorothioate. While it was used on many crops in the past, its use was canceled on over eighty crops in the U.S. in 1991. Parathion usage for U.S. agriculture is estimated at 4-7 million pounds (AI/yr) for the 1992/1993 growing season. It is a class 1 toxin (Danger) and has an oral LD50 in rats of 2 mg/kg and a dermal LC50 in rats of 50 mg/kg.

Similar to most organophosphate insecticides, parathion toxicity involves cholinesterase inhibition. It is absorbed and distributed rapidly throughout the body after exposure through dermal absorption, inhalation or ingestion. Target organ bioactivation of phosphorothionate insecticides to their potent anticholinesterase oxon metabolites (parathion to paraoxon) is extremely important in toxicity because liver and blood provide so much potential protection by a variety of mechanisms, such as the aliesterases which serve as alternate phosphorylation sites (Chambers, 1991). Testing has shown that target site activation of parathion occurs in vivo at sufficient levels to contribute substantially to toxicity (Chambers, 1991). The bioactivation of parathion increases the anticholinesterase potency by about three orders of magnitude. The metabolites are excreted in the urine, and parathion crosses the placental barrier. Parathion is not known to produce delayed neurotoxic effects after exposure (Soliman, 1986; Abou-Donia, 1986).

Parathion given to pregnant rats has caused prenatal and postnatal death of the young. Fetal and infant rats are also known to be more susceptible to parathion than the adults, allowing a toxic dose to be transferred to the developing organism while the pregnant dam is not seriously affected. Parathion is known to cause immunosuppression and hormonal alterations in exposed populations.

References.

Abend, Y., Goland, S., Evron, E., Sthoeger, Z., Geltner, D., *Acute Renal Failure Complicating Organophosphate Intoxication.* Renal Failure 1994; 16(3):415-17.

Abou-Donia, M.B., Abdo, K.M., Timmons, P.R., Proctor, J.E., *Brain Acetylcholinesterase, Acid Phosphatase, and 2',3'-cyclic Nucleotide-3'-Phosphohydrolase and Plasma Butyrylcholinesterase Activities in Hens Treated with a Single Dermal Neurotoxic Dose of S,S,S-tri-n-butyl Phosphorotrithioate.* Toxicology & Applied Pharmacology 1986; 82:461-473.

Bardin, P.G., van Eeden, S.G., Moolman, J.A., Feden, A.P., Joubert, J.R., *Organophosphate and Carbonate Poisoning.* Arch. Intern. Med. 1994; 154:1433-1441.

Bernad, P.G., Saunder, G., *Clinical and Laboratory Evaluation of Patients Exposed to Neurotoxicants.* Clinics in Laboratory Medicine 1990; 10(2):387-402.

Bernad, P.G., *Assessment of Neurotoxic Effects of Exposure to Solvents.* American Occupational Health Conference, Georgia World Congress Center, April 26, 1993.

Burchfiel, J.L., Duffy, F.H., Van Sim, M., *Persistent Effects of Sarin and Dieldrin upon the Primate Electroencephalogram.* Toxicology and Applied Pharmacology 1976; 35(2):365-79.

Cantor, K.P., Blair, A., Everett, G., Gibson, R., Burmeister, L.F., Brown, L.M., Schuman, L., Dick, F.R., *Pesticides and Other Agricultural Risk Factors for Non-Hodgkins Lymphoma Among Men in Iowa and Minnesota.* Cancer Research 1992; 52:2447-2455.

Chambers, J.E., Chambers, H.W., Snawder, J.E., *Target Site Bioactivation of the Neurotoxic Organophosphorus Insecticide Parathion in Partially Hepatectomized Rats*. Life Sciences 1991; 48:1023-1029.

Chanda, S.M., Harp, P., Liu, J., Pope, N., *Comparative Developmental and Maternal Neurotoxicity Following Acute Gestational Exposure to Chlorpyrifos in Rats*. Journal of Toxicology and Environmental Health 1995; 44:189-202.

Chow, E., Seiber, J.N., Wilson, B.W., *Isofenphos and an In Vitro Activation Assay for Delayed Neuropathic Potential*. Toxicology and Applied Pharmacology 1986; 83:178-183.

Davis, J.R., Brownson, R.C., Garcia, R., *Family Pesticide Use in the Home, Garden, Orchard, and Yard*. Archives of Environmental Contamination and Toxicology 1992; 22:260-266.

Davis, J.R., Brownson, R.C., Garcia, Bentz, B.J., Turner, A., *Family Pesticide Use and Childhood Brain Cancer*. Archives of Environmental Contamination and Toxicology 1993; 24:87-92.

Derelanki, M.J., Hollinger, M.A. (eds.), CRC Handbook of Toxicology. Boca Raton, FL: CRC Press, 1995.

Deschamps, D., Questel, F., Baud, F.J., Gervais, P., Dally, S., *Persistent Asthma after Acute Inhalation of Organophosphate Insecticide*. The Lancet 1994; 344:1712.

Duffy, F.H., Burchfiel, J.L., Bartels, P.H., Gaon, M., Sim, V.M., *Long-Term Effects of an Organophosphate upon the Human Electroencephalogram*. Toxicology and Applied Pharmacology 1979; 47(1):161-76.

Ecobichon, D.J., Joy, R.M. (eds.), Pesticides and Neurological Diseases. Boca Raton, FL: CRC Press, 1982.

Eriksson, P, Fredriksson, A., *Neurotoxic Effects of Two Different Pyrethroids, Bioallethrin and Deltamethrin, on Immature and Adult Mice: Changes in Behavioral and Muscarinic Receptor Variables*. Toxicology and Applied Pharmacology 1991; 108:78-85.

Hayes, W.J., Jr. (ed.), Pesticides Studied in Man. Baltimore, MD: Williams & Wilkins, 1982.

Hoskins, B., Ho, I.K., *Tolerance to Organophosphorus Cholinesterase Inhibitors*. In: Chambers & Levi (eds.), Organophosphorus Compounds: Chemistry, Fate and Effects. San Diego, CA: Academic Press, 1992; 285-297.

Husain, K., Pant, S.C., Raza, S.K., Singh, R., Gupta, S.D., *A Comparative Study of Delayed Neurotoxicity in Hens Following Repeated Administration of Organophosphorus Compounds*. Indian J. Physiol. Pharmacol. 1995; 39(1):47-50.

Jamal, G.A., *Neurological Syndromes of Organophosphorus Compounds*. Adverse Drug React. Toxicol. Oxford University Press, 1997; 16(3):133-170.

Jonkman, E.J., et al., *Electroencephalographic Studies in Workers Exposed to Solvents or Pesticides*. Electroencephalography and Clinical Neurophysiology 1992; 82:438-444.

Julka, D., Pal, R., Gill, K.D., *Neurotoxicity of Dichlorvos: Effect on Antioxidant Defense System in the Rat Central Nervous System*. Experimental and Molecular Pathology 1992; 56:144-152.

Kaloyanova, F.P., El Batawi, M.A. (eds.), Human Toxicology of Pesticides. Boca Raton, FL: CRC Press, 1991.

Kaltner, H., Andrae, S., Wittmann, J., *Activity of Cholinesterases in the Japanese Quail Embryo: Effects of Dichlorphos on the Embryonic Development*. Biochemical Pharmacology 1993; 45(1):87-92.

Kaplan, J.G., Lessler, J., Rosenber, N., Pack, D., Schaumburg, H.H., *Sensory Neuropathy Associated with Dursban (Chlorpyrifos) Exposure*. Neurology 1993; 43:2193-96.

Kassa, J., Bajgar, J., *Treatment of the Stressogenic Effect of Dichlorvos*. Sbor. Ved. Praci. LF UK Hradec Kralove 1994; 37: 29-32.

Lemmon, C.R., Pylypiw, H.M., *Degradation of Diazinon, Chlorpyrifos, Isofenphos, and Pendimethalin in Grass and Compost*. Bulletin of Environmental Contamination and Toxicology 1992; 48:409-415.

Marinovick, M., Guizzetti, M., Galli, C.L., *Mixtures of Benomyl, Pirimiphos-methyl, Dimethoate, Disainon and Azinphos-methyl*

Affect Protein Synthesis in HL-60 Cells Differently. Toxicology 1994; 94:173-185.

Mennear, J.H., *Dichlorvos Carcinogenicity: An Assessment of the Weight of Experimental Evidence.* Regulatory Toxicology and Pharmacology 1994; 20:354-361.

Miranda, F., Duffy, F.H., et al., *Letters on Brain Mapping.* Clinical Electroencephalography 1990; 20(3):vii-x.

Moretto, A., Capodicasa, E., Lotti, M., *Clinical Expression of Organophosphate Induced Delayed Polyneuropathy in Rats.* Toxicology Letters 1992; 63:97-102.

Muto, M.A., Lobelle Jr., F., Bidanset, J.H., Wurpel, J.N.D., *Embryotoxicity and Neurotoxicity in Rats Associated with Prenatal Exposure to Dursban.* Vet. Hum. Toxicol. 1992; 34(6):498-501.

Richardson, R.J., *Assessment of the Neurotoxic Potential of Chlorpyrifos Relative to Other Organophosphorus Compounds: A Critical Review of the Literature.* Journal of Toxicology and Environmental Health 1995; 44:135-165.

Richardson, R.J., Moore, T.B., Kayall, U.S., Fowke, J.H., Randall, J.C., *Inhibition of Hen Brain Acetylcholinesterase and Neurotoxic Esterase by Chlorpyrifos In Vivo and Kinetics of Inhibition by Chlorpyrifos Oxon In Vitro: Application to Assessment of Neuropathic Risk.* Fundamental and Applied Toxicology 1993(b); 20:273-279.

Richardson, R.J., Moore, T.B., Kayall, U.S., Randall, J.C., *Chlorpyrifos: Assessment of Potential for Delayed Neurotoxicity by Repeated Dosing in Adult Hens with Monitoring of Brain Acetylcholinesterae, Brain and Lymphocyte Neurotoxic Esterase, and Plasma Butyrylcholinesterase Activities.* Fundamental and Applied Toxicology 1993(a); 21:89-96.

Richter, E.D., Kowalski, M., Leventhal, et al., *Illness and Excretion of Organophosphate Metabolites Four Months After Household Pest Extermination.* Archives of Environmental Health 1992; 47(2):13-138.

Soliman, S.A., Curley, A., Farmer, J., *In Vivo Inhibition of Chicken Brain Acetylcholinesterase and Neurotoxic Esterase in Relation to the Delayed Neurotoxicity of Leptophos and Cyanofenphos*. J. Environ. Pathol. Toxicol. Oncol. 1986; 7(1-2):211-24.

Taylor, P., *Anicholinesterase Agents*. In: Goodman & Gilman, The Pharmacological Basis of Therapeutics, 8th Ed. New York: Permagon Press, 1990; 131-149.

Wagner, S.L., Orwick, D.L., *Chronic Organophosphate Exposure Associated with Transient Hypertonia in an Infant*. Pediatrics 1994; 94(1):94-97.

Webster, R.C., Sedik, L., Melendres, J., et al., *Percutaneous Absorption of Diazinon in Humans*. Fd. Chem. Toxic. 1993; 31(8):69-572.

Chapter 10

CHLORINATED HYDROCARBON PESTICIDES

The gravest defect of Silent Spring *was that it presented ... [an] over-simplified picture of the needs of the interrelated worldwide complex problems of health, food, fiber, wildlife, recreation and human population. It made no mention of the importance of chemicals such as fertilizers and pesticides for producing and protecting our food and fiber crops; nor did it mention that by producing more food per unit of cultivated area, more land would be available for other uses, including recreation and wildlife.*

—Norman Borlaug, Father of the Green Revolution in Agriculture and Nobel Prize Winner, 1970.

§ 10-1. Overview.

The chlorinated hydrocarbon pesticides (also called organochlorine compounds) are widely used in agriculture, forestry, and public health. In agriculture, they are used as insecticides, as acaricides, and as fumigants in a variety of crops, including grains, cotton, vegetables, and fruit orchards. They have dramatically reduced the prevalence of malaria and other diseases that have insect vectors.

The chlorinated hydrocarbons occur in four major chemical groups: 1) cyclodiene series; 2) halogenated aromatic; 3) cycloparaffins; and 4) chlorinated terpenes. (See Table 10.1.)

Table 10.1
Chlorinated Hydrocarbons

Cyclodiene Series

Aldrin
Dieldrin
Endrin
Heptachlor
Isodrin
Endosulfane
Chlordane

Halogenated Aromatics

DDT
Kelthane
Methoxychlor
Chlorobenzylate
Chlorphenesin

Cycloparaffins

Hexachlorocyclohexane
Benzene hexachloride
Lindane

Chlorinated Terpenes

Polychlorocamphenes
Polychloropinenes

The best known of the chlorinated hydrocarbons is DDT. This compound can be detected in fields where it has been applied for more than six months. It persists in the soil for more than ten years and accumulates in living organisms through the food chain. The adverse impact of DDT on the environment provided the impetus for the environmental movement.

§ 10-2. Mode of Entry into the Body.

Chlorinated hydrocarbons can enter the body by inhalation, ingestion, and absorption through the skin. Skin absorption is minimal when the compound is in powder or dust form. In liquid form, however, dissolved in an oil or organic solvent, it is readily absorbed in quantities sufficient to be toxic.

As is the case with many organic solvents, chlorinated hydrocarbons are highly lipophilic and are stored in fat. Because of this property, chlorinated hydrocarbons readily cross cell membranes and accumulate in cells of the central nervous system, liver, kidneys and myocardium. The lipophilic nature of the chlorinated hydrocarbons contributes to their passage through the food chain from contaminated plant foods to animals, including man. Moreover, chlorinated hydrocarbons can remain virtually unchanged in the environment for decades, potentially capable of contaminating food supplies. While chlorinated hydrocarbons have low toxicity compared to organophosphate compounds, their stability and tendency to bioaccumulate increase their potential for toxicity (Bernad, 1989).

A study of contamination of dairy products demonstrated the ability of chlorinated hydrocarbons to accumulate (Stehr-Greer, 1988). The contamination was traced to grain that had been treated with heptachlor. The grain was used in the production of ethyl alcohol at a plant producing the alcohol-gasoline mixture called "Gasohol," but the contamination had spread to a 45-cow family dairy farm. The family had consumed undiluted, contaminated, raw milk products for about 8 months. The highest level of contamination determined in fat biopsies was 89.2 ppm.

The heptachlor fat levels in the dairy farm family members were compared with those of 94 unexposed control subjects who lived in the same area, and with data from the population at large obtained in the Second National Health and Nutrition Examination Survey (NHANES-II). The exposed group was found to have a significantly higher level of insecticide compared to the controls. No neurologic or hepatic symptoms were apparent in the exposed group, however, even in those with the highest serum levels (Stehr-Greer, 1988).

§ 10-3. The Metabolism Factor.

The lack of symptoms in the family group exposed to chlordane may be due to individual differences in rates of metabolism and excretion. In the liver, the cytochrome P450 (a linked microsomal enzyme system) is thought to play a critical role in detoxification. The P450 is the site of many oxidation reactions, such as hydroxylation and sulphoxidation, as well as many conjugation reactions which convert toxic chemicals to water-soluble forms that can be excreted in urine, stool or bile (Steventon, 1988). Genetic differences in the human population are expressed as varying susceptibility to toxins.

In his practice, the author has seen patients exposed only to minimal amounts of chemicals, as judged from serum and sampling, who developed multiple significant symptomatologies, leading to virtual total disability and complete incapacity. Conversely, the author has also had experience with patients who had virtually no symptoms, and indeed had normal neurologic examinations, while a spouse living in the same house and exposed to the same level of chemicals had multiple, often severe, symptoms.

Whether or not an individual becomes symptomatic depends on a number of factors. In addition to genetics, relevant factors may include nutrition, concurrent infections, dose and duration of exposure, total body burden, and general health. Occupational exposure to dieldrin at levels 1,000 times higher than the exposure of the general population, for example, has been tolerated without obvious effect for up to 15 years. Chronic exposure to levels above 0.3 mg/kg/day, however, may cause symptoms. Acute exposure to 20-40 mg/kg/day has been associated with seizure activity followed by recovery. High exposures have been fatal.

§ 10-4. Possible Mechanisms of Neurotoxicity.

The neurotoxicity of chlorinated hydrocarbon pesticides appears to be a function of the blocking of the enzyme sodium-potassium ATPase (Na-K ATPase), particularly by DDT. The blocking of chloride conductance in cells is also thought to be a factor (Stark, 1988). DDT acts on the axons of neurons by interfering with conductance of the NA-K ATPase. Cyclodienes such as chlordane act at the synapse, affecting the release of neurotransmitters and the inhibition of ATPase. Calcium-magnesium ATPase is also affected (Shankland, 1982; Matsumura, 1985; Ecobichon, 1982). An action on the presynaptic terminal enhances the release of neurotransmitters (Shankland, 1982). The cyclodienes appear to have a more direct action on the central nervous system, and considerably less on the peripheral nervous system, than does DDT.

§ 10-5. Neurotoxic Effects.

Chlorinated hydrocarbon insecticides act on the central nervous system. They are associated with excitability, paresthesias, headaches, dizziness, disorientation, and tremor, which can progress to stupor, coma, and convulsions in severe cases. Severe complications involve seizures with hypoxemia, metabolic acidosis, and death (Olanoff, 1983; Demeter, 1978).

Intoxication associated with acute oral exposure usually begins within a period of 45 minutes to several hours. Careless use of the products can result in subacute toxicity over periods of weeks to months. A spill of 1,3-dichloropropene was associated with chronic symptoms for more than 2 years after the incident. The symptoms included fatigue, irritability, headache, chest pain, concentration difficulties, and decreased libido (Flessel, 1978).

§ 10-6. Specific Chlorinated Hydrocarbon Pesticides.

§ 10-6(a). Chlordane.

Chlordane is a pesticide that once had many household and crop uses. In the U.S., it was restricted to termiticide treatments in 1984 and since 1988 it cannot be used at all (except for those products already in circulation) (EPA, 1988c). Chlordane is still manufactured in the U.S. for export, however. Velsicol Chemical Corporation is the sole producer of chlordane. There are many formulations of chlordane, and although more than a hundred chemicals actually comprise technical chlordane, the four main components are heptachlor, cis-chlordane, trans-chlordane, and trans-nonachlor (Cassidy, 1994). Trans-nonachlor is a minor constituent of chlordane, but a long-lived one.

Ingestion is the primary route of exposure to chlordane, unless one lives in a chlordane-treated house or in one of the 12% to 25% of treated houses where chlordane was misapplied (Fenske and Sternback, 1987). It is estimated that between 50% and 75% of an inhaled or ingested dose is absorbed in the human body. Chlordane is distributed quickly within the body and is stored in adipose tissue, primarily as the oxychlordane metabolite. Excretion is slow. Approximately 85% to 90% are excreted in the feces, and 10% in the urine (Hayes and Laws, 1991). The trans-nonachlor component is also lipophilic and has been detected in most of the American adipose tissue surveys since 1983. Human adipose tissue levels appear to have peaked in 1980 and are currently going down.

Surveys done on human adipose tissue obtained during surgery and postmortem examinations have revealed a high incidence of incorporation of chlordane metabolites (Kutz, 1983). The metabolites found include trans-nonachlor, heptachlor epoxide, and oxychlordane. In 1974 and 1975, trans-nonachlor appeared in 96% to 97% of the samples at mean levels of 0.10 to 0.15 ppm. Oxychlordane was found in 92% to 93% at a mean level of 0.11 ppm, and heptachlor epoxide was reported in 92% to 93% at mean levels of 0.08 to 0.09 ppm.

§ 10-6(a)(1). Neurotoxic Effects.

There are many effects from both acute and chronic exposures to chlordane, including systemic effects, immunological effects, neurological effects, reproductive effects, and developmental effects (ATSDR, 1994). Significant neuromuscular effects of chlordane include hyperexcitability in laboratory animals, especially increases in reactivity to removal and handling, tiptoe gait, and increased grip strength. In contrast to increased excitability, motor activity (irritability, hypoactivity, convulsions) decreased in studies of both acute and subacute exposures, which may indicate that the pattern of effects produced by chlordane is different from that produced by psychomotor stimulants. Repeated dosing with chlordane produces cumulative toxicity.

While acute toxicity from chlordane/heptachlor does exist, quantitative data are hard to find. Frequently, the clinical neurotoxicologist does not see the patient until years have passed since the exposure, and the patient may no longer live or work at the site of the exposure. Moreover, the patient's symptoms are often completely misdiagnosed, and the patient may go from one physician to another with no results.

A survey of houses in which chlordane and heptachlor had been used revealed a wide range of neurologic complaints (Spyker, 1989). Sixty-eight patients ranging in age from 2 to 93 years (with a mean of 33 years) from 30 houses in 9 states were included in the study. Symptom frequency was as follows: headache — 67%; GI difficulties — 63%; fatigue — 62%; memory deficits — 57%; personality changes — 54%; decreased attention span — 52%; numbness or paresthesias — 45%; disorientation — 36%; loss of coordination — 30%; dry eyes — 25%; and seizures — 8%. Electromyography (EMG) was abnormal in 5 of 23 patients (22%), current perception threshold was abnormal in 2 of 11 patients (18%), electronystatogram was abnormal in 8 of 13 patients (62%), and abnormalities were observed in psychiatric testing in 9 of 16 patients (56%). Fat biopsy was carried out in 22 patients. The testing showed chlordane/heptachlor metabolites in the 11-73 percentile of adult normals.

Electroencephalography (EEG) has also been useful in the diagnosis of neurotoxic effects of pesticides and other toxins (Bernad, 1988). In cases of chlordane toxicity, the EEG may show several abnormalities. (See Table 10.2.)

Table 10.2
EEG Abnormalities That May Be Associated With Chlordane Toxicity

Bilateral synchronous theta wave activity.
Bilateral synchronous spike and wave complexes interictally.
Excess of slow waves; spike activity, and paroxysmal bursts of delta waves.

During the theoretical progress from a normal to an abnormal neurologic state, damage to the central nervous system may be occurring while the patient is asymptomatic or is experiencing an unusual collection of symptoms that do not fit neatly into any diagnostic category. During this period, the EEG could be a useful tool for evaluating the patient. However, variations in EEG exposure to different chlorinated hydrocarbons may be complicated by synergistic effects of these products which are often used in mixtures (Bernad, 1989).

Chronic and acute exposures may also present varying EEG patterns. Animal studies have shown EEG abnormalities initially on chronic exposure to endrin (Speck, 1958). However, these abnormalities disappeared within several weeks, even with continued exposure to the toxic substance. These results suggest the development of some sort of tolerance.

In his practice, The author has seen 2 patients who were exposed to industrial, technical-grade chlordane after gross misapplication of pesticides in their home. The patients, aged 49 and 54 when they presented, had been initially diagnosed as having a psychiatric condition.

They were hospitalized for 2 days in a hospital psychiatric service, and were released with some abatement of symptoms.

When the patients returned to their home, their symptoms recurred. These included runny nose, blurred vision, and an inability to get along with family members and co-workers. While on vacation, removed from the chemical contamination in their home, they improved.

While the psychiatric interpretation was obvious, it was incorrect. The neurotoxicologic etiology of their symptoms was not considered during their psychiatric care. Not until a year later in 1 case and 3 years in the other, were the environmental causations considered. In these and in other patients in similar environmental situations, exposure in low dosage occurs constantly, resulting in slow accumulation of the pesticide with progressive symptomatology.

Symptoms of acute chlordane poisoning include headache, blurred vision, dizziness, anorexia, fatigue, and seizures. Chronic exposure can lead to a large number of symptoms, including muscle wasting, disorientation, personality changes, memory loss, and decreased attention span.

A woman who worked at a pesticide manufacturing facility spilled an unknown quantity of chlordane on her skirt. Forty minutes later, she became confused and developed convulsions. She was taken to a hospital, but unfortunately the contaminated clothing was not removed. At the hospital, attempts were made to remove the insecticide from her skin, but the convulsions continued, and the woman died a few minutes after her arrival (Derbes, 1955).

In acute, fatal exposures to chlordane in adults, generalized seizures usually occur prior to death (Derbes, 1955). These seizures are sudden and abrupt, occurring without warning, and may be preceded by a period of malaise, general hyperexcitability, and myoclonic jerking.

In his practice, the author has seen a 3-year-old patient who developed an intractable seizure disorder after exposure to industrial chlordane in a house where it was not applied correctly. The exposure occurred from age 5 months to age 11 months. The child developed seizures at age 6 months, and has had a poorly controlled mixed seizure disorder since that time. She has been treated with multiple anticonvulsant medications. A confounding factor was a familial history of febrile convulsions. The child may have had a genetic predisposition to seizures, and the chlordane may have been the precipitating factor. The theoretical basis for this etiology is referred to as the Kindling Model of Seizures.

In another report, a 19-month-old infant who was exposed orally and topically to an unknown quantity of chlordane, developed seizures (Personal Communication, 1988). The seizures were controlled with phenobarbital, and an EEG taken a week later was normal. The serum chlordane concentration was 350 ppb.

Large numbers of people have developed symptoms of chlordane poisoning after the use of chlordane. In 1987, over 250 adults and children were exposed when the wooden apartment building in which they lived and the surrounding soil were sprayed with chlordane (Kilburn, 1995). Neurobehavioral functions were measured in 216 of the adults who had been exposed and in 174 control subjects. Tests included balance, reaction times, digit symbol, verbal recall and trail-making. Performance was significantly impaired in the exposed group compared to the controls. Mood-state scores were elevated, as were respiratory, neurobehavioral, and rheumatic symptoms. Long-term memory, however, was unaffected.

§ 10-6(b). The Cyclodienes.

The cyclodiene compounds aldrin, dieldrin, and endrin are among the most toxic of the chlorinated hydrocarbons. Their molecular structures and overall effects are quite similar.

Dieldrin is a Class I insecticide (Warning) that has many constituents. Dieldrin readily bioaccumulates and biomagnifies in tissue.

The main routes of exposure are through ingestion of contaminated food and drinking water. Dieldrin is extremely lipophilic and has a half-life of approximately 269 days. A 1987 report states that 17% of U.S. water samples were positive for Dieldrin, and garden fruits provided the highest dose of Dieldrin (Hayes, 1957).

Dieldrin has been shown to produce central nervous system toxicity, liver damage, liver cancer, immune suppression, lung cancer, and adverse fetal effects in experimental animals. Dieldrin has also been shown to induce testosterone hydroxylases and to exhibit estrogenic effects on human cells in vitro. Dieldrin crosses the placental barrier and has been measured in fetal blood and placenta at a much higher level than in the maternal blood and uterine muscle (Hayes, 1957; Jager, 1970).

§ 10-6(b)(1). Neurotoxic Effects.

The neurotoxic effects of the cyclodiene compounds are manifestations of effects on the central nervous system. The peripheral nerves are usually not affected. Massive doses would be required to induce effects on the peripheral nervous system (Van den Brecken, 1973).

It has been proposed that the main site of attack of cyclodienes is the synapse, and the primary effect is the intensification of synaptic activity (Joy, 1982). It is also thought that different types of neurons respond in varying degrees, and that there is no special predilection for excitatory or inhibitory synapses, or for any particular neurotransmitter system.

The acute neurotoxicity is usually associated with ingestion of the insecticide, either accidentally, or voluntarily in suicide attempts. An example of the latter was the case of a 23-year-old farmer who drank a Coca-Cola bottle full of an aldrin mixture. He developed generalized seizures 20 minutes after admission to a hospital. The seizures were so severe that he broke his shoulder. He was treated with phenobarbital for the next 4 days, and no further seizures were seen. Symptoms over the next 5 days included restlessness, hyperthermia, tachycardia, hypertension, and a semi-stuporous state. An EEG taken 2.5 weeks after ingestion was abnormal with bursts of high amplitude. His recovery process was slow, and EEGs taken 6 months after the exposure were still abnormal (Spiotta, 1951; Derbes, 1955).

In another acute poisoning, 3 people were exposed when they consumed bread made from flour contaminated with endrin. The patients exhibited bizarre behavior, seizures, and postictal amnesia. They also had tonic-clonic seizures lasting 2 minutes or more (Coble, 1967). A second incident involving flour contaminated with endrin produced poisoning on an epidemic scale: 867 people were hospitalized, and 26 died (Weeks, 1967).

In another incident, two siblings, a 4-year-old male and a 2-year-old female, drank from a bottle containing 5% dieldrin. When the children were found, the 2-year-old girl was dead and the 4-year-old boy was in status epilepticus. He was treated and survived (Garrettson, 1969).

A study of workers exposed to aldrin, dieldrin, and telodrin yielded data suggesting three syndromes associated with these pesticides. The first syndrome was characterized as a convulsive intoxication or seizure with minimal antecedent symptoms. This syndrome was usually associated with a single, very high exposure. The symptoms have generally been associated with highly toxic, but nonpersistent compounds such as endrin. An accumulative intoxication can occur with compounds having a lower acute toxicity but a higher persistence.

A second multi-symptom syndrome was characterized by headache, dizziness, drowsiness, hyperirritability, general malaise, nausea, anorexia, vomiting, muscle twitching, myoclonic jerks, and seizures. This syndrome is also seen in association with chlordane-heptachlor. In these workers, a mild, acute exposure, in itself not significant, may induce an abrupt onset of seizures superimposed upon a subclinical accumulation of intoxication.

The third syndrome was seizure activity associated with a minor increase in insecticide blood level, and possibly in the central nervous system, caused by a mild, acute overexposure. This syndrome suggests a threshold effect, although this has not been proven.

§ 10-6(b)(2). Electrophysiological Testing.

While most data on the use of EEG and other electrophysiologic diagnostic procedures are clinical reports, a few controlled studies have been carried out. In one study, EEG findings from a group of 122 chemical plant workers, who were exposed daily to aldrin, dieldrin, and endrin, were compared with those of 122 office workers (Hoogendam, 1962). EEG abnormalities were found in 20.5% of the chemical plant workers compared to 9.0% in the control group of office workers. Fourteen of the chemical plant workers with EEG abnormalities had convulsions. These workers had specific EEG abnormalities consisting of bilateral synchronous theta wave activity, and occasional bilateral synchronous spike and wave complexes. These specific patterns had a tendency to return to normal within 6 months after removal from exposure to the insecticides.

In this study, the EEG abnormalities associated with exposure to the cyclodienes produced in the plant were very specific. Other studies done at that time failed to reach similar conclusions (Bernad, 1989). Another study of workers exposed to aldrin and dieldrin showed diffuse abnormalities rather than specific findings (Spiotta, 1951). A 1975 study, however, did find specific abnormalities (Gupta, 1975). An excess of slow waves, spike activity, and paroxysmal bursts of delta wave abnormalities were found in the EEGs of 6 patients after chronic consumption of aldrin and benzene hexachloride in wheat.

§ 10-6(c). DDT/DDE.

DDT has the chemical formula $C_{14}H_9C_{15}$, and DDE is $C_{14}H_8C_{14}$. DDT is dichloro diphenyl trichlrorethane, and the principal isomer is 1,1'-(22,2,2-trichloroethylidene)-bis[4-chlorobenzene] (p,p'-DDT). DDT was introduced to the U.S. in 1942 and was distributed widely in the environment as an insecticide. All uses of DDT in the U.S. were canceled in 1973, except for emergency uses and a few other uses permitted on a case-by-case basis only. DDT is, however, still used extensively in the tropics and in developing countries for malaria control, and its long-range transport across the globe is well-documented (Borlaug, 1972).

General exposure to DDT is widespread. DDT is stored in all tissues (its greatest affinity is for fat) and eventually reaches a plateau. It is believed that DDT is metabolized to DDD and then to DDA, which is the main urinary excretion product and not generally found in tissues. Recent studies illustrate an increased susceptibility in the cholinergic muscarinic receptors and a different behavior reaction in animals already exposed to DDT, when again exposed to a similar neurotoxic agent as adults. The study exposed mice to levels of DDT that would be expected during lactation, then exposed them again in adult life to a pyrethrin insecticide. The study noticed an increased sensitivity to the second dose in the exposed animals compared with controls.

Human effects of DDT include headache, nausea, tremors, severe vomiting, and shorter lactation periods in women. p,p'-DDT is a weak estrogen and has been shown to inhibit testicular growth and sexual characteristics in chickens (Ecobichon, 1982). Because mothers excrete DDT/DDE in their breast milk, breast-fed babies are at a greater risk for DDT/DDE exposure than those fed cow's milk or formulas.

§ 10-6(d). Gamma-HCH (Lindane).

Lindane is also known as benzene hexachloride (BHC) and has eight separable steric isomers (Hayes, 1982). It has considerable persistence in the environment and is commonly detected in human breast milk and fat biopsies. All isomers are absorbed via the skin, intestinal tract and lungs (Starr, 1972).

Each of the isomers of BHC is metabolized slightly differently. Studies have shown, however, that most isomers, including B-HCH, produce 2,4-dichlorophenol in the urine of rats, as well as 2,3,4,6-tetrachlorophenol in both its free and conjugated forms.

Lindane is a central nervous system stimulant, the opposite of its beta isomer. It does, however, also induce monooxygenase activity. Lindane binds the GABA receptor binding site in the cerebellum and therefore interferes with GABAergic transmission.

§ 10-6(e). Heptachlor and Heptachlor Epoxide.

Heptachlor is a chlorinated cyclodiene pesticide. It is primarily used for termite control and as a wood treatment in combination with other chemicals such as chlordane. Heptachlor epoxide (HE) is the oxidation product of heptachlor. HE occurs in soil and in or on plants following heptachlor treatments.

Heptachlor is commonly used either with chlordane or directly in the chlordane mixture itself and was first isolated from technical chlordane. Heptachlor epoxide is extremely lipophilic and long-lasting. Due to its widespread use and high volatility it is a common contaminant in whale blubber.

Heptachlor is readily absorbed by the skin, lungs and gastrointestinal tract. It has produced hyperexcitability and decreased motor activity in studies of both acute and subacute exposure. This cyclodiene insecticide is known to alter hormone concentrations during pregnancy and to decrease fertility, and is suspected to cause tumors and blood disorders in exposed human populations. Heptachlor also produces cumulative toxicity (Hayes, 1982).

References.

Bernad, P.G., *The Utility of EEG and Neurophysiologic Techniques After Neurologic Exposure.* Clin. Electroencephalography 1988; 20: Abstract of paper presented at the Meeting of the American Medical EEG Association, October 27-30, Lexington, KY.

Bernad, P.G., *Review: EEG and Pesticides.* Clin Electroencephalography 1989; 20:9-10.

Borlaug, N., *In Defense of DDT and Other Pesticides.* UNESCO Courier, Feb. 1972.

Coble Y, Hildebrandt, P., David, J., et al., *Acute Endrin Poisoning.* JAMA 1967; 202:489.

Demeter, J., Heyndrickx, A., *Two Lethal Endosulfan Poisonings in Man.* J. Anal. Toxicol. 1978; 2:68-74.

Derbes, V.J., Dent, J.H., Forrest, D.N., Johnson, M.D., *Fatal Chlordane Poisoning.* JAMA 1955; 158:1367-1369.

Ecobichon, D.J., Joy, R.M., Pesticides and Neurobiological Diseases. Boca Raton, Fl: CRC Press, Inc., 1982: 121-142.

Flessel, P., Goldsmith, J.R., Kahn, E., et al., *Acute and Possible Long-Term Effects of 1,3-Dichloropropene — California.* 1978; 27:50-55.

Garrettson, L.K., Curley, A., *Dieldrin — Studies in a Poisoned Child.* Arch. Environ. Health. 1969; 19:814.

Gupta, P.C., *Neurotoxicity of Chronic Chlorinated Hydrocarbon Insecticide Poisoning: A Chemical and Electroencephalographic Study in Man.* Indian J. Med. Res. 1975; 63:601-606.

Hayes, W.J., Jr., *Dieldrin Poisoning in Man.* Public Health Report 1957; 72:1087.

Hayes, W.J., Jr. (ed.), Pesticides Studied in Man. Baltimore, MD: Williams & Wilkins, 1982.

Hoogendam, I., Versteeg, P.J., De Vlieger, M., *Electroencephalograms in Insecticide Toxicity.* Arch. Environ. Health. 1962; 4:92-100.

Jager K.W., Aldrin, Dieldrin, Endrin, and Telodrin — An Epidemiological and Toxilogical Study of Long-Term Occupational Exposure. Amsterdam: Elsevier Publishing. 1970.

Joy, R.M., *Mode of Action of Lindane, Dieldrin, and Related Insecticides in the Central Nervous System.* Neurobehavioral Toxicol. Teratol. 1982; 4:813-823.

Kilburn, K.H., Thornton, J.C., *Protracted Neurotoxicity from Chlordane Sprayed to Kill Termites.* Environ. Health Perspect. 1995; 103:690-694.

Kutz, F.W., *Chemical Exposure Monitoring.* Research Review 1983; 85:277-292.

Matsumura, F., Toxicology of Insecticides. New York: Plenum Press, 1985: 140.

Olanoff, L.S., Bristow W.J., Colcolough, J., Jr., *Acute Chlordane Intoxication.* 1983; 20:291-306.

Shankland, D.L., *Neurotoxic Action of Chlorinated Hydrocarbon Insecticides.* Neurobehavioral Toxicol. Teratol. 1982 4:805-811.

Speck, L.B., Maaske, C.A., *The Effects of Chronic and Acute Exposure of Rats to Endrin.* AMA Arch. Industr. Health. 1958; 18:268.

Spiotta, E.J., *Aldrin Poisoning in Man.* Arch. Ind. Hyg. Occup. Med. 1951; 4:560-566.

Spyker, D.A., Bond, R.R., Jylkka, M., Bernad, P.G., *Subacute Home Chlordane Poisoning: Fact or Fallacy.* Vet. Hum. Toxicol. 1989; 31:356 (Abstract 108).

Stark, L.G., Albertson, T.D., Joy, R.M., *Effects oif Hexachlorocyclohexane Isomers on the Acquisition of Kindled Seizures.* Neurobehavioral Toxicol. Teratol. 1988; 8:487-491.

Starr, H.G., Clifford, N.J., *Acute Lindane Intoxication – A Case Study.* Arch. Environ. Health 1972; 24:374.

Stehr-Greer, P.A., Burse, V.W., Wohlleb, J.C., *Persistence of Heptachlor in Serum of People Consuming Contaminated Dairy Products.* Lancet 1988; 11:570-571.

Steventon, G., William, A.V., Waring, R.H., et al., *Xenobiotic Metabolism in Motorneuron Disease.* Lancet 1988; ii:644-647.

Van den Brecken, J., Akkermans, LM.A., Van Lange, R.G., *The Effect of DDT and Dieldrin on Skeletal Muscle Fibers.* Eur. J. Pharmacology 1973; 21:89.

Weeks, D.E., *Endrin Food Poisoning. A Report on Four Outbreaks Caused by Two Separate Shipments of Endrin-Contaminated Flour.* Bull. WHO 1967; 37:499-512.

Whelan, E.M., Toxic Terror: The Truth Behind the Cancer Scares. Buffalo, NY: Promethius Books, 1993.

Chapter 11

THE ROLE OF NUTRIENTS

Perhaps the essential difference between the pessimist and the realist is that the former bows his head in resignation to the inevitability of evil, while the latter sees the darkness of experience as a challenge to him to fashion new lights which will conquer the shadows — new lights of science and medicine and law, to bind up the wounds and restrain the beast in the whims of Nature and of human nature.

—Joshua Loth Liebman, *Hope for Man* (1966).

§ 11-1. Overview.

Diet can have profound effects on both the central and peripheral nervous systems. Deficiencies or excesses in vitamin and mineral intake can result in nervous system symptoms and signs similar to those of exposure to chemicals such as solvents and insecticides. Vitamin and mineral deficiencies have been noted in patients presenting with symptoms of chemical exposure (Johnson, 1989). In some instances, a mineral and/or vitamin deficiency, as well as deficiencies of certain amino acids and fatty acids, can exacerbate the effects of chemical exposure. In medicolegal situations, it is conceivable that a plaintiff in a tort may deliberately avoid certain vitamins or minerals in an attempt to multiply the effects of a toxic exposure or to simulate its effects.

Vitamins and minerals are required for the operation of the detoxification systems in body cells that change toxic substances into less toxic molecules that can be safely excreted in urine and bile. These chemical changes are expedited by specific enzymes, which are proteins that act as catalysts. Without enzymes, the biotransformation of toxic materials, and practically all other chemical reactions that occur in a living organism, would not occur fast enough to keep it alive. Enzymes accelerate these reactions by factors of at least a million. Many enzymes require vitamins and minerals as cofactors in order to function properly. On the other hand, heavy metals, such as cadmium, aluminum, and mercury, can inactivate enzymes.

Detoxification occurs in two phases. Phase I detoxification occurs through oxidation, reduction, and/or hydrolysis. In many instances, one or more or a combination of these processes is all that is required. Phase I is also referred to as the cytochrome P-450 monooxygenase system. The basic process of Phase II is conjugation, which is chemical combination with another molecule. The resulting conjugates are excreted safely in bile and eliminated in feces.

Glutathione is one of the major conjugating substances in Phase II. Glutathione is a tripeptide, a compound composed of 3 amino acids: glutamic acid, cysteine, and glycine. A deficiency in glutathione can impair the body's detoxification system. Thus, a diet deficient in these 3 amino acids may adversely affect detoxification, possibly exacerbating the effects of exposure to a neurotoxin. Zinc is required as a cofactor for glucoronic acid to function properly in the detoxification process. Thus, a zinc deficiency could also intensify the effects of toxic exposure.

Glutathione is constantly recycled, and niacin (vitamin B_3) is an essential cofactor for the recycling process. Also required for recycling are the enzymes glutathione reductase and glutathione peroxidase. As cofactors, the former requires riboflavin (vitamin B_2), while the latter requires selenium.

Other Phase II conjugators include 3'-phosphoadenosine, 5'-phosphosulfate (PAPS) and glucoronic acid, which require cysteine and zinc respectively. The amino acids cysteine and glycine alone are capable of conjugating chemicals. Phase II conjugators such as glutathione, PAPS, and cysteine all contain sulflhydryl groups, implying that sufficient dietary sulfur is important for maintaining the detoxification system.

Once a chemical has been absorbed into the bloodstream, biotransformation can occur through many different biochemical pathways. Many substances are metabolized into alcohols which are subsequently changed to aldehydes. Aldehydes, in turn, can be changed into an acidic form that can be safely excreted in the urine. In another possible pathway, the chemical is changed from alcohol to chloral hydrate. Often referred to as "knock-out drops" or a "Mickey Finn," chloral hydrate is used as a sedative. An accumulation of chloral hydrate in the body can induce symptoms of sedation. The chloral hydrate step can occur when the detoxification system is overloaded or if there is insufficient enzyme to change the chemical to an aldehyde.

The enzyme catalyzing the step from the alcohol to the aldehyde form is alcohol dehydrogenase. It requires a specific amount of zinc as a cofactor in order to function. If there is insufficient intake of zinc, the biotransformation of alcohol may not be fast enough to avoid accumulation of chloral hydrate. If the detoxification system is overloaded, there can be a delay in processing the toxin, which can damage cells and tissues, including those of the nervous system. The products of alternate pathways, such as chloral hydrate, can also be damaging.

Which detoxification pathway a toxin goes through depends on several factors, including:

- Genetics;
- Nutrient levels;
- Total load; and
- Detoxification damage.

The synthesis of enzymes is controlled by genes. Some individuals fail to inherit certain genes, and are thus lacking in the enzymes synthesized by the missing genes. Possible manifestations of genetic disease include adverse reactions to substances that are harmless to the general population. Certain levels of nutrients (vitamins, minerals, amino acids, and essential fatty acids) are required for enzymes to operate. Iron and molybdenum are required for the operation of aldehyde oxidase, the enzyme that catalyzes the step from aldehyde into an acid. Magnesium is required as a cofactor by more than 300 enzymes.

Because of the increasing use of chemicals in industry and agriculture, the chemical load in individuals tends to be quite high, depending upon location and occupation. The detoxification system itself can be damaged by chemicals that have not been metabolized, or that have been metabolized in alternate pathways. Other problems stem from our eating habits and the way we prepare foods. Vitamins and minerals are often poured down the drain with cooking water. Frequent consumption of fast foods can result in accumulation of possibly harmful additives, as well as increased blood pressure and blood cholesterol levels. Processed foods often have poor nutritional value and contain large amounts of salt, and many have preservatives, including phosphates, which can interfere with the absorption of calcium.

§ 11-2. Nutrient Deficiency and Overdose.

Deficiency diseases usually involve both the peripheral and central nervous systems. Patients with deficiency diseases usually present with non-neurologic signs of malnutrition, such as wasting, skin and mucous membrane lesions, and circulatory problems (Victor, 1994). While deficiency diseases may occur in pure form, they often occur in various combinations.

§ 11-3. Free Radicals and Antioxidants.

Free radicals are highly reactive chemicals bearing an unpaired electron (Lohr, 1995). Some free radicals are formed during some of the biochemical reactions in the detoxification process. The formation of free radicals, however, is not limited to detoxification pathways. They are also formed as a result of the routine cellular oxidative metabolism of both endogenous and exogenous compounds (Keaney, 1995). Once they are released, free radicals can enter into a number of reactions that can damage or destroy cell membranes and the interiors of cells. Free radicals have been associated with the pathogenesis of atherosclerosis (Keaney, 1995), arthritis, Alzheimer's disease (Smith, 1995; Frölich, 1995), cancer (Rogers, 1990; Borolongan, 1996), neuropsychiatric disorders (Lohr, 1995; Cadet, 1994), Parkinson's disease (Frölich, 1995; Evans, 1993), gastroduodenal disease (Phull, 1995), and aging (Greenstock, 1993).

The formation of free radicals is often referred to as "oxidative stress." This term is not entirely accurate, however, since many of the biochemical reactions that contribute to oxidative stress are not oxidative in nature (Keaney, 1995). The production of the free radical superoxide anion (O_2^-), for example, is often thought of as oxidative stress even though it usually functions in reduction, the opposite of oxidation.

Antioxidants are compounds that limit the actions of free radicals by neutralizing, or "scavenging," the destructive oxidants. Antioxidants can be classified into two major groups: enzymatic and nonenzymatic.

Enzymatic antioxidants are the main form of intracellular antioxidant defense. They include superoxide dismutase (SOD), catalase, and glutathione peroxidase. Many enzymatic antioxidants require cofactors. Glutathione peroxidase, for example, requires selenium, and SOD requires zinc.

Nonenzymatic antioxidants include transferrin, albumin, and ceruloplasmin. The low-molecular weight antioxidants are water-soluble compounds, including vitamin C (ascorbic acid), thiols and bilirubin. The lipid-soluble or lipoprotein-associated antioxidants include vitamins A and E, ubiquinol-10, lycopene, 17 β-Estradiol, thyroxine, and catecholamines (Keaney, 1995).

The beneficial effects of antioxidants in a variety of applications have been demonstrated by clinical experience and many studies. Epidemiologic studies of the 1980s and 1990s suggested an association between the intake of antioxidant vitamins and reduced risk of coronary disease (Riersmam, 1989; Rimm, 1993; Stampfer, 1993). The mechanisms of this protection are unknown. However, it is suspected that the antioxidants may help to preserve normal endothelial function. The role of the endothelium in blood vessels is the regulation of vascular tone and platelet activity. The control is regulated to a large extent through the release of endothelium-derived relaxing factor (EDRF), which is impaired in patients with coronary heart disease or coronary risk factors. Because increased oxidative stress has been linked to impaired action of EDRF and to the loss of dilation of the blood vessel (Keaney, 1993; Keaney, 1995a), it has been postulated that antioxidants may help to preserve normal endothelial function (Levine, 1996).

In a study of patients with coronary artery disease, Levine found that 2 grams of ascorbic acid produced marked improvement in blood vessel dilation 2 hours after administration, reversing endothelial vasomotor dysfunction in the patients (Levine, 1996). In a review, K. Gey of the Vitamin Unit at the University of Berne in Switzerland noted that epidemiologic studies have indicated an association between poor plasma levels of all essential antioxidants and increased relative risk of cancer and heart disease (Gey, 1993). Low levels of carotene have been seen in some cancer patients, and vitamin E deficiencies have been detected in patients with ischemic heart disease.

Two large epidemiologic studies reported in 1993 provided evidence of a significant role for vitamin E in reducing the risk of coronary heart disease in men and women (Stampfer, 1993; Rimm, 1993). The study of women began in 1980 with 87,245 female nurses, aged 34 to 59 years, who were free of diagnosed cardiovascular disease and cancer. The subjects filled out dietary questionnaires about their consumption of vitamin E and other nutrients. In the 8-year follow-up, there were 552 cases of major coronary disease. Women with a high intake of vitamin E supplements for a period of 2 years had a profound and statistically significant lower relative risk of coronary disease than did women not taking the supplements or taking them for a shorter period of time. Also the reduction in risk was seen only in the subjects who took supplements, not in those with a high dietary intake of vitamin E (Stampfer, 1993).

The men's study started in 1986 with 39,910 male health professionals ranging in age from 40 to 75 years (Rimm, 1993). All subjects were free of diagnosed coronary heart disease, diabetes, and hypercholesterolemia. The subjects filled out questionnaires about their intake of vitamin E, vitamin C, carotene, and other nutrients. The subjects were followed for 4 years, during which time there were 667 cases of coronary disease. Men who took vitamin E supplements had a much lower risk for coronary heart disease than did men with low or no intake. The inverse relationship between coronary heart disease and the use of vitamin E supplements was maintained after adjusting for variables such as higher health consciousness among men who took vitamin supplements. A moderate reduction was found in men with increasing intake of dietary vitamin E. The vitamin E content of foods varies with methods of cooking, processing and storage. Carotene intake was associated with a lower risk for coronary disease among men who were current or former smokers than among those who had never smoked. Vitamin C intake was not associated with lower risk for coronary disease.

The Zutphen Study was an epidemiologic investigation of the effect of dietary flavonoids and antioxidant vitamins on the incidence of stroke (Keli, 1996). A group of 552 men aged 50 to 69 was examined first in 1970 and followed for 15 years. Men with a high intake of flavonoid antioxidants had a 73% lower risk of stroke during the 15 years of follow-up examination. Beta-carotene intake, independent from flavonoid intake, was associated with a 46% lower stroke risk.

Antioxidants are known to play a key role in the healing of wounds (Martin, 1996). Wound healing occurs in three phases: inflammation, cellular proliferation, and remodeling. During the inflammatory phase, white blood cells migrate to the wound site. Neutrophils release proteases and reactive oxygen compounds in the area, which help to kill bacteria, but also may have adverse effects on surrounding tissues. Antioxidants at the site may be inactivated or depleted during the proliferative phase. Fibroblasts produce collagen, which is needed for wound repair, and vitamin C is required for the production of collagen. A decrease in collagen at the wound site will increase healing time.

The cause of Alzheimer's disease is not yet fully established. The disease is characterized by atrophy of the cerebral cortex (Rowland, 1995). Histopathology (biopsy) is the only definite diagnostic technique for Alzheimer's disease. However, clinical diagnosis has a high degree of accuracy if dementia is established by clinical examination and confirmed by neuropsychologic tests (Rowland, 1995). A genetic basis is strongly suggested, since there is a higher concordance of Alzheimer's disease in monozygotic twins than in dizygotic twins. Although the question is still quite controversial, there is mounting evidence that free radicals are involved in the pathogenesis of neurodegenerative diseases, such as Alzheimer's disease (Smith, 1994; Smith, 1994a; Smith, 1995; Smith 1995a; Smith, 1995b; Yan, 1994) and Parkinson's disease (Frölich, 1995; Evans, 1993).

Both senile plaques and neurofibrillary tangles must be found to make a diagnosis of Alzheimer's disease (Adams, 1997). Senile plaque is found throughout the cerebral cortex and hippocampus, and the number of plaques per microscopic field correlates with the severity of intellectual loss. Senile neuritic plaques are spherical microscopic lesions that are best seen with Bielschowsky stain. Neurofibrillary tangles are fibrillary intracytoplasmic structures within the neurons and, like the plaques, are also seen with the Bielschowsky stain. Electron microscopy shows paired helical filaments. Although neurofibrillary tangles are not specific to Alzheimer's disease, they occur first in the hippocampus, particularly in region CA1 and subiculum, and eventually throughout the cerebral cortex (Rowland, 1995).

Any proposed mechanism must take into account the conversion of normal cellular proteins into the insoluble, aggregated fibrillar proteins found in the lesions (Smith, 1995). Oxidative stress is associated with the formation of carbonyls from proteins, lipids, and carbohydrates. Several carbonyl-related lesions have been described in association with Alzheimer's disease lesions, suggesting that the modifications, which are likely results of oxidative stress, could play a role in the development of Alzheimer's (Yan, 1994). Iron may also be involved in the neuronal damage associated with Alzheimer's disease. The accumulation of iron in neurons with neurofibrillary tangles is possibly a result of the enzyme heme oxygenase and could have serious pathological consequences. Iron mediates a variety of redox reactions involving hydrogen peroxide which result in the production of more reactive oxidative compounds. The increased concentration of aluminum in neurons filled with neurofibrillary tangles stimulates iron-induced peroxidation of lipids (Good, 1992; Gutteridge, 1985). In addition, elevated iron levels could result in increased protein modifications by reducing sugars. These protein modifications have been identified in association with senile plaques and neurofibrillary tangles (Wolff, 1989; Smith, 1994; Yan, 1994; Vitek, 1994; Ledesma, 1994).

Free radical damage is different from other Alzheimer's pathology in that it can be ameliorated with antioxidants and free radical scavengers. The role of iron in the pathogenesis of Alzheimer's disease suggests that treatments which lower iron levels may be helpful.

There is a growing body of evidence supporting a possible role of free radicals in the pathogenesis of Parkinson's disease (Evans, 1993; Adams, 1991). Parkinson's disease is characterized by specific and progressive destruction of the nigrostriatal dopaminergic neurons. Evidence supporting a role of free radicals in Parkinson's disease includes the association of the formation of 6-hydroxydopamine, a neurotoxin, with the oxidative metabolism of dopamine. The findings of decreased concentrations of the antioxidant glutathione peroxidase in the substantia nigra compared to other parts of the brain, and the reduction of nigral glutathione peroxidase in Parkinson's disease, also suggest a role for free radicals. The discovery of increased iron in the substantia nigra of Parkinson's patients provides another clue. Iron may have a pathogenic role in causing damage of lipid peroxidative tissue by the formation of hydroxyl radicals. Also, the preferential expression of the CuZnsuperoxide dismutase gene in the substantia nigra suggests that the region is particularly susceptible to oxidative stress.

The possibility of the involvement of free radicals in Parkinson's disease has prompted the use of antioxidants in treatment. Studies of the use of vitamins C and E have shown that high doses of these vitamins can slow the rate of progression of the disease (Evans, 1993; Lieberman, 1992).

§ 11-4. Minerals.

Minerals are various metals that are essential nutrients. Some — such as calcium, sodium, potassium, and magnesium — are required in relatively large amounts. Other are required in such small amounts (less than 1 μg/g of wet weight) that they are referred to as "trace elements." While inadequate dietary intake can be the cause of deficiency, syndromes associated with deficiency can occur even when the amount of a mineral in the diet is abundant. Other causes of deficiency include various metabolic disorders and malabsorption syndromes in which the mineral cannot be absorbed from the intestine in sufficient quantities. Interactions between metals can also cause deficiencies. Calcium can decrease the absorption of zinc. On the other hand, use of zinc supplements in excess of 10 times the recommended daily allowance can cause a copper deficiency (Falchuk, 1994).

§ 11-4(a). Calcium.

Sources of calcium include milk, cheese and other dairy products, broccoli, and dark green leafy vegetables, such as collard and turnip greens (NAS, 1989). For most adults in the United States, the average daily intake of calcium is about 0.6 to 0.8 grams a day. However, many people take supplementary calcium for a variety of reasons. Calcium is involved in many vital processes, including bone formation and heart function. Calcium deficiency or excess, therefore, can have serious consequences. The metabolism of calcium is complex, involving interactions with phosphorous, vitamin D, parathyroid and other hormones.

In the average adult body there are about 1 to 2 grams of calcium, 98% of which is in bone. Much of the remaining 2% is in the extracellular fluid (ECF) and blood plasma. However, the small amount of calcium in the ECF is critical for a variety of functions (Holick, 1994). A reduction in the concentration of calcium (as free calcium ions) results in neurologic symptoms such as increased neuromuscular irritability and tetany. Symptoms and signs include paresthesias in the limbs and around the mouth, anxiety, irritability, seizures, bronchospasm, and spasms in the hands and feet (Holick, 1994).

While insufficient dietary intake can result in low calcium levels (hypocalcemia) in the body, low calcium can also be the result of the interaction of many factors. Hypocaclemia can be chronic or transient. Causes of chronic hypocalcemia include excess magnesium, hyperparathyroidism, and vitamin D deficiency. Transient hypocalcemia is often asymptomatic and can be due to many causes including kidney failure, burns, and medications such as heparin and glucagon. Neurologic symptoms of chronic hypocalcemia include muscle spasms, facial grimacing, and, in extreme cases, convulsions and spasm of the larynx (Potts, 1994).

Hypercalcemia, an overabundance of calcium, can also stem from many causes, including parathyroid gland dysfunction, cancers, kidney failure, high turnover of bone tissue, and various vitamin D imbalances (Potts, 1994). Hypercalcemia is often asymptomatic, and when symptoms and signs are present, they vary with the type of hypercalcemia. Neurologic symptoms associated with parathyroid-related hypercalcemia, for example, include fatigue, weakness in the proximal muscles, and muscle atrophy. A frequently employed treatment is surgical removal of one or more of the small parathyroid glands located in the thyroid gland. Neuromuscular disease usually resolves completely after the surgery (Potts, 1994).

§ 11-4(b). Magnesium.

Magnesium is involved in almost every phase of the detoxification pathway. It is a cofactor for more than 300 enzymes. It is also a cofactor for enzymes that catalyze the synthesis and breakdown of hormones and other brain chemicals. Consequently, magnesium deficiency can manifest in a variety of symptoms indicative of nervous system disorders, many of which are similar to those associated with chemical exposure. Magnesium deficiency has been associated with neck and back pain. Injections of magnesium have provided relief for chronic back pain (Rogers, 1990b). Other nervous system symptoms associated with magnesium deficiency include anxiety, panic disorder, fine tremors, muscle spasms, Raynaud's spastic vessels (cold white fingers), general nervousness, cardiac arrhythmias, and fatigue (Rea, 1986). It has been estimated that about 80% of the United States population are deficient in magnesium.

§ 11-4(c). Sodium.

Sodium is an extremely important nutrient, and its excess or deficiency can have profound effects on the health of an individual. Sodium is ubiquitous in nature and on the supermarket shelf and deli counter. The major sources of sodium are salt and processed foods containing salt. Such familiar foods as lunch meats, frankfurters, ham, bacon, sausage, cheeses, pickles, and olives are all rich in sodium, as are baking powder and soda, food additives such as monosodium glutamate, and some antacids.

The metabolism of sodium is closely related to water. The amount of sodium in the body depends on the balance of dietary intake of sodium and its excretion in urine. In a normal healthy person the balance is maintained even in the face of abrupt, but not too lengthy episodes of over- or underconsumption of sodium. The balance is also aided by thirst. Generally accompanying the consumption of salty foods, thirst causing a person to drink water, which helps to restore the balance. A mechanism involving the hypothalamus, the posterior pituitary gland (neurohypophysis), and the kidneys is also involved in maintaining water/sodium equilibrium (Levinsky, 1994).

Hypernatremia, the excessive sodium condition, can occur through water loss or sodium gain. The water loss can be through the skin, lungs, or kidneys. Hypernatremia can have devastating effects on the central nervous system because of dehydration of brain cells. Manifestations include altered mental state, twitching, seizures, and dulling of senses. Stupor and coma may also occur. In severe cases, the effects may be irreversible. High mortality rates are seen in children and adults (Levinsky, 1994; DeVita, 1993).

Hyponatremia, sodium deficiency, usually occurs as combined water and sodium deficits. It is also referred to as volume depletion. Hyponatremia can be due to many causes, including kidney failure, inappropriate secretion of antidiuretic hormone from the posterior pituitary, excessive water consumption, and various hormonal imbalances. Manifestations include loss of gastrointestinal fluids, acute kidney failure, reduced skin turgor, dry mouth, and reduced armpit sweating (Levinsky, 1994).

§ 11-4(d). Potassium.

Sources of potassium include fruits, particularly oranges, grapefruit, prunes, apples, pears, peaches and bananas; vegetables, particularly broccoli, carrots, tomatoes, and potatoes; and milk, fish, shellfish, turkey, and cooked oatmeal (NAS, 1989). Potassium is involved in the transport of materials into and out of cells through the expenditure of energy, and thus plays a vital role in many life functions. The kidneys maintain potassium balance in normal, healthy individuals.

Hyperkalemia, excessive potassium, can result from a number of causes. Inadequate excretion of potassium may be caused by acute or chronic kidney failure, disorders of the adrenal cortex, and certain medications, such as nonsteroidal anti-inflammatory agents, angiotensin converting enzyme inhibitors, beta blockers, and the type of diuretic that inhibits the excretion of potassium (spironolactone, amiloride, triamterene). Alteration of serum potassium levels is seen in crush injuries to tissues, insulin deficiency, metabolic disorders, and as an effect of drugs, including arginine and digitalis. Excessive intake can also induce hyperkalemia. This occurs most often from excessive use of potassium supplements, which are frequently prescribed to counteract the potassium-wasting effects of thiazide diuretics. If a patient switches from a thiazide to a diuretic (such as spironolactone) that inhibits potassium excretion, and continues out of habit to take potassium supplements, the patient could develop hyperkalemia (Levinsky, 1994).

Manifestations of hyperkalemia include cardiac arrhythmias, which could advance to ventricular fibrillation and death if the hyperkalemia is not corrected. Occasionally, peripheral muscles may also be affected by weakness which becomes progressively worse, advancing to quadriplegia and respiratory paralysis.

Hypokalemia, the deficiency of potassium, can be caused by insufficient dietary intake, thiazide diuretics, gastrointestinal disorders resulting in vomiting and diarrhea, anatomical disorders, and certain surgeries. Excessive licorice ingestion, excessive glucocorticoid (Cushing's disease), certain antibiotics, magnesium depletion, and kidney dysfunctions involving a number of complex metabolic interactions can also cause hypokalemia.

The most prominent manifestations of hypokalemia are neuromuscular. Some patients complain of muscle weakness, particularly in the lower limbs. In severe cases, total paralysis, including respiratory paralysis, may occur. Electrocardiogram abnormalities may also develop. Rapid reduction of potassium could result in cardiac arrest. Kidney dysfunctions associated with hypokalemia can cause excessive urination and thirst (Levinsky, 1994).

§ 11-4(e). Zinc.

Dietary sources of zinc include meat, shellfish, poultry, cheese, and whole grains. Zinc deficiency can be manifested in the nervous system by psychological disturbances. Non-neurologic manifestations include growth retardation, alopecia and immunologic disorders. In addition to inadequate dietary intake, deficiency syndromes can be caused by malabsorption syndrome, metabolic disorders, and interactions with other minerals. Excess fiber, for example, can retard the absorption of zinc (NAS, 1989).

Zinc acts as an antioxidant in helping to neutralize the effects of free radicals. Zinc is also believed to preserve the activity of some important enzymes by protecting them against oxidation. Zinc is required as a cofactor for alcohol dehydrogenase, the enzyme necessary to converting alcohol to aldehyde. Insufficient intake or absorption of zinc could result in the accumulation of chloral hydrate, with detrimental effects on the central nervous system.

§ 11-4(f). Chromium.

Chromium is an essential trace element that promotes insulin function, the maintenance of normal blood sugar metabolism, and the lowering of blood cholesterol levels (Mertz, 1959; NAS, 1989; Urberg, 1987; Urberg, 1988). The major source of biologically active chromium is brewer's yeast, which contains many chromium compounds. Mertz determined that the most biologically active form of chromium was a complex of nicotinic acid (niacin) and chromium, which complex he termed glucose tolerance factor (GTF) (Mertz, 1976). Urberg found that combined chromium and niacin exhibited synergy and effected greater improvement in glucose tolerance and lowering of cholesterol than did chromium or niacin alone (Urberg, 1987; Urberg, 1988). The combination has also been found to increase binding of insulin to white blood cells.

The niacin-chromium combination also has greater bioavailability than chromium alone, which is poorly absorbed. About 0.5% to 2% of chromium chloride, a form of chromium frequently utilized in supplements, is absorbed compared to about 10% to 25% of the combination (Mertz, 1976; Anderson, 1985). The combination consists of one or more chromium atoms bound to either an oxygen or nitrogen atom of one or more molecules of niacin. This structure enables the formation of more chemical complexes, thus increasing the biological activity compared to inorganic forms, such as chromium chloride (Anderson, 1981).

§ 11-4(g). Manganese.

Manganese is necessary for the proper function of glutathione synthease, the enzyme required for the synthesis of glutathione, the major Phase II detoxification conjugator. In the brain, glutamine synthease is needed for the production of glutamine. Glutamine, in turn, is required for conversion to the neurotransmitters glutamate and gamma amino butyric acid (GABA). While trace amounts of manganese are required, large amounts of inhaled manganese can be highly neurotoxic. Miners in several countries have suffered from manganese madness, a disorder characterized by numerous neurological problems, including hallucinations, bizarre behavior and emotional instability (Politis, 1980). Chronic manganese toxicity can also lead to neurological signs similar to those of Parkinson's disease.

The adrenal gland enzyme choline acetyl transferase requires manganese for its operation. The enzyme catalyzes the formation of acetylcholine, which determines the firing rate of nerve impulses.

Manganese toxicity has occurred in association with nutritional supplements and parenteral nutrition (Fell, 1996). Nervous system disorders were found in a group of children receiving long-term parenteral nutrition, which included manganese at the then-recommended dose (1.0 μmol/kg for patients under 10 kg and 0.8 μmol/kg for those over 10 kg) in a prepared solution. Two patients had a movement disorder characterized by dystonic limb movements and abnormal posturing. These two patients had the highest whole blood manganese concentrations (1700 and 1840 nmol/l). Abnormalities in cranial MRI scans consistent with basal ganglia damage were found in these and other patients with the highest blood manganese levels. While the abnormalities may be at least partially reversible in adults, the long-term effects on the developing brain are not known. Parkinsonism in association with the accumulation of manganese in the blood during parenteral nutrition has also occurred (Ejama, 1992, via Fell, 1996). Liver disease has also been seen in patients with extremely high manganese levels.

§ 11-4(h). Selenium.

Selenium is an essential trace element occurring naturally in rock and soil. Animal studies have shown a correlation between high blood selenium levels and a lower risk of cancer (Freshwater Foundation, 1993). These studies have encouraged the widespread use of selenium supplements. Selenium deficiency can result in cardiomyopathy, congestive heart failure, and degeneration of the striated muscle in the heart. Excessive selenium or toxicity can cause alopecia, abnormal nails, emotional instability and lassitude. Selenium is a component of the antioxidant enzyme glutathione peroxidase, which is involved in the control of oxygen metabolism, particularly the chemical breakdown of water (Falchuk, 1994). There is some evidence that selenium may prevent a dangerous mutation of Coxsackie virus which causes a paralytic illness similar to polio.

§ 11-4(i). Aluminum.

Aluminum is present in trace amounts in the form of aluminum salts in a variety of processed foods. Aluminum has been suspected of having a role in Alzheimer's disease, but conclusive evidence is lacking. There is also evidence that aluminum may be involved in other brain disorders (Freshwater Foundation, 1992). Significant neurobehavioral effects from aluminum consumption have been seen in mice. The onset of these effects was accelerated when the aluminum was ingested with a citrate found in citrus fruit. Disruption of three brain functions was revealed by a standard behavioral test battery.

After 5 weeks on the high-aluminum diet, mice demonstrated lower grip strength and fewer startle responses to a loud noise. When fed the aluminum without the citrate, the effects took 12 weeks to develop (Golub, 1992). An accumulation of aluminum was found in the brains of the animals. The enhancement of the effects by citrate suggests that the aluminum salts found in soda pop, orange juice, wine coolers and reconstituted lemon juice might be a significant source of the metal.

§ 11-4(j). Iron.

Major sources of dietary iron include meats, dairy products, and green leafy vegetables such as spinach. Iron has many functions in the body. It is vital for the production of hemoglobin, which carries oxygen in blood erythrocytes to all parts of the body. Iron deficiency can result in anemia. Iron-deficiency anemia is not so much a disease in itself as a sign of many other diseases. Iron deficiency can be due to insufficient dietary intake or to conditions that impede the absorption of iron. Iron deficiency is also associated with many conditions that cause an increase in iron loss. Bleeding in the gastrointestinal tract is a major cause of iron deficiency Oral iron supplementation is often effective in preventing and alleviating the effects of iron loss (NAS, 1989).

§ 11-4(k). Copper.

Copper is an essential trace element. The normal daily intake of copper is 2 to 5 mg. The usual amount of copper in a normal human body ranges from 100 to 150 mg (Warren, 1960, via Walshe, 1995). While it is found in most tissues, copper is most highly concentrated in the pigmented nuclei of the brain in adults.

Dietary copper deficiency is virtually unknown in humans. It is sometimes seen in premature infants, but does not appear to involve the central nervous system (Walshe, 1995). Severe copper deficiency is seen in Menkes disease, a genetic disorder that is manifested soon after birth by a syndrome that includes cerebral and cerebellar degeneration and a decline in mental development. The disease generally progresses to focal and generalized seizures, and spastic paraplegia. Biochemically it is characterized by very low concentrations of copper and caeruloplasm, a serum protein containing copper. The copper deficiency is thought to be the basis of the failure of myelination (Walshe, 1995).

Wilson's disease (hepatolenticular degeneration) is an inherited disease associated with an excess of copper in the brain and liver. The symptoms vary widely, and the disease is often misdiagnosed as other obscure neurologic syndromes. The disease can be broadly classified into four major categories: pseudosclerotic, Parkinsonian, choreic, and dystonic. Pseudosclerotic is most common in adults. In some patients, neurologic symptoms can be severe, including bizarre spontaneous movements, epileptiform seizures, dystonia and contractures. Although the sensory cortex often has concentrations of copper as high as those found in motor control centers, the sensory motor system is not damaged. The disease is treatable in many patients (Walshe, 1995).

§ 11-4(l). Iodine.

Sources of iodine include fish, shellfish, and seaweed products (NAS, 1989). This mineral is vital for the synthesis of thyroid hormones secreted by the thyroid gland. Iodine deficiency in adults is associated with hypothyroidism, which can result in goiter, a condition characterized by enlargement of the thyroid gland. The use of iodized salt has helped to lower the incidence of goiter. Hypothyroidism is associated with many other conditions including cancers, congenital, and endocrine disorders. Thyroid hormone has a number of functions, including the maintenance of appropriate rates of metabolism (Wilson, 1994).

Hypothyroidism in adults is associated with myxedema. Manifestations of myxedema include weakness, fatigue, lethargy, dry, coarse skin, swelling in the hands, face, and extremities, arthralgia, paresthesias, constipation, muscle cramps, and memory deficit and hearing problems in the elderly. The condition is treatable with thyroid replacement therapy and can usually be prevented by sufficient iodine intake, either dietary or supplemental. Iodine deficiency in infants and young children may result in cretinism, a condition characterized by the same signs and symptoms as myxedema and by mental and growth retardation as well.

Hyperthyroidism, excessive thyroid hormone, has not been associated with excessive intake of iodine. The most common hyperthyroid condition is Graves' disease, which is probably an autoimmune disorder. Its most obvious manifestation is exophthalmos, a bulging outward of the eyes which can be so severe that they appear to be ready to pop out. Other manifestations include nervousness, tremor, emotional instability, and muscle weakness.

§ 11-4(m). Fluorine.

Fluorine is a mineral occurring naturally in water in some localities. Its major function is maintaining the structure of the teeth. It may also have a role in maintaining bone. Taken long-term as fluoride compounds added to water or dentifrices, fluorine helps to prevent dental caries. Excessive fluoride in drinking water can cause mottling of the teeth.

§ 11-5. Vitamin Deficiency and Excess.

Except for subacute combined degeneration of the spinal cord associated with vitamin B_{12} deficiency and the ophthalmologic manifestations of Wernicke's disease associated with thiamine deficiency, it is difficult to assign symptoms to the deficiency of one particular vitamin (Victor, 1994). The B vitamins are particularly important in neurologic disease. Many clinicians advise obtaining B vitamin serum levels, especially vitamin B_{12}, in any patient presenting with distal paresthesias and others symptoms of peripheral neuropathy (Schilling, 1995).

§ 11-5(a). Vitamin B_6 (Pyridoxine).

Ellis and Presley suggested an association between vitamin B_6 and carpal tunnel syndrome in 1972 (Ellis, 1973). Since that time, several additional reports suggesting this relationship have appeared (Folkers, 1978; Ellis, 1981; Ellis, 1990). Excessive vitamin B_6 ingestion may result in intoxication and a sensory polyneuropathy similar to that seen with its deficiency (Victor, 1994).

Pure pyridoxine deficiency is extremely rare (Wilson, 1994). However, pyridoxine therapy frequently results in drug interactions. Many drugs act as pyridoxine antagonists, including isoniazid, penicillamine, cycloserine, and carbonyl reagents. (Wilson, 1994; Santoro, 1991; Nisar, 1990).

Pyridoxine has been associated with a syndrome involving sensory ataxia and dysfunction of the dorsal root ganglia of the spinal cord

(Schaumberg, 1983, via Goetz, 1985). This syndrome has been seen in some patients consuming 2 grams or more daily, particularly among women taking megadoses of the vitamin for premenstrual tension and edema. Symptoms include paresthesia, hyperaesthesia, bone pain, muscle weakness, and fasiculation, most marked in the extremities and usually bilateral (Dalton, 1987). The symptoms come on gradually. Iatrogenic sensory neuropathy has been seen in association with high-dose pyridoxine therapy for pyridoxine-dependent epilepsy (McLachlan, 1955). This disease is a genetic disorder of pyridoxine metabolism. The patient will develop convulsions and brain damage and will die if not treated from infancy with high doses (up to 2,000 mg a day) of pyridoxine. Some patients develop a sensory neuropathy in association with the treatment.

Neurotoxicity was observed in association with dosages of 1 or 3 grams of pyridoxine administered to healthy volunteers (Berger, 1992). Concurrent sensory symptoms and abnormalities in quantitative sensory threshold (QST) measurement were observed in all subjects. Symptoms appeared earlier in subjects receiving higher doses, suggesting the existence of a dose-percent relationship for pyridoxine-induced neuropathy. The results also suggest that QST is a sensitive measurement for early peripheral neuropathy.

§ 11-5(b). Vitamin B_{12} (Cobalamin).

Vitamin B_{12} is a complex organometallic compound with chemical characteristics similar in some respects to heme, a constituent of hemoglobin. Unlike hemoglobin, however, vitamin B_{12} cannot be synthesized in the human body and must be obtained from dietary sources. Foods of animal origin, such as meat and dairy products, are the only sources of this vitamin. The current minimum daily requirement is 2.5 μg. Insufficient intake is the usual cause of vitamin B_{12} deficiency, but other factors may also be involved, including various malabsorption syndromes. Infestation with the fish tapeworm *Diphyllobothrium latum,* which absorbs the vitamin in the host's intestine, can also result in vitamin B_{12} deficiency. Certain bacteria can rob the patient of vitamin B_{12} in a condition called blind loop syndrome (Babior, 1994). Some vegetarians must take vitamin B_{12} supplements.

Vitamin B_{12} deficiency can involve the blood, and the gastrointestinal and nervous systems. While the blood (anemia) and gastrointestinal manifestations are treatable, those of the nervous system do not always respond fully to treatment. The typical neurologic manifestation of vitamin B_{12} deficiency is a sensory neuropathy that begins in the feet and lower legs (Schilling, 1995). Demyelination is an early pathologic sign and is followed by degeneration of axons and eventually neuronal death. Anatomic sites of involvement include the spinal cord, peripheral nerves, and cerebrum. Among the early signs and symptoms of nervous system involvement are numbness and paresthesias, ataxia, and weakness. The senses of vibration and proprioception (position) may be weakened. Loss of proprioception may be described by the patient as difficulty with walking. While neurologic involvement can be expected to be bilateral, unilateral neuropathy, or bilateral involvement with asymmetrical neuropathy, has been observed (Schilling, 1995). Disturbances of mental function vary from mild irritability to severe dementias or psychosis. Psychiatric patients are frequently screened for vitamin B_{12} deficiency when hematologic and other neurologic factors are not evident. However, low vitamin B_{12} levels in these patients do not necessarily imply a deficiency, particularly in the absence of hematologic and neurologic symptoms. Further evaluation is usually required to confirm vitamin B_{12} deficiency in this situation (Brett, 1994).

Nervous system disease may occur without the low blood hemoglobin and red blood cell counts characteristic of anemia. In other cases, anemia may become evident later in the course of the disease. The absence or delay of hematologic symptoms often results in misdiagnosis. The delay is thought to be more common in patients who take supplements containing folic acid. In some patients, however, neurologic disease may be accompanied by severe anemia. Because dividing cells require vitamin B_{12}, a sore mouth and tongue is another common sign of deficiency (Schilling, 1995).

Vitamin B_{12} deficiency has been misdiagnosed as multiple sclerosis and as other nervous system disorders, including diabetic neuropathy, amyotrophic lateral sclerosis, and Guillain-Barré syndrome (Schilling, 1995). Misdiagnosis is more likely to occur when anemia is absent. There may also be an association of unknown etiology between vitamin B_{12} deficiency and multiple sclerosis (Gruener, 1994). Some patients with multiple sclerosis have pernicious anemia and similar disorders. Because the neurologic damage associated with vitamin B_{12} deficiency is progressive, misdiagnosing vitamin B_{12} deficiency can result in delayed treatment and possible irreversible neurologic damage.

While treatment is not always successful, the peripheral neuropathy associated with vitamin B_{12} deficiency is eminently treatable. Treatment is usually administered by injection.

§ 11-5(c). Vitamin B_1 (Thiamine).

Thiamine was one of the first vitamins to be specifically associated with a disease — beriberi. Thiamine deficiency is associated with three types of nervous system involvement: peripheral neuropathy, Wernicke's encephalopathy (cerebral beriberi), and the Korsakoff syndrome.

Peripheral neuropathy is characterized by symmetric impairment of motor, sensory, and reflex function seen mainly in the distal segments of limbs. The condition may or may not be painful. (Victor, 1994). An inflammation of the myelin sheath is a major pathologic sign. Symptoms of Wernicke's encephalopathy include nystagmus, palsies of the rectus muscles of the eye which can lead to unilateral or bilateral paralysis of the eye muscles (ophthalmoplegia and ataxia). The ataxia of Wernicke's disease may be so severe that the patient cannot walk or stand without support. Though the condition improves with treatment, in many cases the patient is left with a wide and uncertain gait. Progressive mental deterioration may also occur, leading to a global confusional state that may result in coma or death. Wernicke's encephalopathy is sometimes seen in association with anorexia (Tan, 1994).

Thiamine replacement usually results in improvement, although Korsakoff syndrome (also referred to as Korsakoff's psychosis) may occur. Korsakoff syndrome is characterized by retrograde amnesia, impaired learning ability, and confabulation (the filling in of memory gaps with imaginary events). Complete or partial recovery is seen only in about 50% of patients. Korsakoff syndrome can be thought of as a later stage of the same clinical process as Wernicke's disease.

Thiamine deficiency is prevalent among alcoholics, so much so that it is difficult to make a clinical distinction between the neuropathy of alcoholism and that of thiamine deficiency. Thiamine deficiency occurs in alcoholics because of the displacement of food by alcohol, the alcohol-induced increased demand for thiamine, and impaired absorption of thiamine from the intestine. It has been established that Wernicke's encephalopathy in alcoholics is due to thiamine deficiency rather than to the direct neurotoxic effects of alcohol. Reduced activities of enzymes dependent on thiamine have been observed in the brains of alcoholics who do not have Wernicke's disease (Leoville, 1995).

Low thiamine levels have been associated with Alzheimer's type dementia (Gold, 1995). In a study comparing thiamine levels in Alzheimer's patients and a control group of patients with other forms of dementia, it was found that significantly more patients with Alzheimer's had low plasma thiamine levels than patients in the control group. However, levels of thiamine in red blood cells did not correlate with a diagnosis of Alzheimer's disease. According to the investigators, the latter result suggests that current methods of evaluating thiamine status relying on assays of enzyme activity in red blood cells are not accurate indicators of thiamine levels in the central nervous system.

In some studies, high-dose thiamine therapy (3-8 gm/day) in patients with suspected Alzheimer's disease has been associated with mild improvement in cognitive function (Mastrogiacomo, 1996; Meador, 1993). The transport of free thiamine across the blood-brain barrier is dependent on its conversion to thiamine diphosphate (TDP) by the enzyme pyrophosphokinase (PPK). TDP is the predominant form of thiamine in the brain. Thiamine as TDP is an essential cofactor for three key enzymes involved in brain energy metabolism (Mastrogiacomo, 1996). In an autopsy study, Mastrogiacomo demonstrated that the levels of free thiamine and its monophosphate ester were normal in brain tissue of Alzheimer's victims. However, levels of TDP were reduced by 18% to 21% in all three cortical brain areas examined.

§ 11-5(d). Vitamin B_2 (Riboflavin).

Major sources of riboflavin include meats, fish, poultry, whole and enriched grains, legumes, and dark green vegetables such as spinach and asparagus (Bates, 1987; NAS, 1989). Riboflavin occurs in the forms of the coenzymes flavin mononucleotide (FMN) and flavin adenine dinucleotide (FAN). These coenzymes are required for various oxidation-reduction reactions and are essential for the structure of the enzyme succinate dehydrogenase, which is instrumental in the release of energy in the cell. Manifestations of riboflavin deficiency include sore throat, swelling and soreness in the mucous membranes of the mouth, cheliosis (dryness, flaking, and fissuring of the lips and angles of the mouth), glossitis, and a form of anemia (Bates, 1987).

§ 11-5(e). Vitamin B_3 (Niacin).

Niacin is the term used to describe nicotinic acid and those of its derivatives. Niacin is an essential component of nicotinamide adenine nucleotide (NAD) and of nicotinamide adenine dinucelotide phosphate (NADP). Pellagra, the niacin-deficiency disease, was once endemic in the American South and other parts of the world, and is generally associated with excessive consumption of corn (maize) and millet. However, the etiology is more complex than that of a simple nutritional deficiency. It may involve an imbalance in dietary amino acids. With improvement in nutritional education, pellagra has become a rare disease in the United States.

Pellagra is generally characterized by dermatitis, diarrhea, and dementia. The mental manifestations of pellagra are rather vague, including fatigue, insomnia, and apathy. The disease may progress to an encephalopathy characterized by disorientation, hallucinations, confusion, loss of memory, and organic psychosis. Paresthesia and polyneuritis are often present, but are the results of other dietary deficiencies.

Niacin overdose is sometimes seen in people who are overzealous in their consumption of supplements. Paresthesias and muscle weakness have been observed in women taking doses approaching 120 milligrams a day for periods of about 6 months (Wilson, 1994).

§ 11-5(f). Folic Acid.

Fruits and vegetables are the major dietary source of this vitamin. It is synthesized by some species of bacteria as well as by plants. The minimum daily requirement is generally around 50 μg, but may be increased manyfold during pregnancy and other periods of increased metabolic demand. While the role of folic acid in the pathogenesis of nervous system disease is controversial and not fully understood, a link is now well-established between the chances of fetal neural tube defects and folic acid intake before and during pregnancy (Dickinson, 1995; MRC, 1991; Wald, 1994). A 1993 study definitely established a correlation between the daily intake of folic acid and a dose-related decline in risk (Whirler, 1993).

In adults, folate deficiency is associated with, and may have a causal relationship to, some nueropsychiatric disorders (Dickinson, 1995, Botez, 1976; Gray, 1989). These disorders, some of which may resemble typical subacute combined degeneration of the spinal cord (SACD), are often dramatically relieved by the administration of 5 to 10 mg of folic acid daily (Botez, 1976). Folic acid supplementation may also reduce the incidence of premature birth (Baumslag, 1970), cleft palate (Peer, 1958), and primitive neuroectodermal brain tumors in children (Bunin, 1993).

Dietary supplementation with folic acid can be quite beneficial, and folic acid itself is harmless in most situations. However, it is suspected of masking the effects of vitamin B_{12} deficiency and possibly causing neurologic damage when there is a deficiency of vitamin B_{12} (Dickinson, 1995).There is, however, considerable controversy over this issue, and a controlled trial of the rate of neurologic deterioration in pernicious anemia (PA) with or without folic acid in humans is obviously unethical. What is known is based on clinical data and animal studies. The dose of folic acid may be a critical factor. In one series, it was noted that 2 PA patients receiving 50 mg of folic acid daily deteriorated neurologically, while only 1 of 5 patients receiving 75 mg intramuscularly once weekly experienced such deterioration (Editorial, 1947; Berk, 1948). Some clinicians use periconceptual administration of tablets rather than food fortification, particularly in elderly patients, because of the possibility of irreversible neurologic damage in the presence of vitamin B_{12} deficiency (Rush, 1994).

Animal studies with the fruit bat *Rousettus aegyptiacus,* which requires vitamin B_{12} at levels 5 to 15 times that of humans on a weight-to-weight basis, have also provided evidence of neurologic damage associated with administration of folic acid in vitamin-B_{12}-deficient organisms (Van Tonder, 1975; Van der Westhuyzen, 1982). In bats made vitamin-B_{12}-deficient, administration of folic acid was associated with neurologic damage so severe that the affected animals could not fly (Van der Westhuyzen, 1982). This investigation, however, has been criticized on the basis of faulty technique and lack of controls (Dickinson, 1995).

In addition to vitamin B_{12} deficiency, the administration of folic acid may also be detrimental in the context of epilepsy (Dickinson, 1995). Some anticonvulsant drugs, such as phenytoin, may induce a megaloblastic anemia that is responsive to folate. Thus, if an epileptic patient is in the early stages of developing PA and receives folic acid, the symptoms of SACD could possibly be masked. Failure to administer vitamin B_{12} in this situation could conceivably allow neurologic deterioration to occur (Dickinson, 1995). It has been suggested that seizures may be made more severe if folic acid is administered to epileptic patients with megaloblastic anemia, because folic acid reduces serum phenytoin levels (Reynolds, 1967). This possible effect of phenytoin has been disputed (Hunter, 1969; Norris, 1971). Inadvertent administration of folic acid can occur with the use of over-the-counter multivitamin preparations.

§ 11-5(g). Pantothenic Acid.

Pantothenic acid is a component of coenzyme A, an important metabolic molecule. It is involved in the metabolism of proteins, carbohydrates, and fats in a way that is not completely understood. Pantothenic acid is present in many foods, and is synthesized by intestinal bacteria as well.

Pantothenic acid deficiency has recently been associated with the pathogenesis of acne vulgaris (Leung, 1995). Improvement approaching complete cure has been obtained by replacement therapy with the vitamin. A case has been documented of successful therapy of dilated cardiomyopathy with pantothenic acid (Ostman-Smith, 1994). Large doses produced a dramatic and sustained improvement in cardiac function.

§ 11-5(h). Biotin.

Biotin is required for the action of an important class of enzymes called carboxylases. Inside cells, biotin enters into chemical reactions resulting in the formation of four enzymes that catalyze the incorporation of bicarbonate into acetyl coenzyme A (acetyl-CoA). Acetyl-CoA represents a vital step in the cascade of chemical reactions involved in the release of energy in the cell. Manifestations of biotin deficiency include a dermatitis about the mouth, alopecia, and ataxia. In children, biotin deficiency can result in developmental delay. Deficiency can occur after prolonged consumption of raw egg white. In the intestine, the egg white binds with biotin, preventing its absorption. It can also occur in individuals lacking an enzyme called biotinidase (Wilson, 1994).

§ 11-5(i). Vitamin A.

Vitamin A is a fat-soluble vitamin essential for normal growth, vision, and reproduction and maintenance of epithelial cells, which line the inner surfaces of organs such as the bronchial tubes. Vitamin A is used in the treatment of acne and other dermatologic disorders. Excessive intake of vitamin A has been directly associated with neurotoxicity. In high doses, vitamin A accumulates, and can induce increased intracranial pressure syndrome (pseudotumor cerebri).

Symptoms of vitamin A deficiency include night blindness, which is the earliest symptom of deficiency. Other early manifestations include dry conjunctiva, and gray, foamy plaques. These early manifestations respond well to vitamin A therapy. A typical regimen is 30,000 IU for a week. If not treated, vitamin A deficiency may cause degenerative changes in the retina, ulceration and necrosis of the cornea, possibly leading to perforation, endophthalmitis, and permanent blindness (Wilson, 1994).

Dietary vitamin A excess is rare in most parts of the world. In arctic regions, pseudotumor cerebri occurs among populations that eat polar bear liver. Vitamin A intoxication is most often associated with consumption of large doses of supplements. Motivated by reports in the popular press of vitamin A's cancer prevention properties, some individuals may take 100,000 or even 200,00 IU daily, while the recommended daily allowance is 5,000 IU. At 100,000 IU daily, intoxication develops over a period of months, while at 200,000 IU, intoxication may develop in a few weeks (Goetz, 1985). Acute vitamin A toxicity from a single large dose is characterized by dizziness, headache, abdominal pain and vomiting (Wilson, 1994).

Signs and symptoms of vitamin A toxicity include erythema, itching, anoxia, and swelling of the liver and spleen. The earliest signs of increased intracranial pressure include headaches, blurred vision, transient obscured vision, and paresis of the sixth cranial nerve. The neurologic symptoms are similar to those of other disorders. Dermatologic symptoms, swollen organs, and a history of excessive vitamin A ingestion help to establish the diagnosis (Goetz, 1985).

§ 11-5(j). Vitamin C (Ascorbic Acid).

Sources of vitamin C include citrus fruits and dark green leafy vegetables. Vitamin C is added to many processed foods such as bottled juices. Scurvy, the most common syndrome associated with vitamin C deficiency, is rare in most parts of the world today. It is still found, however, among urban poor. Scurvy results in a reduction of collagen formation, and is usually manifested at first in dermatologic symptoms. Direct neurologic involvement is usually limited to emotional disturbances and convulsions late in the course of the disease. Treatment with vitamin C usually results in rapid resolution.

The utilization, transport, and uptake of vitamin C in the body are influenced by its metabolites. The level of these metabolites may not rise to significant levels until large quantities of vitamin C are consumed. Some oral vitamin C supplements are produced to incorporate metabolites such as threonate. The synergistic action of the vitamin and its metabolites serves to expedite and maximize the absorption and utilization of vitamin C. The combination of the vitamin and its metabolites has been shown to be more effective than vitamin C alone in preventing scurvy in rats and in elevating white blood cell levels.

§ 11-5(k). Vitamin D.

Overdose of the fat-soluble vitamin D is not directly associated with neurotoxicity, but neurologic symptoms can occur as secondary effects to those of the vitamin. Excessive vitamin D can induce bone demineralization and degeneration, which could, in turn, lead to spinal cord compression. The effects on bone may alter calcium balance, resulting in general weakness, cramps, muscle aches, and mild metabolic encephalopathy. Trigeminal neuralgia and adverse effects on the membranes covering the brain and spinal cord (meninges) have also been reported. Impairment of kidney function could lead to secondary encephalopathy and coma (Goetz, 1985).

§ 11-5(l). Vitamin E (Alpha Tocopherol).

Vitamin E is found in soybean, sunflower, corn, and cottonseed oils, germ of whole grains, fish liver oils, and nuts (NAS, 1989). Vitamin E deficiency is associated with a rare neurologic polyneuropathy and pigmentary retinopathy, developing after a prolonged intestinal malabsorption disorder of childhood. The syndrome consists of a spinocerebellar degeneration accompanied by malabsorption (Victor, 1994; Satya-Murti, 1986; Sokol, 1989). Vitamin E deficiency is also seen in children with chronic gall bladder dysfunction (cholestatic hepatobiliary disease). Symptoms and signs include ataxia, loss of tendon reflexes, ophthalmoparesis, proximal muscle weakness, and decreased sensory function. Neurologic function generally improves after long-term vitamin E therapy. True vitamin E toxicity appears to be limited to people receiving anticoagulant therapy and to premature infants receiving parenteral vitamin E therapy. Most people can take relatively large doses over extended periods with no apparent ill effect. Some complain of headaches and gastrointestinal upset (Wilson, 1994).

§ 11-5(m). Carnitine.

The major sources of dietary carnitine are red meat for adults and human milk for infants. About 75% of the body's carnitine requirements is obtained from dietary sources. The remaining 25% is synthesized in the body. The amino acids lysine and methionine are required for the synthesis (Engel, 1986; Di Donato, 1994). Carnitine performs a vital function in energy supply by controlling the inflow of long-chain fatty acids into the mitochondria, the cell components in which energy release takes place. Carnitine also facilitates the oxidation of pyruvate, a step in the energy-release process, and prevents the accumulation of acyl coenzyme A, a substance which could destabilize the cell membrane, possibly resulting in cell death (Bremer, 1983; Uziel, 1988).

Although there is still some controversy over the classification of carnitine deficiency disease, there is wide agreement that the disease can be either primary or secondary, and occurs in three forms that affect either the heart, muscles, or liver (Di Donato, 1994; Engel, 1994). Primary carnitine deficiency (PCD) is a group of disorders affecting carnitine metabolism, rather than a single disease entity. There is a strong genetic component in the etiology of these disorders. Manifestations include muscle weakness, enlarged liver, and a cardiomyopathy that can be fatal if not treated. Plasma carnitine levels as low as 10% of normal have been detected. High levels of blood ammonia, hypoglycemia, accumulation of fat in skeletal muscle, and elevations in liver enzymes have also been observed (Di Donato, 1994).

Treatment with oral L-carnitine has been effective in many patients. Muscle strength has improved, and metabolic disorders have resolved. However, many patients do not respond to this therapy (Carpenter, 1984; Di Donato, 1994). Carnitine supplementation or replacement therapy has been shown to be dramatically effective (Di Donato, 1994). Typical regimens are 2 to 6 mg of oral L-carnitine a day. Heart function and muscle strength return to normal or improve, and hypoglycemic attacks disappear. Patients on long-term replacement therapy can usually lead a normal life, but untreated patients may die of heart failure at an early age.

Secondary carnitine deficiency (SCD) is due to a number of causes. As is the case with PCD, there is controversy over the classification of these disorders. A condition referred to as organic aciduria can lead to SCD. Other conditions associated with SCD include respiratory metabolism defects, and hemodialysis. It has been suggested that an important cause of the depletion of carnitine from tissue and body fluids in SCD is a metabolic block that causes excessive accumulation of acyl-coenzyme A in the mitochondria. This leads to a series of biochemical events culminating in the loss of carnitine from cells. Symptoms are similar to those of PCD. Some therapeutic success has been achieved with valproate and pivampcillin (Karpati, 1975). Therapy with L-carnitine has also been effective. Results of L-carnitine replacement therapy have been mixed (Di Donato, 1994).

§ 11-6. Other Nutrients.

We are currently in a period of intense research into the effects of nutrients on general health and well-being. Some of this research has uncovered previously unknown benefits of well-known nutrients such as vitamins and minerals. Other work has focused on natural substances not previously considered to be nutrients. As might be expected, there is considerable controversy over the value of these substances in human nutrition.

§ 11-6(a). *Ginko biloba.*

Ginko biloba is a tree native to China and the Far East. It was discovered by Western botanists as a fossil, and thought to be extinct, before it was discovered as a living plant in China. Fossil records of *G. biloba* go back at least 200 million years. In China, where *G. biloba* has been used medicinally for thousands of years, it is thought to improve circulation to the brain. Whole leaf and extract of *G. biloba* are now being used in Western countries. Evidence from studies suggests that *G. biloba* increases blood flow to the brain and acts as an antioxidant. It is claimed to increase mental clarity, memory, alertness, and intellectual capacity, as well as to alleviate hearing problems, allergies, and the effects of stroke. In a recent study, mildly to severely demented outpatients with Alzheimer's disease or multi-infarct dementia were given an extract of *Ginko biloba* commonly used in Europe. The resulting data suggest that this extract is capable of stabilizing and, in a substantial number of cases, improving the cognitive performance and the social functioning of demented patients (LeBars, 1997).

§ 11-6(b). Ginseng.

Ginseng is thought to have properties similar to those of *Ginko biloba*. It has been used for thousands of years in the East for medicinal purposes and as a general sort of tonic to improve energy and feelings of well-being. In recent years, it has seen increasing use in the West.

Studies have shown that it can have a wide range of benefits, including increased stamina in athletes increased concentration in radio operators improvement of lymphocyte immune function in elderly subjects and reduction of fasting blood glucose and body weight in patients with type II diabetes mellitus. Animal studies have demonstrated a variety of effects including increased adaptability to stress decreased aggressive behavior decreased learning time and stabilization of sleep in sleep-deprived rats. Ginseng has been linked to breast pain and tenderness as well as occasional vaginal bleeding. The explanation is that it may contain small amounts of estrone, estrodiol and estriol.

§ 11-6(c). Melatonin.

Although supplemental melatonin is believed to be beneficial in a number of ways, the full range of its physiological actions is not known (Lipartiti, 1996). Melatonin, a hormone secreted by the pineal gland, is known to modulate gonadal function, and it has a role in regulating biological or circadian rhythm. Data from a growing number of studies indicate that circadian rhythms are a fundamental regulatory system that has potent influences on behavior and physiology at all stages of life, including fetal life (Rivkees, 1997). After birth, the circadian system matures, with day-night rhythms in activity and hormone secretion developing between 1 and 3 months.

Several disorders of the circadian system are now recognized. These include jet lag, excessive daytime sleepiness (Roth, 1996), delayed sleep-phase syndrome, advanced sleep-phase syndrome, and other sleep disorders (Dawson, 1996). It is believed that episodes of cardiovascular disease are more likely to occur in the morning (Buff, 1997). Treatments that have been tried include naps, surgery, and various devices, as well as pharmacotherapy with antidepressants, stimulants such as amphetamines, pemoline, or newer, safer agents such as modafinil (Roth, 1996; Duncan, 1996).

In recent years, melatonin has been proposed as a therapeutic alternative for circadian disorders (Kendler, 1997). Because of its hypnotic effect, it has been used to mitigate insomnia in the elderly. Reductions in melatonin secretion have been associated with aging, as well as a number of disorders, including Alzheimer's disease, and diabetes. A causative effect of melatonin in these disorders, or any therapeutic effect of melatonin in their treatment, has not yet been demonstrated, however. Some studies indicate that adjuvant therapy (in addition to an anticancer drug) may be of benefit in the treatment of some cancers (Lissoni, 1997; Lissoni, 1996; Lissoni, 1995; Cos, 1996).

References.

Adams, J.D., Odunze, I.N., *Oxygen Free Radicals and Parkinson's Disease*. Free Rad. Biol. Med. 1991; 10:161-69.

Adams, R.D., Victor, M., Ropper, A., Principals of Neurology, 6th Ed. New York: McGraw-Hill, 1997.

Anderson, R., *Nutritional Role of Chromium*. Sci. Tot. Envir. 1981; 17:13-29.

Anderson, R., Kozlovsky, A., *Chromium Intake, Absorption and Excretion of Subjects Consuming Self-Selected Diets*. Am. J. Clin. Nutr. 1985; 41:1177-83.

Babior, B.M., Bunn, H.F., *Megaloblastic Anemias*. In: K.J. Isselbacher, E. Braunwald, J.D. Wilson, J.B. Martin, A.S. Fauci, D.L. Kasper (eds.), Harrison's Principles of Internal Medicine. New York: McGraw-Hill, Inc., 1994.

Baumslag, N., Edelstein, T., Metz, J., *Reduction of the Incidence of Prematurity by Folic Acid Supplementation in Pregnancy*. Br. Med. J. 1970; i:16-17.

Bates, C.J., *Human Riboflavin Requirements, and Metabolic Consequences of Deficiency in Man and Animals*. World Rev. Nutr. Diet 1987; 50:215.

Berger, A.R., Schaumberg, H.H., Schroeder, C., et al., *Dose Response, Coasting, and Differential Fiber Vulnerability in Human Toxic Neuropathy: a Prospective Study of Pyridoxine Neurotoxicity*. Neurology 1992; 42:1367-70.

Berk, L. Bauer, J.L., Castle, W.B., *Folic Acid: A Report of 12 Patients Treated with Synthetic Pteroylglutamic Acid*, with *Comments on the Current Literature*. South Afr. Med. J. 1948; 22:604-11.

Borolongan, C.V., Kanning, K., Poulos, S.G., et al., *Free Radical Damage* and *Oxidative Stress in Huntington's Disease.* J. Fla. Med. Assoc. 1996; 83:335-41.

Botez, M.I., Cadotte, M., Beaulieu, R., et al., *Neurologic Disorders Responsive to Folic Acid Therapy.* Canad. Med. Assoc. J. 1976; 115:217-23.

Bremer, J., *Carnitine Metabolism and Function.* Physiol. Rev. 1983; 63:1420.

Brett A.S., Roberts, M.K., *Screening for Vitamin B_{12} Deficiency in Psychiatric Patients*. J. Gen. Intern. Med. 1994; 9:522-24.

Buff, D.D., Calikyan, R., Neches, R.B., Bavli, S.Z., *Circadian Patterns in the Onset of Cardiogenic Acute Pulmonary Edema.* Clin. Cardiol., 1997; 20:261-264.

Bunin, G.R., Kuijten, R.R., Bukley, J.D., et al., *Relation Between Maternal Diet and Subsequent Primitive Neuroectodermal Tumors in Young Children*. N. Engl. J. Med. 1993; 329:536-41.

Cadet, J.L., Kahler, L.A., *Free Radical Mechanisms in Schizophrenia and Tardive Dyskinesia.* Neurosci. Biobehav. Rev. 1994; 18:457-67.

Carpenter, S., Karpati, G., Pathology of Skeletal Muscle. New York: Churchill Livingstone, 1984.

Cos, S., Verduga, R., *Effects of Melatonin on the Proliferation and Differentiation of Human Neuroblastoma Cells in Culture.* Neurosci. Lett. 1996; 216:113-116.

Dalton, K., Dalton, M.J., *Characteristics of Pyridoxine Overdose Neuropathy Syndrome*. Acta Neurol. Scand. 1987; 76:8-11.

Dawson, D., Armstrong, S.M., *Chronobiotics — Drugs That Shift Rhythms*. Pharmacol. Ther. 1996; 69:15-36.

DeVita, M.V., Michelis, M.P., *Perturbations in Sodium Balance. Hyponatremia*. Clin. Lab. Med. 1993; 13:135.

Dickinson, C.J., *Does Folic Acid Harm People with Vitamin B_{12} Deficiency?* Q. J. Med. 1995; 88:357-364.

Di Donato, S., *Disorders of Lipid Metabolism Affecting Skeletal Muscle: Carnitine Deficiency Syndromes, Defects in the Catabolic Pathway, and Channarin Disease.* In: A.G. Engel, C. Franzini-Armstrong, Myology, 2d Ed. New York: McGraw-Hill, Inc., 1994: 1587-1609.

Duncan, W.C., Jr., *Circadian Rhythms and the Pharmacology of Affective Illness.* Pharmacol. Ther. 1996; 71:253-312.

Engel, A.G., *Carnitine Deficiency Syndromes and Lipid Storage Myopathies.* In: A.G. Engel, B.Q. Banker (eds.), Myology. New York: McGraw-Hill, Inc., 1986: 1663-1696.

Editorial, *A Warning Regarding the Use of Folic Acid.* N. Engl. J. Med. 1947; 237:713-15.

Ejama, A., Imamura, T., Nakamura, S., et al., *Manganese Intoxication During Parenteral Nutrition.* Lancet 1992; 339:426.

Ellis, J., Folkers, K., Levy, M., et al., *Therapy with Vitamin B_6 with and Without Surgery for Patients Having the Idiopathic Carpal Tunnel Syndrome.* Res. Commun. Chem. Pathol. Pharmacol. 1981; 33:331-344.

Ellis, J., Folkers, K., *Clinical Aspects of Treatment of Carpal Tunnel Syndrome with Vitamin B_6.* Ann. N.Y. Acad. Sci. 1990; 585:302-20.

Ellis J.M., Presley, J., Vitamin B_6, the Doctor's Report. New York: Harper and Row, 1973.

Engel, A.G., Franzini-Armstrong, C., Myology, 2d Ed. New York: McGraw-Hill, 1994.

Evans, P.H., *Free Radicals in Brain Metabolism and Pathology.* Br. Med. Bull. 1993; 49:577-87.

Falchuk, K.H., *Disturbances in Trace Element Metabolism.* In: K.J. Isselbacher, E. Braunwald, J.D. Wilson, J.B. Martin, A.S. Fauci, D.L. Kasper (eds.), Harrison's Principles of Internal Medicine. New York: McGraw-Hill, Inc., 1994.

Fell, J.M.E., Reynolds, A.P., Meadows, N., *Manganese Toxicity in Children Receiving Long-Term Parenteral Nutrition*. Lancet 1996; 347:1218-21.

Folkers, K., Ellis, J., Watanabe, T., et al., *Biochemical Evidence for a Deficiency of Vitamin B_6 in the Carpal Tunnel Syndrome Based on a Crossover Clinical Study*. Proc. Natl. Acad. Sci. USA 1978; 75:3410-3412.

Freshwater Foundation, *Selenium Study Uses New Cancer Map*. Health and Environment Digest 1993; 7:5-6.

Freshwater Foundation, *Aluminum Suspicion Growing*. Health and Environment Digest 1992; 6:6.

Frölich, L., Riederer, P., *Free Radical Mechanisms in Dementia of Alzheimer Type and the Potential for Antioxidative Treatment*. Arzneimittelforschung 1995; 45(3A):143-46.

Gey, K.F., *Prospects for the Prevention of Free Radical Disease, Regarding Cancer and Cardiovascular Disease*. Br. Med. Bull. 1993; 49:679-99.

Goetz, C.G., Neurotoxins in Clinical Practice. Jamaica, N.Y.: Spectrum Publications, 1985.

Gold, M., Chen, M.F., Johnson, K., *Plasma and Red Blood Cell Thiamine Deficiency in Patients with Dementia of the Alzheimer's Type*. Arch. Neurol. 1995; 52:1081-86.

Golub, M.S., Toxicology and Applied Pharmacology, 1992; (January):314.

Good, P.F., Perl, D.P., Bierer, L.M., Schmeidler, J., *Selective Accumulation of Aluminum and Iron in the Neurofibrillary Tangles of Alzheimer's Disease*; *a Laser Probe (LAMMA) Study*. Ann. Neurol. 1992; 31:286-92.

Gray, G.E., *Nutrition and Dementia*. J. Am. Diet. Assoc. 1989; 89:1036-38.

Greenstock, C.L., *Radiation and Aging: Free Radical Damage, Biological Response and Possible Antioxidant Intervention*. Med. Hypotheses 1993; 41:473-82.

Gruener, D.M., Shakin Kunkel, E.J., Snyderman, D.A., *Dietary Vitamin B_{12} Deficiency in a Patient with Multiple Sclerosis*. Gen. Hosp. Psychiatry 1994; 16:224-228.

Gutteridge, J.M., Quinlan, G.J., Clark, I., Halliwell, B., *Aluminum Salts Accelerate Peroxidation of Membrane Lipids Stimulated by Iron Salts*. Biochim. Biophys. Acta 1985; 835:441-47.

Holick, M.F., Krane, S.M., Potts, J.T, Jr., *Calcium, Phosphorous and Bone Metabolism; Calcium-Regulating Hormones.* In: K.J. Isselbacher, E. Braunwald, J.D. Wilson, J.B. Martin, A.S. Fauci, D.L. Kasper (eds.), Harrison's Principles of Internal Medicine. New York: McGraw-Hill, Inc., 1994.

Hunter, R., Barnes, J., Matthews, D.M., *Effects of Folic-Acid Supplement on Serum-Vitamin B_{12} Levels in Patients on Anticonvulsants.* Lancet 1969; ii:666-67.

Institute of Food Technologists, *Vitamin E: A Scientific Status Summary by the Institute of Food Technologists' Expert Panel on Food Safety and Nutrition and the Committee on Public Information.* Nutr. Rev. 1977; 35:57-62.

Johnson, A., Rea, W.J., *Review of 200 Cases in the Environmental Control Unit.* Presented at the Seventh International Symposium on Man and His Environment in Health and Disease, February 25-26, 1989, Dallas.

Karpati, G., Carpenter, S., Engel, A.G., et al.., *The Syndromes of Carnitine Deficiency*. Neurology 1975; 25:16.

Keaney, J.F., Jr., Gaziano, J.M., Xu, A., et al., *Dietary Antioxidants Preserve Endothelium-Dependent Vessel Relaxation in Cholesterol-Fed Rabbits.* Proc. Natl. Acad. Sci. USA 1993; 90:11880-11884.

Keaney, J.F., Vita, J.A., *Atherosclerosis, Oxidative Stress, and Antioxidant Protection in Endothelium-Derived Relaxing Factor Action.* Prog. Cardiovasc. Dis. 1995; 38:129-54.

Keaney, J.F., Xu, A., Cunningham, D.C., et al., *Dietary Probucol Preserves Endothelial Function in Cholesterol-Fed Rabbits by Limiting Vascular Oxidative Stress and Superoxide Production.* J. Clin. Invest. 1995a; 2520-29.

Keli, S.O., Hertog, M.G.L., Feshens, E.J.M., Kromhout, D., *Dietary Flavonoids, Antioxidant Vitamins and Incidence of Stroke*. Arch. Intern. Med. 1996; 154:637-42.

Kendler, B.S., *Melatonin: Media Hype or Therapeutic Breakthrough?* Nurse Pract. 1997; 66-67, 71-72, 77.

LeBars, P.L., et al., *A Placebo-Controlled, Double Blind, Randomized Trial of an Extract of Ginko Biloba for Dementia*. JAMA, Vol 278. 1997; 16:1327-1332.

Leoville, J., Butterworth, R.F., *Reduced Activity of Thiamine-Dependent Enzymes in Brains of Alcoholics in the Absence of Wernicke's Encephalopathy*. Alcohol Clin. Exp. Res. 1995; 19:1073-77.

Ledesma, M.D., Bona, C., Colac, C., Alveoli, J., *Analysis of Microtubule- Associated Protein Tau Glaciation in Paired Helical Filaments*. J. Biol. Chem. 1994; 269:21614-19.

Leung, L.H., *Pantothenic Acid Deficiency as the Pathogenesis of Acne Vulgaris*. Med. Hypotheses 1995; 44:490-92.

Levine, G.N., Free, B., Callers, S., *Ascorbic Acid Reverses Endothelial Vasomotor Dysfunction in Patients with Coronary Artery Disease*. Circulation 1996; 93:1107-13.

Levinsky, N.G., *Fluids and Electrolytes*. In: K.J. Isselbacher, E. Braunwald, J.D. Wilson, J.B. Martin, A.S. Fauci, D.L. Kasper (eds.), Harrison's Principles of Internal Medicine. New York: McGraw-Hill, Inc., 1994.

Lieberman, A., *Emerging Perspectives in Parkinson's Disease*. Neurology 1992; 42 (Supp. 4).

Lipartiti, M., Franceschini, D., Zanoni, R., et al., *Neuroprotective Effects of Melatonin*. Adv. Exp. Med. Biol. 1996; 398:315-321.

Lissoni, P., Cazzaniga, M., Tancini, G., *Reversal of Clinical Resistance to LHRH Analogue in Metastatic Prostate Cancer by the Pineal Hormone Melatonin: Efficacy of :LHRH Analogue Alone*. Eur. Urol. 1997; 31:178-181.

Lissoni, P. Brivio, O., Brivio, F., et al., *Adjuvant Therapy with the Pineal Hormone Melatonin in Patients with Lymph Node Relapse Due to Malignant Melanoma.* J. Pineal. Res. 1996; 21:239-242.

Lissoni, P., Barni, S., Brivio, F., et al., *Treatment of Cancer-Rlated Thrombocytopania by Low-Dose Subcutaneous Interleukin-2 Plus the Pineal Hormone Melatonin,* J. Biol. Regul. Homeost. Agents. 1995; 9:52-54.

Lohr, J.B., Browning, J.A., *Free Radical Involvement in Neuropsychiatric Illnesses.* Psychopharmacol. Bull. 1995; 31:159-65.

Manzoor M., Runcie, J., *Folate-Responsive Neuropathy.* Presse Medicale 1994; 23:131-37.

Martin, A., *The Use of Antioxidants in Healing.* Dermatol. Surg. 1996; 22:156-60.

Mastrogiacomo, F., Betterdorff, L., Grisar, T., Kish, S.J., *Brain Thiamine, Its Phosphate Esters, and Its Metabolizing Enzymes in Alzheimer's Disease.* Ann. Neurol. 1996; 39:585-91.

McLachlan, R.S., Brown, W.F., *Pyridoxine Dependent Epilepsy with Iatrogenic Sensory Neuropathy.* Can. J. Neurol. Sci. 1995; 22:50-51.

Mertz, W., Schwarz, K., *Relation of Glucose Tolerance Factor to Impaired Intravenous Glucose Tolerance of Rats on Stock Diets.* Am. J. Physiol. 1959; 196:614-18.

Mertz, W., *Effects and Metabolism of Glucose Tolerance Factor.* In: The Nutrition Foundation, Present Knowledge in Nutrition. Washington: The Nutrition Foundation, 1976; 36:365-72.

MRC Vitamin Study Research Group, *Prevention of Neural Tube Defects: Results of the Medical Research Council Vitamin Study.* Lancet 1991; 338:131-37.

National Academy of Sciences Committee on Diet and Health, Diet and Health Recommendations to Reduce Chronic Disease Risk. Washington: National Academy Press, 1989.

Nisar, M., Watkin, S.W., Bucknall, R.C., Agnew, R.A., *Exacerbation of Isoniazid Induced Peripheral Neuropathy by Pyridoxine.* Thorax 1990; 45:419-20.

Norris, J.W., Pratt, R.F., *A Controlled Study of Folic Acid and Epilepsy*. Neurology 1971; 21:659-64.

Ostman-Smith, I., Brown, G., Johnson, A., Land, J.M., *Dilated Cardiomyopathy Due to Type II X-Linked 3-Methylglutaconic Aciduria: Successful Treatment with Pantothenic Acid*. Br. Heart J. 1994; 72:349-53.

Peer, L.A., Strean, L.P., Walker, J.C., Jr., *Study of 400 Pregnancies with Birth of Cleft-lip Palate Infants*. Plast. Reconstr. Surg. 1958; 22:442-49.

Phull, P.S, Green, C.J., Jacyna, M.R., *A Radical View of the Stomach; the Role of Oxygen-Derived Free Radicals and Anti-Oxidants in Gastroduodenal Disease*. Eur. J. Gastroenterol. Hepatol. 1995; 7:265-74.

Politis, M.J., Schaumberg, H.H., Spencer, P.S., *Neurotoxicity of Selected Chemicals*. In: Experimental and Clinical Neurotoxicology. Baltimore: Williams and Wilkins, 1980.

Potts, J.T., Jr., *Diseases of the Parathyroid Gland and Other Hyper- and Hypocalcemic Disorders*. In: K.J. Isselbacher, E. Braunwald, J.D. Wilson, J.B. Martin, A.S. Fauci, D.L. Kasper (eds.), Harrison's Principles of Internal Medicine. New York: McGraw-Hill, Inc., 1994.

Rea, W.J., *Magnesium Deficiency and Chemical Sensitivity*. Clinical Ecology 1986; 4.

Reynolds, E.H., *Effect of Folic Acid on the Mental State and Fit-Frequency of Drug-Treated Epileptic Patients*. Lancet 1967; i:1086-88.

Riersmam, R.A., Wood, D.A., Macintyre, C.C.H., et al., *Low Plasma Vitamin E and C and Increased Risk of Angina in Scottish Men*. Ann. N.Y. Acad. Sci. 1989; 570:291-95.

Rimm, E.B., Stampfer, M.J., Ascherio, A., et al., *Vitamin E Consumption and the Risk of Coronary Heart Disease in Men*. N. Engl. J. Med. 1993; 328:1450-56.

Rivkees, S.A., *Developing Circadian Rhthmicity. Basic and Clinical Aspects*. Pediatr. Clin. North Am. 1997; 44:467-487.

Rogers, S.A., *A Practical Approach to the Person with Suspected Indoor Air Quality Problems*. Indoor Air '90, Fifth International Conference on Indoor Air Quality and Climate, Toronto, Ontario, 1990a; 5:435-349.

Rogers, S.A., Tired or Toxic? Syracuse, N.Y.: Prestige Publishing, 1990b.

Rowland, L.P. (ed.), Merrit's Textbook of Neurology, 9th Ed. Baltimore, MD: Williams & Wilkins, 1995.

Roth, T., Roehrs, T.A., *Etiologies and Sequelae of Excessive Daytime Sleepiness*. Clin. Ther. 1996; 18:562-576.

Rush, D., *Perioconceptional Folate and Neural Tube Defect.* Amer. J. Clin. Nutr. 1994; 59:511S-15S.

Santoro L., Ragno, M., Nucciotti R., et al., *Pyridoxine Neuropathy. A Four-Year Electrophysiological and Clinical Follow-Up of a Severe Case.* Acta Neurol. (Napoli) 1991; 13:13-18.

Satya-Murti, S., et al., *The Spectrum of Neurologic Disorders from Vitamin E Deficiency.* Neurology 1986; 36:917.

Schaumberg, M.D., Kaplan, J,., Weindbank, M.D., et al., *Sensory Neuropathy from Pyridoxine Abuse: A New Megavitamin Syndrome.* N. Engl. J. Med. 1983; 309:445-448.

Schilling, R.F., Williams, W.J., *Vitamin B_{12} Deficiency: Underdiagnosed, Overtreated?* Hosp. Prac. 1995.

Smith, M.A., Taneda, P.L., Richey, S., et al., *Advanced Maillard Reaction End Products Are Associated with Alzheimer Disease Pathology*. Proc. Natl. Acad. Sci. 1994; 91:5710-14.

Smith, M.A., Perry, G., *Free Radical Damage, Iron, and Alzheimer's Disease.* J. Neurol. Sci. 1995; 134 (Supp.) 92-94.

Smith, M.A., Kutty, R.K., Richey, S.D, et al., *Heme-Oxygenase-1 Is Associated with the Neurofibrillary Pathology of Alzheimer's Disease*. Am. J. Pathol. 1994a; 145:42-47.

Smith, M.A., Sayre, L.M., Monnier, V.M., Perry, G., *Radical Aging and Alzheimer's.* Trends Neurosci. 1995a; 374:16.

Smith, M.A., Rudnicka-Nawrot, P.L., Richey, D., et al., *Carbonyl-related Posttranslational Modification of Neurofilament Protein in the Neurofibrillary Pathology of Alzheimer's Disease*. J. Neurochem. 1995b; 64:2660-66.

Sokol, R. J., et al., *Vitamin Deficiency E Neuropathy in Children with Fat Malabsorption: Studies in Cystic Fibrosis and Chronic Cholestasis*. Ann. N.Y. Acad. Sci. 1989; 570:156.

Stampfer, M.J., Hennekens, C.H., Manson, J.E., et al., *Vitamin E Deficiency and the Risk of Coronary Disease in Women*. N. Engl. J. Med. 1993; 328:1444-49.

Tan, G. H., Farnell, G.F., Hensrud, D.D., Litin, S.C., *Acute Wernicke's Encephalopathy Attributable to Pure Dietary Thiamine Deficiency*. Mayo Clin. Proc. 1994; 69:849-50.

Urberg, M., Zemel, M.B., *Evidence for Synergism Between Chromium and Nicotinic Acid in the Control of Glucose Tolerance in Elderly Humans*. Metabolism 1987; 36:896-99.

Urberg, M., et al., *Hypercholesterolemic Effects of Nicotinic Acid and Chromium Supplementation*. J. Fam. Prac. 1988; 27:303-06.

Uziel, G., Gravaglia, B., Di Donato, S., *Carnitine Simulation of the Pruvate Dhydrogenase Complex (PDHC) in Human Muscle Mitochondria*. Muscle Nerv. 1988; 11:270.

Van der Westhuyzen, S.V., Fernandes-Costa, F., *Cobalamin Inactivation by Nitrous Oxide Produces Severe Neurological Impairment in Fruit Bats; Protection by Methionine and Aggravation by Folates*. Life Sci. 1982; 31:2001-10.

Van Tonder, S.V., Metz, J., Green, R., *Vitamin B_{12} Metabolism in the Fruit Bat (*Rousettus aegypticus*). The Induction of Vitamin B_{12} Deficiency and its Effect on Folate Levels*. Br. J. Nutr. 1975; 34:397-410.

Victor, M., Martin, J.B., *Nutritional and Metabolic Diseases of the Nervous System*. In: K.J. Isselbacher, E. Braunwald, J.D. Wilson, J.B. Martin, A.S. Fauci, D.L. Kasper (eds.), Harrison's Principles of Internal Medicine. New York: McGraw-Hill, Inc., 1994.

Vitek, M.P.K., Bhattacharya, J.M., Glendenning, E., *Advanced Glaciation End Products Contribute to Amyloidosis in Alzheimer Disease*. Proc. Natl. Acad. Sci. 1994; 91:4766-70.

Wald, N.J., Bower, C., *Folic Acid, Pernicious Anemia and Prevention of Neural Tube Defects*. Lancet 1994; 343:307.

Walshe, J.M., *Copper: Not Too Little, Not Too Much, but Just Right.* Journal of the Royal College of Physicians of London 1995; 29:280-288.

Warren, P.J., Earl, C.J., et al., *The Distribution of Copper in Human Brain*. Brain 1960; 83:709-717.

Whirler, M.M., Shapiro, S., Mitchell, A.A., *Periconceptional Folic Acid Exposure and Risk of Concurrent Neural Tube Defects.* JAMA 1993; 269:1257-61.

Wilson, J.D., *Vitamin Deficiency and Excess.* In: K.J. Isselbacher, E. Braunwald, J.D. Wilson, J.B. Martin, A.S. Fauci, D.L. Kasper (eds.), Harrison's Principles of Internal Medicine. New York: McGraw-Hill, Inc., 1994.

Wolff, S.P., Bascal, Z.A., Hunt, J.V., *Autoxidative Glycosylation: Free Radicals and Glaciation Theory.* In: J.W. Baines, V.M. Monnier (eds.), The Maillard Reaction in Aging, Diabetes, and Nutrition. New York: Alan R. Liss, 1989; 259-75.

Yan, S.D., Chen, X., Schmidt, J., et al., *Glycated Tau Protein in Alzheimer's Disease: A Mechanism for Induction of Oxidant Stress.* Proc. Natl. Acad. Sci. 1994; 91:7787-91.

Chapter 12

OTHER TOXIC AGENTS

We would know nothing at all about chronic risk attributable to most toxic substances if scientists had not detected and evaluated them. Our response to such risks, therefore, must be based on a set of scientific findings. Science, however, is hardly ever unambiguous or unanimous, especially when the data on which definitive science must be founded scarcely exists.

—W.D. Ruckelshaus, *"Risk, Science & Democracy,"* Science Tech. (1985).

§ 12-1. Gases.

Substances discussed in this section occur as gases in normal conditions of temperature and pressure, and enter the body through inhalation. While vapors that emanate from solvents also enter the body through inhalation, they occur as liquids in normal conditions of temperature and pressure. Toxic gases that cannot be seen and have no odor are particularly dangerous. Carbon monoxide, for example, an odorless and colorless gas, is responsible for over half of the poisoning fatalities reported annually in the United States (McKay, 1956).

§ 12-1(a). Carbon Monoxide.

Among the many causes of hypoxia and anoxia seen by physicians, inhalation of carbon monoxide is perhaps the most common aside from asphyxia (Baker, 1983). Carbon monoxide may build up in the home as the result of a defective furnace, cracked heat exchanger, blocked chimney, malfunctioning space heater, or improperly ventilated fireplace or wood stove (Perera, 1995). One author noted that over 95% of the carbon monoxide cases studied had been caused by domestic appliances (Durin, 1987).

The affinity of carbon monoxide for hemoglobin is approximately 250 times that of oxygen. A 1% concentration of this gas in inspired air is usually fatal to a resting adult in 30 to 40 minutes, while children, with their higher respiratory rate, and active adults will die more rapidly. Fortunately, carboxyhemoglobin is dissociable by oxygen and thus a rational basis for therapy exists. One of the most common diagnostic signs of carbon monoxide poisoning is a cherry-red discoloration of the skin and mucous membranes. This discoloration, however, was found in only 1% of the cases in a particular study of 100 carbon monoxide poisoning patients (Turner, 1995).

Blood levels which measure the percentage of blood saturation with carboxyhemoglobin are a valuable diagnostic tool. Table 12.1 shows symptoms produced by various percentages of carbon monoxide in blood. In many cases, administering 100% oxygen is more practical than using hyperbaric oxygen therapy (Balzan, 1995).

Table 12.1
Symptoms That Correlate to Blood Saturation Levels of Carbon Monoxide

Percentage of Blood Saturation	Symptoms
0-10	None
10-20	Tightness across forehead, possible headache
20-30	Headache, throbbing in temples
30-40	Severe headache, weakness, dizziness, dimness of vision, nausea, vomiting and collapse
40-50	Same as 30-40, with more possibility of fainting and collapse, increased pulse and respiration
50-60	Fainting, increased pulse and respiration, coma with intermittent convulsions
60-70	Coma with intermittent convulsions, depressed heart action and respiration, possible death
70-80	Weak pulse and slowed respiration, respiratory failure and death

The onset of carbon monoxide poisoning may be either sudden or gradual, depending on the concentration and period of exposure. In the treatment of the chronic or gradual form of poisoning, the most important factors are avoiding further exposure and taking a thorough rest. In the treatment of acute carbon monoxide poisoning, the most important thing is to get the gas out of the blood as rapidly as possible, thus decreasing the possibility of serious aftereffects or loss of life through failure of the heart and respiration. As soon as the patient begins to breathe air in which there is no carbon monoxide, the process of eliminating the gas from the blood will begin naturally. However, this normal elimination process is slow and often has serious effects. It requires possibly 8 to 15 hours to reduce the carbon monoxide hemoglobin to 10% of the total hemoglobin. Inhalation of pure oxygen will remove the carbon monoxide from the blood 4 or 5 times faster. The use of oxygen alone in an oxygen therapy unit is common practice. Oxygen is usually readily available owing to its general use in industry.

§ 12-1(a)(1). Neurotoxic Effects.

Victims of acute carbon monoxide poisoning commonly present with headache and nausea. Muscle weakness, dizziness, and confusion are also seen. The patient's condition may advance to stupor, unconsciousness, and death. In some cases, the patient may be awake and aware of surroundings, but will be unable to move because of muscle weakness. (Kindwall, 1994).

There is still much that is unknown about the effects of chronic exposure, or delayed effects of acute exposure. Delays in diagnosis of up to 5 years have been reported (Kelafant, 1996). Encephalopathy and peripheral neuropathy have also been reported.

§ 12-1(b). Ethylene Oxide.

Ethylene oxide is used in the manufacture of a number of products, including polyester fibers for fabrics, film, plastic bottles, and antifreeze. It is also used to sterlilize laboratory equipment that is not heat-resistant. Chronically exposed laboratory workers have developed persistent neurological and psychological impairment (Crystal, 1988).

Acute encephalopathy and peripheral neuropathy have been associated with ethylene oxide at concentrations of 700 ppm and above. Subacute poluneuropathy with bilateral footdrop have been seen at occupational exposures (Finelli, 1983). Electromyography revealed denervation potentials. These patients improved 4 to 7 months after removal from exposure. Nerve biopsies of exposed patients have shown axonal neuropathy, mild Schwann cell change, and damage to unmyelinated fibers (Kuzuhara, 1983).

Long-term exposure has been associated with a chronic encephalopathy characterized by a decline in intellectual abilities. EEG slowing, headache, and peripheral neuropathy have also been seen (Salinas, 1981). Hospital workers have been affected. Workers exposed in hospital supply facilities where they were chronically exposed to ethylene oxide were found to be cognitively impaired. Ten workers were found to have hypoactive reflexes, and poor performance on tests of psychmotor speed (Klees, 1990; Kilburn, 1985).

§ 12-1(c). Formaldehyde.

Formaldehyde is a gas, but it is used as a water solution called formalin. The commercial solution, which may contain 35% to 50% formaldehyde by weight, also contains methanol as a preservative. It is also sold in a polymerized solid form called paraformaldehyde or trioxane. The gas has a strong odor, and the solution has a strong and penetrating odor that most people find irritating.

The major use of formaldehyde today is the manufacture of the resins urea-formaldehyde, phenol-formaldehyde, acetal-formaldehyde, and melamine-formaldehyde. These resins have a number of uses, including finishes for wrinkle-resistant textiles, and adhesives in the manufacture of particle boards and plywoods. Formaldehyde is also used as a tissue preservative, germicide, and embalming fluid.

§ 12-1(c)(1). Toxic Effects.

Exposure to formaldehyde can result in a wide range of effects, including irritation of mucous membranes, skin irritation, and respiratory disturbances. There is some evidence that it may be a carcinogen in long-term exposure, but the data are not considered to be conclusive (Stayner, 1994). Neurotoxic effects are sometimes seen in histology technicians. Symptoms include dizziness, lightheadedness, equilibrium disturbances, mood alterations, concentration problems, and memory deficits (Kilburn, 1985; Kilburn, 1987).

§ 12-1(d). Hydrogen Sulfide.

Hydrogen sulfide is a colorless gas with a foul odor. It is a dangerous, acute-acting toxin that can cause instant death in high concentrations. Hydrogen sulfide is used in petroleum refining, rayon manufacture, tanning, processing of protein wastes, and in various laboratory applications. Hydrogen sulfide is a product of decay, and is thus a potential hazard of liquid manure systems used for the efficient recycling of energy-rich animal wastes. The use of these systems is increasing. These systems have been associated with the deaths of animals and farm workers. In one incident, farm workers died after entering manure tanks that had been recently emptied (Zenz, 1994). It is generally recommended that workers entering a closed space containing a manure tank wear self-contained air packs and safety harnesses.

At low concentrations of about 200 ppm, hydrogen sulfide depresses the nervous system. Individuals exposed at these concentrations may lose consciousness. Neurological symptoms associated with acute hydrogen sulfide poisoning include dizziness, headache, lightheadedness, headaches, sleep disturbances, fatigue, weakness in the extremities, spasms, convulsions, and delirium (Wasch, 1989).

§ 12-1(e). Nitrous Oxide.

Nitrous oxide, also called laughing gas, is commonly used as a dental anesthetic. Because of its euphoric effects, it has been abused.

Nitrous oxide is associated with a neuropathy that is primarily distal and follows a radicular pattern. Both sensory and motor nerves are usually affected. A sign referred to as "reverse l'Hermitte" is often characteristic of nitrous oxide neuropathy. This sign involves a tingling sensation passing up from the toes to the neck after flexing the neck. The syndrome varies from one patient to another. There may be a gradually progressive disorder starting with paresthesias and numbness in the extremities, which may be accompanied by clumsiness and gait disturbance. There may also be loss of sphincter control.

Abnormalities in nerve conduction studies and sural nerve biopsy are often characterized by the degeneration of axons (Layzer, 1978)

In some patients, symptoms and signs of upper motor neuron disease may be observed. This disorder may occur in addition to the neuropathy. The syndrome is similar to the subacute degeneration seen in vitamin B_{12} deficiency. Nitrous oxide has been shown to inactivate certain enzymes requiring vitamin B_{12} for their operation, resulting in a disorder similar to vitamin B_{12} deficiency in the presence of sufficient quantities of the vitamin (Chanarin, 1982). Animal studies have suggested that exposure to nitrous oxide for 2 months can result in the inactivation of vitamin-B_{12}-dependent enzymes to a degree that would be attained after 3 to 5 years of a vitamin-B_{12}-deficient diet (Dinn, 1978).

Some studies have shown that dentists and dental assistants exposed to nitrous oxide have a greater rate of neuropathy than those not exposed (Brodsky, 1981). However, some investigators believe that most neuropathy associated with nitrous oxide stems from abuse rather than from its usual use in dental practice (Layzer, 1978).

§ 12-1(f). Methylene Chloride.

Methylene chloride, also known as dichloromethane or methyl chloride, is used as a degreaser, a refrigerant, a paint solvent and stripper, and a solvent for polymers. It is also used as an aerosol propellant.

Methyl chloride is metabolized to carbon monoxide, which can be measured in the blood as carboxyhemoglobin. The half-life of carboxyhemoglobin resulting from methyl chloride exposure is 13 hours as compared to 5.3 hours for carbon monoxide inhaled directly (Ratney, 1974). It is estimated that about 600 ppm of methylene chloride in the atmosphere may lead to a carboxyhemoglobin concentration of about 12%. The carboxyhemoglobin level could therefore be used as an indicator for setting occupational standards (Holmberg, 1994).

Reported neurologic effects of methyl chloride exposure include depression, gair ataxia, tremor, seizures, headache, vertigo, and impaired vision (Gross, 1979; Rapkero, 1979; Putz-Anderson, 1981). Methyl chloride has also been associated with peripheral neuropathy (Gross, 1979). The narcotic effect of methyl chloride may continue and increase up to 48 hours after removal from the source of exposure. Signs of a generalized encephalopathy may be present, including apathy, somnolence, and agitation. Focal areas of brain damage, particularly in the frontal and parietal lobes have been reported in patients with symptoms of methyl chloride intoxication (Rapkero, 1979).

§ 12-2. Therapeutic Drugs.

All therapeutic drugs have side effects, and the nervous system is a frequent target. The Food and Drug Administration (FDA) requires that drug companies reveal all known side effects of the drugs they manufacture. Full disclosure statements are put into the box or other package in which the product is sold. These statements are accessible to the public in publications, such as *Physicians Desk Reference* (PDR), which are available in almost every public library.

Anyone who reads a disclosure statement will be confronted with a long list of side effects for the drug in question. The side effects list is based on reports from trials and from clinical use of the drug. The listing is usually divided into body systems. The inclusion of a side effect in the disclosure statement does not mean that every patient using the drug will suffer from that side effect. With a given drug, some side effects are more likely to occur than others, but every patient reacts differently to a medication, in ways that are generally not possible to predict. In addition to side effects, the disclosure statement may include warnings about particular problems associated with the drug, as well as contraindications and drug interactions.

As is the case with any therapy, the decision to use a drug is based on a risk/benefit ratio. For some patients, the use of a high-risk drug may be justified. Most anti-cancer drugs, for example, have dangerous side effects. However, when their use has the potential to prolong life and/or improve the quality of life, the risk may be acceptable.

§ 12-2(a). Neurologic and Psychtropic Drugs.

As might be expected, drugs that target the nervous system are more likely to have nervous system side effects. However, side effects in the nervous system are by no means limited to drugs that target the nervous system. The following sections discuss side effects associated with some of the more commonly used neurologic and psychotropic drugs.

§ 12-2(a)(1). Anticonvulsants.

These drugs are primarily used for the control of epilepsy. They are also used for treating neuropathies and similar syndromes, as well as dystonias and dyskinesiasa. Toxicity associated with these drugs may be acute, subacute, or chronic. Since therapy with these agents is often lifelong, minimization of their side effects is essential.

§ 12-2(a)(1)(i). Phenytoin.

Phenytoin, one of the most effective anticonvulsants, has been in use for more than 50 years. It can, however, induce serious side effects in the nervous system even at low doses. There appears to be little correlation between the dose of phenytoin and the onset of side effects, but blood levels have been associated with certain side effects. (See Table 12.2.) Blood levels are useful in establishing a dosage range that is likely to result in the best therapeutic effect with the fewest side effects.

Table 12.2
Phenytoin Blood Levels and Associated Neurologic Side Effects

Blood Level (μg/mL)*	Side Effect
20	Nystagmus
30	Slurred speech, ataxia
40	Mental changes, vestibulocerebellar changes and vertigo

*These levels are approximations.

A rare toxic syndrome associated with phenytoin involves various involuntary movements, including facial grimaces, flailing "throwing" arm motions, and choreic tongue movements. This syndrome has been associated with phenytoin blood levels of 30% to 90%. It is most frequent in patients who experienced anoxic encephalopathy with extrapyramidal signs early in life. These movement disorders are usually reversible with drug cessation (Klawans, 1975).

Some reported side effects do not correlate with blood levels. Mild neuropathies may occur after long-term treatment with phenytoin. Age also appears to be a factor. When the syndrome is clinically apparent, the neuropathy is bilateral and mostly sensory. Loss of deep tendon reflexes in the lower limbs may also occur. They syndrome can sometimes be detected with EMG when symptoms are not apparent (Swift, 1981). Cerebellar degeneration and mental deterioration are rare, irreversible toxic effects of phenytoin that do not seem to be associated with blood levels of the drug.

§ 12-2(a)(1)(ii). Carbamazepine.

This drug has side effects similar to those of phenytoin. Most of the reported neurologic side effects are mild and transient. (See Table

12.3.) A non-neurologic side effect is bone marrow suppression, which usually requires discontinuation of the drug. Because carbamazepine is frequently used as adjunctive therapy to phenytoin and other anticonvulsant drugs, it is often not possible to determine if it is the causative agent.

Table 12.3
Carbamazepine Neurologic Side Effects

Ataxia
Nystagmus
Diplopia
Involuntary movement disorders
Respiratory depression*
Increased seizure activity*
Myoclonus with asterixis*
Hyporeflexia*
Hyperreflexia*

*Occurs with acute overdose.

Carbamazepine is thought to have less depressive effect than other anticonvulsant drugs, and is a frequent choice for patients with depression and mood and behavioral disorders. The drug itself, however, has been associated with depression and irritability (Masland, 1982).

§ 12-2(a)(1)(iii). Valproic Acid.

This agent has seen increased use over the past decade in the treatment of absence seizures and other forms of epilepsy. As is the case with carbamazepine, it is often used in conjunction with other anticonvulsants, thus making it difficult to determine which drug is responsible for adverse effects. Patients taking valproic acid and phenobarbital should be watched carefully, because valproic acid tends to increase blood phenobarbital levels, possibly resulting in excessive sedation (Bruni, 1980).

The most serious adverse effect of valproic acid is a potentially lethal hepatotoxic reaction, first manifested by increases in certain liver enzymes. These increases may be transient, but in some patients may lead to liver failure. The hepatotoxicity may be accompanied by tremor with asterixis, encephalopathy, and increased seizures. However, these adverse effects may occur in the absence of liver toxicity at therapeutic doses of valroic acid. (Nattson, 1981; Masland, 1982).

§ 12-2(a)(2). Psychotropic Medications.

Psychotropic drugs have become some of the most commonly prescribed medications. These drugs are frequently lumped by the general public into two generalized categories: "uppers" (antidepressants), and "downers" (anti-anxiety drugs and tranquilizers). Considerable controversy surrounds the use of these drugs. Some say they are overused and are producing a drugged society. Others maintain that these drugs are an effective and inexpenisve way of dealing with the mental problems that inevitably result from our competitive, fast-paced way of life. Despite the widespread use of these drugs, possible side effects and drug interactions should be considered carefully before prescribing.

§ 12-2(a)(2)(i). Neuroleptic Agents (Tranquilizers).

Several classes of neuroleptics are currently in use. (See Table 12.4.) The phenothiazine group is the largest. Neuroleptic agents are associated with several potentially serious adverse effects, including encephalopathy, neuroleptic malignant syndrome, dystonias, akathasia, Parkinsonism, and tardive dyskinesia.

Table 12.4
Neuroleptic Agents

Phenothiazines:

Piperazinyl

- Butaperizine
- Fluphenazine
- Perphenazine
- Perchloroperazine
- Thiopropazate
- Trifluoperazine

Aminoalkyl

- Chlorpromazine
- Triflupromazine

Thioxanthenes:

- Chlorprothixene
- Thiothixene

Other:

- Clozapine
- Haloperidol

Encephalopathy: Neuroleptics readily cross the blood-brain barrier and affect the nervous system at various levels. They may lower the seizure threshold and may exacerbate previously existing epilepsy. The drugs can cross the placenta, and infants of mothers who are regular users of neuroleptics may exhibit depressive behavior and apnea.

Neuroleptic Malignant Syndrome: The most prominent symptom of this syndrome is hyperthermia, which can resemble heat stroke. Other neurologic symptoms include dysarthria, abnormal eye movements, opisthotonic spasm, and seizures. Additional symptoms include those reflective of autonomic dysfunction, such as diaphoresis, unstable blood pressure, tachycardia, and tachypnea.

Parkinsonism: Parkinsonism is one of the more frequent adverse effects associated with neuroleptoic agents. The symptoms are practically indistinguishable from those of true Parkinson's disease, and include rigidity, tremor, bradykinesia, and postural reflex abnormalities. The patient may have difficulty rolling over in bed or getting up from a chair. Movements are slow, and walking is difficult. Balance is poor and the patient may be in danger of falling. The symptoms usually start in the second to fourth week of therapy. Drug-induced Parkinsonism is usually reversible with cessation of the drug, but because phenothizines are cleared from the body slowly, the symptoms may persist for a few weeks (Simpson, 1977). Administration of an naticholinergic drug is helpful and may help limit the Parkinsonian symptoms to a few weeks.

Dystonias: Dystonias are likely to be seen early in the course of therapy with neuroleptics. When administered by injection, a single dose of a phenothiazine *or* haloperidol can result in symptoms. Clinical symptoms frequently involve the eyes and neck. The patient may complain of inability to move the eyes in a vertical plane. In some instances the eyes remain staring upward. There may be pain associated with the fixed eye position or with attempts to move the gaze to a different plane. The patient may exhibit abnormal posture, including a backward spasm of the head and neck.

Drugs associated with dystonias also tend to be associated with parkinsonism. As is the case with drug-induced Parkinsonism, anticholinergic drugs will help to reduce the chances of developing dystonias. Acute administration of anticholinergic drugs by injection may relieve the dystonia in a matter of minutes, but it may be necessary to continue oral anticholinergic drugs for a few days.

Akathisia: Akathisia is a syndrome charaterized by severe restlessness, often accompanied by a subjective feeling of anxiety. It is most likely to occur in the first few days of therapy, and, as with dystonias and drug-induced Parkinsonian disease, anticholinergic drugs may reverse the syndrome. If anticholinergic drugs are not used, withdrawal of the neuroleptic may result in resolution of the symptoms. Akathisia is generally self-limiting, and it may be possible to stop the anticholinergic therapy. However, akathisia may persist indefinitely.

Tardive Dyskinesias: Tardive dyskinesias are characterized by abnormal, involuntary movements. The symptoms most often start in the face and tongue and then progress to the trunk and extremities. The diaphragm may also be affected, resulting in speech and breathing difficulties. The symptoms are usually first noticed when the dosage of the neuroleptic is decreased or when the medication is stopped.

In some patients, the symptoms may worsen following withdrawal of the neuroleptic. This is usually a short-term effect. While tardive dyskinesias are often reversible and may remit spontaneously, the effects may linger. Residual effects may be apparent in about half the patients with tardive dyskinesia (Hersohn, 1972).

§ 12-2(a)(2)(ii). Antianxiety Agents (Anxiolytics).

The two major classes of anxiolytics are the benzodiazepines and meprobromate, which is its own class and is no longer widely used. The benzodiazepines are some of the most heavily prescribed drugs in the world, and include such familiar names as diazepam (Valium), and chlordiazepoxide (Librium). Although this class of drugs is generally safe when used at therapeutic doses, a number of neurologic side effects, some life-threatening, have been associated with them.

Neurologic symptoms include drowsiness, excitability, exacerbation of neurotic depression, antisocial behavior, temper outbursts, and hallucinations. Neurologic symptoms may also occur on withdrawal of the drugs, as well as during therapy (Greenblatt, 1974; Hollister, 1961). The anticholinergic effects of dry mouth, tachycardia, and dilated pupils are often seen in the first few days or weeks of therapy.

Addiction has been a major problem with the benzodiazepines. Withdrawal symptoms can be quite severe if the patient's intake has been 100 mg or more daily for more than a month. Withdrawal symptoms include anorexia, nausea, apprehension, confusion, and hallucinations.

§ 12-2(a)(2)(iii). Antidepressant Drugs.

Several classes of antidepressant drugs are currently available (see Table 12.5), and, in response to demand, pharamaceutical companies are constantly developing new ones. The hope is to make an agent that has as few side effects as possible by making the drug specific for a particular receptor on the neuron. Today's antidepressant drugs are much improved over earlier ones, but neurologic side effects still occur. Side effects include dry mouth, dizziness, gastrointestinal symptoms, and blurred vision.

Table 12.5
Major Classes of Antidepressant Drugs

Tricyclic Agents:
- Amitriptyline
- Amoxapine
- Clomipramine
- Desipramine
- Imipramine
- Nortriptyline
- Trimipramine

Serotonergic Reuptake Blockers:
- Fluoxetine
- Fluvoxamine
- Sertriline
- Trazodone
- Zimetidine

Tetracyclic Agents:

Maprotiline
Minaserin
Oxaprotiline

Other:

Alprozolam
Bupropion
Buspirone

---

§ 12-3. Plants and Fungi.

There are scores of wild and domesticated plants, including house plants, that can have neurotoxic effects if ingested. Fortunately, most plants would have to be eaten in large quantities for the effects to be life-threatening. Mushrooms, which are the fruiting bodies of fungi, are another matter. Some can cause convulsions, hallucinations, and death if consumed even in small quantities. Plants are the most common source of ingested poisons in children.

§ 12-3(a). Mushroom Poisoning.

Of the 5,000 U.S. mushroom species, only 2% are poisonous. The most common problem associated with mushrooms is allergic reaction. Anaphylaxis has also been reported. Poisoning from mushrooms sold in a store or served in a restaurant is exceedingly rare. As the popularity of foraging for wild mushrooms grows, however, so will the incidence of poisonings due to the inability to distinguish toxic from nontoxic mushrooms. Most poisonous mushrooms resemble edible mushrooms at some point in their growth. Unfortunately, some mushroom hunters rely on folklore to distinguish safe from poisonous species. There is no simple, reliable way to distinguish poisonous from nonpoisonous mushrooms. Mushrooms can be classified on the basis of taxonomic features, but classification by their toxins is most useful for consideration of their toxicity.

Almost all fatal mushrooms are species in the genus amanita. The classic example is *Amanita Phalloides* ("destroying angel"). This mushroom was thought to be a strictly European variety, but was found growing in the United States in 1970 (Parish, 1986). This poisonous variety is found primarily in western coastal states.

The principal toxin of the amanita group is a complex protein containing heptapeptides and octapeptides. Amatoxins are thought to be the major toxins responsible for the symptoms and pathology due to ingestion of *Amanita Phalloides*. Amatoxins are potent inhibitors of protein synthesis, leading to cell death. They cause hepatorenal toxicity and gastrointestinal symptoms. The symptoms occur within 6 to 24 hours. There is a 20%-30% mortality rate. After liver failure, liver transplantation may be necessary.

The hallucinogenic indoles are the most significant group of mushrooms for neurotoxic effects. As the name implies, they can induce vivid, sometimes terrifying hallucinations. Long-term psychic disturbances may result. Symptoms can start as soon as 30 minutes after ingestion. Early symptoms include hyperkinetic movements, laughter, mydriasis (dilated pupils that do not react to light), blurred vision, muscle weakness, increased peristalsis, and cramps.

The muscarine group includes species of Boletus and Clitocybe, which are commonly seen on lawns. Their toxins produce peripheral cholinergic effects such as bradycardia, miosis, and blurred vision. Muscarine poisoning can be distinguished by the triad of perspiration, salivation, and lacrimation.

The coprine group is toxic only if it is consumed with ethanol. Coprine blocks the action of the enzyme acetaldehyde dehydrogenase, which is involved in the metabolism and detoxification of alcohol. If the enzyme is blocked, there is an accumulation of aldehyde. Early neurologic symptoms include blushing and paresthesia in the hands and feet. If the patient is not treated, the symptoms may progress to vertigo, weakness, visual disturbances, and coma. The poisoning is of rapid onset, but usually of short duration with a favorable prognosis (Klein, 1982).

§ 12-3(b). Poisonous Plants.

Plants containing anticholinergic alkaloids are frequently associated with toxic effects, particularly among teenagers who eat or smoke the leaves to get high. The resulting syndrome is often referred to as "red as a beet, dry as a bone, and mad as a hatter." Members of this group include belladonna, henbane, and jimsonweed. Symptoms include dry mouth, dilated pupils, delirium, hallucinations, convulsions, and, in severe cases, coma possibly leading to death.

Poison hemlock is one of the most dangerous plants in North America. It is called "fool's parsley" because of its resemblance to that food plant. The root has been mistaken for wild parsnip. Symptoms of poisoning include muscular weakness, trembling, vomiting, agitation, and dilated pupils. In severe cases, there may be stupor, paralysis, prostration, convulsions, and coma. Fatalities have occurred.

Plants used as medications can also be toxic. Foxglove (*Digitalis purpurea*) is used for treating some types of heart disease. The flower is attractive and produces a sweet nectar. Children have been poisoned, sometimes fatally, from sucking the nectar. Symptoms include irregular heartbeat, slow pulse, dizziness, respiratory arrest, and coma.

The saponin glycosides are natural soaps. Included in this group are buckeye, ginseng and pokeweed. Pokeweed, also called inkberry, is one of the most common causes of plant poisoning in North America. The plant is ubiquitous, growing in empty lots and fields. It produces bluish-purple berries, the squeezings of which children sometimes drink as "grape juice." Symptoms include slow breathing, tremor and syncope. Fatalities have been reported.

The solanum family includes several plants referred to variously as "deadly nightshade," "bittersweet," "climbing nightshade," and "Jerusalem cherry." These plants can be quite dangerous, causing respiratory paralysis, muscle weakness, and convulsions.

§ 12-4. Animal Toxins.

Many animals, both vertebrate and invertebrate, have evolved venoms for defense and for getting food. Humans coming into contact with these animals are sometimes injured by their venoms. Animals that produce toxins include snakes, lizards, spiders, scorpions, hymenoptera (bees, wasps, hornets, etc.) and other insects, and a rich variety of sea animals ranging from the jellyfish to stingrays and other fish. Only about 50 fatalities associated with animal toxins are recorded each year in the United States, but there is considerable morbidity, causing absence from work and lost productivity.

Snakes descend from lizards of some kind, but the precise mode of origin is obscure. There is evidence that snakes passed through a burrowing stage in the early history of their evolution. A burrowing ancestry is particularly suggested by the structure of their eye, which differs from that in typical lizards. There are no scleral ossicles or cartilages in a snake's eye, and accommodation is brought about in a manner unusual for reptiles, involving displacement of the lens. The visual cells include cones of a peculiar type, which have been derived from rods. Other developments include the degeneration of the ear structure. The eardrums, tympanic membranes and Eustachian tubes are absent. It seems unlikely that snakes can hear airborne sounds at all well, though they are sensitive to ground vibrations transmitted through the bones of the jaw. Snakes show many other interesting peculiarities, the most obvious being the complete absence of limbs. Locomotion is by lateral undulation of the body, which exerts pressure on surrounding objects and pushes the snake forward. The skull is modified, permitting an enormous gape and the swallowing whole of large prey. The two halves of the lower jaw are united only by ligaments. The brain is enclosed in a very strong and compact bone. The family Elapidie contains the cobras, kraits and coral snakes, all highly poisonous, with small and relatively non-movable fangs at the front of the maxilla. The hood of the cobra is expanded by the long cervical ribs and may serve to warn potential bite victims. The family Viperidae consists of the vipers of the old world and the rattlesnakes of the new world. These two families are distinguished by the presence of a sensory pit on either side of the head between eye and nostril. It is highly sensitive to temperature changes and helps the snake to detect warm-blooded prey. Rattlesnakes are noted for their caudal appendages, which rattle voluntarily as a warning. These snakes are highly poisonous, though the bite is seldom fatal to man. Only about 20 people a year die from snakebite in the United States.

Fewer than 10% of the known species of snakes are venomous. Venomous species in the United States include rattlesnakes (several varieties), water moccasins, copperheads, and coral snakes. The venoms of most species of snakes contain mixtures of toxic proteins and enzymes. These venoms are predominately neurotoxic. Milking venom from poisonous snakes (e.g., Asian Cobra, Naja Naja) for antivenin is a hazardous endeavor, which can result in neurological catastrophe, including paralysis. A patient bitten while milking a snake may have to be intubated and saved by cobra antivenin (Clemet, 1979; Goldfrank, 1994).

References.

Annau, Z., *The Neurobehaviroal Toxicity of Trichloroethylene.* Neurobehavioral Toxicol. and Teratol. 1981; 3: 417-424.

Baker, Baber, *Carbon Monoxide Intoxication.* Chemical Neurology, Vol II, 1983;11-15.

Baker, E.L., Fine, L.J., *Solvent Neurotoxicity: The Current Evidence.* J. Occup. Med. 1986; 28(2):126-129.

Balzan, M.V., Caciottolo, J.M., *The Dangers of Carbon Monoxide.* Letters to the Editor, N. Engl. J. Med. March 30, 1995: 894.

Bernad, P.G., Newell, S., Spyker, D.A., *Neurotoxicity and Behavior Abnormalities in a Cohort Chronically Exposed to Trichloroethylene.* Vet. Hum. Toxicol. 1987; 29(6).

Brodsky, J.B., Cohen, E.N., Brown, B.W., et al., *Exposure to Nitrous Oxide and Neurologic Disease Among Dental Professionals.* Anesth. Analg. 1981; 60:297-299.

Bruni, J., Wilder, B., Perchalski, R.J., et al., *Valproic Acid and Plasma Levels of Phenobarbital.* Neurology 1980; 30:94-97.

Campos-Outcalt, D., *Trichloroethylene: Environmental and Occupational Exposure.* Am. Fam. Phys. 1992; 46(2): 495-500.

Chanarin, I., *The Effects of Nitrous Oxide on Cobalamins, Folates, and Other Related Events.* Re. Toxicol. 1982; 20:179-213.

Clement, J.F., Pietrusko, R,G., *Pit Viper Snake Bite Envenomation in the U.S.* Clinical Toxicol. 1979; 14:515.

Crystal, H.A., Schaumburg, H.H., Grober, E., *Cognitive Impairment and Sensory Loss Associated with Chronic Low-Level Ethylene Oxide Exposure.* Neurology 1988; 38:567-569.

Dinn, J., McCann, S., Wilson, P., et al., *Animal Model for Subacute Combined Degeneration.* Lancet 1978; ii:1154-1155.

Durin, C., *Carbon Monoxide Poisoning Presenting with Focal Epileptiform Seizures.* Lancet 1987.

Estrin, W.J., Bowler, R.M., Lash., Becker, C.F., *Neurotoxicological Evaluation of Hospital Sterilizer Workers Exposed to Ethylene Oxide.* J. Clin. Toxicol. 1990; 28:1-20.

Feldman, R.G., White, R.F., Currie, J.N., Travers, P.H., Lessell, S., *Long-Term Follow-Up After Single Toxic Exposure to Trichloroethylene.* Am. J. Ind. Med. 1985; 8:119-126.

Feldman, R.G., Mayer, R.M., Taub, A., *Evidence for Peripheral Neurotoxic Effect of Trichloroethylene.* Neurology 1970; 20:599-606.

Finelli, P.F., Morgan, T.F., Yaar, I., Granger, C., *Ethylene Oxide-Induced Polyneuropathy: A Clinical and Neurophysiological Study.* Arch. Neurol. 1983; 40:419-421.

Goldfrank, L.R., et al. (eds.), Goldfrank's Toxicologic Emergencies, 5th Ed. Norwalk, CT: Appleton & Lange, 1994.

Greenblatt, D.J., Shrader, R.I., *Benzodiazepines.* N. Engl. J. Med. 1974; 291:1011-1013.

Gross, J.A., *Ethylene Oxide Toxicity.* Neurology 1979; 29:978-983.

Hersohn, H.L., Kennedy, P.F., McGuire, R.J., *Persistence of Extra-Pyramidal Disorders and Psychiatric Relapse After Long-Term Phenothiazine Therapy.* Br. J. Psychiatry 1972; 120:41-50.

Hollister, L.E., Motzenbecker, F.P., Degan, R.O., *Withdrawal Reactions from Chloridazepoxide.* Psychopharmacology 1961; 2:63-68.

Holmberg, B., Zenz, C., Dodson, V.N., *The Polymer Industry. Sulfide.* In: C. Zenz, O.B. Dickerson, E.P. Horvath (eds.), Occupational Medicine, 3d Ed. St. Louis: Mosby, 1994: 719-753.

Kelafant, G.A., *Encephalopathy and Peripehral Neuropathy Following Carbon Monoxise Poisoning from a Propane-Fueled Vehicle.* Am. J. Ind. Med. 1996; 30:765-768.

Kilburn, K.H., Warshaw, R., Boylen, C.T., *Pulmonary and Neurobehavioral Effects of Formaldehyde Exposure.* Arch. Environ. Health. 1985; 40:254-260.

Kilburn, K.H., Warshaw, R., Thornton, J.C., *Formaldehyde Impairs Memory, Equilibrium, and Dexterity in Histology Technicians: Effects Which Persist for Days After Exposure.* Arch. Environ. Health. 1987; 42:117-120.

Kindwall, E.P., *Carbon Monoxide.* In: C. Zenz, O.B. Dickerson, E.P. Horvath (eds.), Occupational Medicine, 3d Ed. St. Louis: Mosby, 1994: 447-452.

Klawans, H.L., Goetz, C.G., Bergen, D., *Levodopa-Induced Myoclonus.* Arch. Neurol. 1975; 32:331-334.

Klees, J.F., Lash, A., Bowler, R.M., *Neuropsychologic "Impairment" in a Cohort of Hospital Workers Chronically Exposed to Ethylene Dioxide.* J. Clin. Toxicol. 1990; 28:21-28.

Klein, A.E., *Were Toxic Plants or Mushrooms on the Menu?* Patient Care 1982; 165-230.

Kuzuhara, S., Kanazawa, I., Nakanishi, T., Egashira, T., *Ethylene Oxide Polyneuropathy.* Neurology 1983; 33:377-380.

Layzer, F.B., Fishman, R.A., Schaefer, J.A., *Neuropathy Following Abuse of Nitrous Oxide.* Neurology 1978; 28:504-506.

Masland, R.L., *Carbamazepine Neurotoxicity.* In: D.M. Woodbury, J.K. Penry, C.E. Pippenger (eds.), Antiepileptic Drugs. New York: Raven Press, 1982: 521-531.

McKay, A.J., *Carbon Monoxide Poisoning.* N. Engl. J Med. 1956; 272:252.

Nattson, R.H., Cramer, J.A., *Tremor Due to Sodium Valproate.* Neurology 1981; 31:114-115.

Parish, R., Doering, P., *Treatment of Amanita Mushroom Poisoning: A Review.* Vet. Hume. Toxicol. 1986; 28:318-322.

Perera, R.D., *The Dangers of Carbon Monoxide.* Letters to the Editor, N. Engl. J. Med. 1995.

Plessner, W., *Ober Trigeminuserkankung Infolge von Trichloroathylenevergiftung.* Neurol. Zbl. 1915; 34:916.

Putz-Anderson, V., Setzer, J.V., Croxton, J.S., Phipps, F.C., *Methyl Chloride and Diazepan Effects on Performance.* Scand. J. Work Environ. Health. 1981; 7:8.

Rapkero, J.D., Lasley, S.M., *Behavioral Neurologic Effects of Methyl Chloride: A Review of the Literature.* CRC Crit. Rev. Toxicol. 1979; 6:283-302.

Ratney, R.S., Wegman, D.H., Elkins, H.B., *In Vivo Conversion of Methylene Chloride to Carbon Monoxide.* Arch. Environ. Health. 1974; 28:233.

Salinas, E., Sasich, L., Hall, D.H., et al., *Acute Ethylene Oxice Intoxication.* Drug Intell. Clin. Pharm. 1981; 15:385-388.

Salvini, M., Binaschi, S., Riva, M., *Evaluation of the Psychophysiological Functions in Humans Exposed to Trichloroethylene.* Br. J. Ind. Med. 1971; 28:293-295.

Simpson, G.M., *Neurotoxicity of Major Tranquilizers.* In: L. Roisin, H. Shiraki, N. Grcevic (eds.), Neurotoxicology. New York: Raven Press, 1977: 1-7.

Stayner, L., Ward, E., Petsonk, E.L., *Formaldehyde Sulfide.* In: C. Zenz, O.B. Dickerson, E.P. Horvath (eds.), Occupational Medicine, 3d Ed. St. Louis: Mosby, 1994: 666-667.

Swift, T.R., Gross, J.A., Ward, C., Crout, B.O., *Peripheral Neuropathy in Epileptic Patients.* Neurology 1981; 31:826-831.

Turner, M., *The Dangers of Carbon Monoxide.* Letters to the Editor, N. Engl. J. Med. 1995.

Wasch, H.H., Estrin, W.J., Yip, P., et al., *Prolongations of the P-300 Latency Associated with Hydrogen-Sulfide Exposure.* Arch. Neuro. 1989; 46:902-904.

Young, J.Z., The Life of Vertebrates, 2d Ed. New York: Oxford University Press, 1965.

Zenz, C., Cordasco, E.M., *Hydrogen Sulfide.* In: C. Zenz, O.B. Dickerson, E.P. Horvath (eds.), Occupational Medicine, 3d Ed., St. Louis: Mosby, 1994: 675-677.

EPILOGUE

Just as man cannot live without dreams, man cannot live without expectations. If dreams reflect the past, hope summons the future.

—Elie Wiesel, *From the Kingdom of Memory: Reminiscences* (1995).

How would man exist if God did not need him, and how would you exist? You need God in order to be, and God needs you — for that is the meaning of your life.

—Martin Buber, *I and Thou* (1923).

Over the last 100 years, humankind has seen a series of remarkable technological advances. The synthetic chemical industry has experienced perhaps the most striking progress, in that over 70,000 synthetic chemical products have been developed and are in use today. These chemical products are evident in the earth's air, water and soil.

The human central and peripheral nervous systems serve as sensitive indicators of chemical toxicity exposure, and the effects on the human body of daily exposure to chemicals are only beginning to be understood. This publication has covered only a few of the more commonly encountered substances. The author expects that subsequent editions of this text will be published to expand and update the materials included, and to incorporate the most relevant and pertinent studies and clinical information available.

INDEX

A

B

D

E

F

G

H

V

X

Z

NEUROTOXICOLOGY: A CLINICAL SOURCEBOOK

1999 Supplement

By

PETER G. BERNAD
M.D., M.P.H., F.A.C.P

LEXIS®
LAW PUBLISHING
Charlottesville, Virginia

Place in pocket of bound volume.

ISBN 0-327-01487-3

6606610

SUMMARY OF CONTENTS

TABLE OF CONTENTS

CHAPTER 1

NEUROTOXIC EXPOSURE

CHAPTER 4

LABORATORY ANALYSIS

CHAPTER 7

VOLATILE SOLVENTS

CHAPTER 8

METALS

CHAPTER 9

ORGANOPHOSPHATE INSECTICIDES

CHAPTER 11

THE ROLE OF NUTRIENTS

CHAPTER 12

OTHER TOXIC AGENTS

CHAPTER 13

COMPLEMENTARY AND ALTERNATIVE MEDICINE (CAM)

CHAPTER 14

FORENSICS

ACKNOWLEDGEMENT

The author would like to thank Gerald E. Saunders, Jr., and Desere Segal for their superlative efforts in assisting with this supplement.

Chapter 1

NEUROTOXIC EXPOSURE

§ 1-1. Overview of Toxicity.

Page 3. Add at end of § 1-1:

Chemicals continue to be a part of everyday life. Global wind patterns carry all types of airborne chemicals and particulate matter from volcanic eruptions, oil well fires, oil spills, chemical plant explosions, radon, nuclear fallout, electromagnetic radiation, and contamination in local environments. The human population is exposed to chemicals in air, water, foods, household products, manufacturing sites of production, cosmetics, and drugs which potentially have neurotoxic effects. The Environmental Protection Agency (EPA) TSCA inventory of chemicals manufactured or imported in the United States includes more than 65,000 substances with annual increases (NRC, 1984). Estimates of one subset of substances that are neurotoxic includes a large percentage of the more than 500 registered pesticide ingredients which affect the nervous system of exposed biological systems. Nervous system effects have been reported in 167 of the 588 chemicals listed by the American Conference of Governmental Industrial Hygienists. One prominent researcher ranks neurotoxicity as one of the top 10 leading workplace disorders. In fact, one million workers are exposed to 200 chemicals each day, one-third of which may have adverse effects on the nervous system. Because of the increasing number of chemicals in the ambient atmosphere, there is growing scientific, regulatory, and public interest in determining the potential neurotoxic effect (risk assessment) of these substances (Anger, 1984; Anger 1990).

§ 1-2. What Are Neurotoxins?

Page 7. In the last sentence of the third complete paragraph, replace "$_c$NOS" with "one form of NOS" and replace "$_n$NOS" with "another form of NOS".

§ 1-5. Relating a Substance to a Toxic Effect.

§ 1-5(a). Evaluating Neurotoxicity.

Page 14. Add new subsection after § 1-5(a):

§ 1-5(a)(1). Governmental Agency Guidelines.

Risk assessment has been defined by the National Research Council (NRC, 1983) to include four components: hazard identification-examining whether a chemical has an effect by qualitative parameters of dose-response relationships, route, and duration of exposure; dose-response assessment — a quantitative measurement of no observed adverse effect level (NOAEL) and lowest observed adverse effect level (LOAEL) for each study and type of effect as well as the benchmark dose approach (BMD) adopted by the Environmental Protection Agency (EPA) to provide more quantitative dose-response relationships when adequate information on chemicals is available; exposure assessment — the identification of human populations exposed or potentially exposed with frequencies, magnitude, and duration of exposure to the agent; and, risk characterization — the hazard characterization, dose-response analysis, and exposure assessment combined to quantify a measure of neurotoxicity (EPA, 1995; EPA, 1998).

Risk assessment can be misleading, however. For instance, although the EPA blames bad air quality for the increase in asthma figures for air pollution, levels appear to have steadily declined during the time the disease skyrocketed. In fact, one medical journal reported that asthma was increasing in countries with the least air pollution. One should therefore conclude that environmental issues of neurotoxicity can take on political "spins." The environmental lobby has increased its influence and presence in the public domain and the media. Health care providers are urged to remain vigilant in their scientific approach to issues of neurotoxic exposure (NYT, 1998 J30).

On April 30, 1998, the EPA released its latest work on neurotoxicity entitled, *Guidelines for Neurotoxicity Risk Assessment.* It was developed as an interoffice development program by a Technical Panel of the Risk Assessment Forum composed of Agency scientists whose selected drafts were peer-reviewed internally and subsequently by experts in universities, industry, environmental groups, and other government agencies. In particular, these guidelines are intended as a template for the evaluation of agents that have potential neurotoxic effects. These state-of-the-art guidelines are published in part to bridge gaps in methodology, risk assessment, and data, although the agency recognizes the need for new research and analysis that will lead to better assessment of the neurotoxic effects of chemicals (63 FR 26926-26954).

§ 1-7. Twenty-First Century Diseases.

§ 1-7(e). Chronic Fatigue Syndrome.

Page 21. Replace section title with the following:

§ 1-7(e). Chronic Fatigue Immune Dysfunction Syndrome (CFIDS) and Chronic Fatigue Syndrome (CFS).

Page 22. Add at end of § 1-7(e):

A decade of research has been conducted on CFS, no definitive tests exist for CFIDS. Often misdiagnosed because it is frequently unrecognized and resembles other disorders including mononucleosis, multiple sclerosis (MS), fibromyalgia (FM), Lyme disease, post-polio syndrome, and autoimmune diseases such as lupus (Understanding CFIDS, 1998). In about one-third of cases, the onset of CFS follows a bout with gastrointestinal, respiratory, or some other acute infection with flu-like symptoms (i.e., mononucleosis). About 20 to 40 percent of patients do not experience depression or other psychiatric illness.

However, most patients seeking medical care for CFIDS usually suffer from depression or overwork. The primary objective in psychological and laboratory screening is to exclude possible other clinical diagnosis. Although CFIDS can be treated with antidepressant therapy evidence suggests that it may be resistant to selective serotonin reuptake inhibitor antidepressants (Medical Board California — Action Report). CFIDS may turn out to be a latent infection that would be treatable with antibiotics.

Approximately 200,000 to 500,000 adults in the United States are thought to suffer from CFIDS. Most are women between the ages of 25 to 45, but men and children are also affected. Chronic Fatigue Syndrome has also been called the neurasthenia of this time (Psychosomatics, Vol. 31). Although CFIDS has multiple nonspecific symptoms at least one study found that a subtle deficiency of the stress hormone cortisol exists. Additionally, disturbances of immunologic function has been ascribed to CFIDS. The anomalies include depressed natural killer (NK) cell activity and modest increases in the number of activated circulating immune complexes. However, such changes have been known to follow emotionally challenging experiences. CFIDS has not been shown definitively to be associated with any specific opportunistic infection or the development of neoplasms, but neither has an underlying infectious etiology been entirely excluded.

The etiology of CFIDS continues to be poorly understood. The International CFS Study Group published a new definition of CFIDS in the December 1994 issue of the *Annals of Internal Medicine*. The new definition replaces the first case definition in 1978 and subdivides the syndrome into groups for research studies as well as nonresearch clinicians. Internationally, CFIDS symptomatology is known as myalgic encephalomyelitis, postviral fatigue syndrome, epidemic neuromyasthenia, chronic fatigue and immune dysfunction syndrome (NIH Publication No. 97-484).

Page 24. Add new subsections § 1-7(j) and § 1-7(k) after § 1-7(i):

§ 1-7(j). Attention Deficit Hyperactivity Disorder (ADD) (ADHD).

Attention Deficit Hyperactivity Disorder (ADD) (ADHD) is a behavioral syndrome that is often characterized by disruptive behavior, episodes of rage, hyperactivity or lack of it, inattention, distractibility, impulsivity, and destructive behavior. Most children with the disorder also have anxiety, depression, and disruptive conduct. In the 1980s, it was thought that estimates of ADHD in the general population ranged from 2% to 5%. Given the fact that in 1993 over 2 million children were treated for ADHD, the percentage of the population affected with ADHD could be higher. Boys are usually diagnosed with ADHD more often than girls possibly due to overdiagnosis. Some boys are just plain aggressive in behavior without the diagnostic criterion ADD (Well-Connected, 1997).

Although children are affected in larger numbers, adult diagnoses are on the rise. Slightly over 220,000 adult prescriptions were written for Ritalin® in 1992; estimates for 1997, however, have been over 700,000. On the other hand, the number of prescriptions is obscured by the actual number of adults who meet the criteria for ADHD. According to one study, 32% of adults did not meet the criteria, and another 36% met some of the criteria but did not have ADHD in childhood (Well-Connected, 1997).

Diagnosis of ADHD can be complex. A number of associated diseases are related to ADD, including: Oppositional Deficit Disorder, characterized by refusal of the child to follow directions; Pervasive Development Disorder, a rare syndrome involving autistic-type behavior such as hand flapping, slow social development, speech and motor problems, as well as repetitive statements; Primary Disorder of Vigilance, an inherited syndrome characterized by poor attention and concentration and an inability to stay awake; and, Bipolar Disorder (Manic Depression) with episodic cycles of depression and mania with potential problems such as rapid speech (some people seem to talk on and on), irritability, and disconnected often simultaneously. In the future, some think that ADHD will be the general syndrome for a number of other syndromes such as those mentioned.

Other diagnoses that mimic symptomatology of ADHD are lead poisoning, genetic abnormalities such as Tourette's syndrome (50% of patients with Tourette's also have ADD), Posttraumatic Stress Disorder, and other medical conditions such as eye and ear problems, and hyperthyroidism. To determine the exact diagnosis is a challenge for the most informed health provider and can only be assessed with a thorough medical history (Well-Connected; BRAINTRAC).

A detailed history of the patient must be completed before diagnosing ADHD. Extensive questioning of the mother must accompany a reasonable assessment of the mother's diet while pregnant with the child. These responses should be matched to a standardized check list for ADHD in DSM-IV.

Diagnostic Criteria For Attention-Deficit Hyperactivity Disorder

A. Either 1 or 2:

1. Should have 6 or more of the following symptoms of inattention, persisting for at least 6 months to a degree that is maladaptive and inconsistent with developmental level.
   a. Often fails to give close attention to detail, makes careless mistakes.
   b. Often has difficulty sustaining attention in tasks or play.
   c. Often does not seem to listen when spoken to directly.
   d. Often does not follow through and fails to finish tasks.
   e. Has difficulty organizing tasks and activities.
   f. Avoids or dislikes tasks requiring sustained mental effort.
   g. Often loses things necessary for tasks or activities.
   h. Is often easily distracted by extraneous stimuli.
   i. Is often forgetful in daily activities.

2. Should have 6 or more of the following symptoms of hyperactivity-impulsivity persisting for at least 6 months to a degree that is maladaptive and inconsistent with developmental level.
   a. Often fidgets or squirms when sitting.

b. Has difficulty remaining seated when required to do so.
c. Often runs about or climbs excessively in inappropriate situations.
d. Has difficulty playing quietly.
e. Is often "on the go," acts as if "driven by a motor."
f. Often talks excessively.
g. Often blurts out answers to questions before they have been completed.
h. Has difficulty awaiting turn.
i. Often interrupts or intrudes on others.

B. Onset of some symptoms before the age of seven.

C. Symptoms occur in two or more settings (for example, home and school).

D. Clear evidence of significant impairment in social or academic functioning.

E. Not caused by a pervasive development disorder or another other psychologic disorder, including anxiety or depression.

Diagnostic and Statistical Manual of Mental Disorders: 4th Rev., Washington, D.C., American Psychiatric Association

Maternal smoking during pregnancy, infant and child malnutrition, diet, as well as genetics may have an affect on ADHD. Ongoing research has indicated genetic mechanisms such as those that affect the gene for the D4 receptor for dopamine may be involved in ADD. Extroversion and novelty-seeking may result from this alteration. Imaging techniques used to scan the brain have detected distinct differences in the right side of the brain of ADHD children compared to those who do not have the condition ADHD. Three areas of the brain appear to be smaller in ADHD, the caudate nucleus, the globus pallidus, and the prefrontal pallidus located near the midpoint of the brain. The latter two areas accelerate or isolate the signals coming from the prefrontal cortex. Abnormalities in this region may impair a person's ability to control impulsive actions. Other neurotransmitters in this region, including norepinephrine, also have effects on behavior.

Psychoneurometric testing may include WISC-R, Bender Gestalt, and EEG. Brain scans using the following techniques are recommend to evaluate the patient: Magnetic Resonance Imaging (MRI), or single photon emission computed tomography (SPECT). Laboratory tests are generally not recommended unless there is a suspicion of toxicity or other medical problem. Stimulants such as Methylphenidate (Ritalin®) are good management therapy for ADHD. Dexedrine, similar to Ritalin®, and Adderall® (another amphetamine) are also used. Cylert® (pemoline) is another agent that is used. Physicians prescribing drugs for ADHD-affected children caution that the time when the medication is taken by the child is important because if taken in the morning the drug can wear off near the end of the school day eliciting a disruptive response in the child. After school, a mild dose should be given to prevent rebound. Side effects of stimulants include nervousness and sleeplessness, irritability, withdrawal, depression, hallucinations, and lack of spontaneity. Some children, about 9%, also experience tics and jerks though a lower dosage may cause these effects to subside. Symptoms of overdose include muscle twitches, sweating, breathing difficulties, confusion, and vomiting. Ritalin® has proven to be a safe and effective regimen for ADHD although it has caused liver damage in mice (BRAINTRAC, 1992; Well-Connected, 1997; Gadow, 1999). Off-label use of newer medications may also be a potential benefit.

§ 1-7(k). Gulf War Syndrome.

Shortly after the Gulf War, many soldiers complained of an illness characterized by tiredness, difficulty concentrating, muscle and joint pain, diarrhea, breathing problems, and skin rashes (Brown, 1998). According to one report, however, the physical complaints known as "Gulf War Syndrome" are common to army veterans who never went to Iraq, Kuwait or Saudi Arabia. Epidemiologists from the Centers for Disease Control and Prevention (CDC) in Atlanta surveyed Air Force units in 1995 and found that 45% of Gulf War veterans had chronic physical complaints. Those who reported illness showed nothing unusual upon physical examination or analysis of lab specimens.

A Department of Defense report on the 11th Marines also concluded that out of eighteen reported alerts for chemical exposure incidences, assessment of exposure to any chemical warfare agent (CWA) was determined to be unlikely. However, the data show that in many instances the equipment proved to be unreliable, often registering false positives caused by carbon smoke exposure and large droplet petroleum fallout from oil well fires and battlefield contaminants such as vehicle exhaust. Also, the study was compromised by the fact that many witnesses could recall little about some of the alerts. Protective gear was donned during most alerts, including cases when soldiers smelled (or felt on their skin) sulfur, hydrogen sulfide after the bombing of an enemy site, or CS, a riot control agent used in nuclear/biological/chemical (NBC) training. One veteran reported being exposed to sarin. Notable throughout the report are the effects of wind speed and direction which could have led to the misleading reports. Regarding visual sightings, several accounts reported a suspicious unknown white cloud that hovered several kilometers above troops (DOD, October 1998).

During the Gulf War, soldiers were also exposed to depleted uranium (DU) that was used to reinforce tank armor and munitions. Depleted uranium is a byproduct of the process by which naturally occurring uranium is "enriched" by adding isotopes taken from other uranium. The leftover uranium, which is drained of 40% of its original radioactivity, is known as depleted uranium. Thirty-three veterans have been documented as injured from friendly fire involving depleted uranium. Soldiers in or around vehicles struck by DU munitions were possibly exposed through four mechanisms: inhalation, ingestion, direct wounding, and contamination of wounding. Higher than normal levels of uranium have been detected in the urine of veterans with DU fragments still embedded in their bodies. Although 25 individuals have been diagnosed with kidney damage, no evidence exists for heavy metal or radiological toxicity. Babies fathered by these soldiers from 1991 to 1997 have had no birth defects (DOD, July, 31, 1998).

A 1998 news release reported the possibility of emergent health effects caused by exposure of U.S. troops to more than 600 oil wells fires set during the war by retreating Iraqi forces. The fires burned for more than nine months in 1991 and released known pollutants that in sufficient quantify can cause adverse health effects in humans (DOD, November 5, 1998). There is at least one diagnosis of exposure to a mustard product during the Gulf War (McAllister, 1998).

According to research by Duke University and the University of Texas Southwest Medical Center, the Gulf War syndrome might have been caused by exposure to ordinarily harmless chemicals that together may cause nerve damage. It would appear at this time that no single agent has been found to be definitively responsible for all of the symptoms associated with Gulf War syndrome.

§ 1-8. Potentially Toxic Products.

§ 1-8(a). Phen-Fen.

Page 24. In first line of § 1-8(a), replace "phenfluramine (Fen)" with "fenfluramine (Fen)".

Pages 25. Add at end of § 1-8(a):

The anorectic agents, phentermine and fenfluramine (often labeled Phen-Fen therapy) did not prove to be the wonder drug for weight loss its manufacturer hoped it to be due to its adverse effects. Approximately 14 million prescriptions were written for Phen-Fen from 1995 through September 1997 when the drugs were pulled from the market by the FDA after patients taking the medication exhibited a higher rate of valvular disease and pulmonary hypertension. Since the recall, 12% to 25% of those prescribed for the diet therapy either alone or in combination have developed valvular heart disease. The number of people who demonstrated side effects appears to decline with time, however. Some physicians think this might suggest that in mild cases the valvular disease might plateau or even get better, though in severe cases the condition could deteriorate (Stapleton, 1998). It is thought that phentermine induces weight loss via presynaptic release of norepinephrine and dopamine as well as by blocking their uptake. Dexfenfluramine is thought to initiate its anorectic effect by blocking presynaptic serotonin release and uptake (Lew, 1998; Am. J. Psychiatry, 1987).

Phen-Fen therapy has also been shown to have neuropsychological effects. Episodes of mania have been reported with use of fenfluramine, 60mg/d, and phentermine 15 mg/d for treatment of morbid obesity without history of depression. The patient demonstrated auditory hallucinations, reduced sleep, pressured speech and grandiose delusions that "God was explaining the universe to her." The symptoms appeared on two separate occasions within two weeks of starting Phen-Fen therapy. Mania was induced by dexfenfluramine in a patient with a history of bipolar disorder two weeks after being prescribed the drug. The patient exhibited distinct mood cycles, with rapid onset and escalation of anger, rage and even homicidal thoughts toward her mother, labile mood with easy shifts into fearfulness, and out-of-control temper. In this case, alcohol was consumed by the patient. Weight loss was reported by the patient but not the psychotic episode for fear of being taken off the medication. The drug was discontinued, and her mixed manic rapid cycling state improved after discontinuance of the drug. Episodes of psychotic behavior has also been reported in a patient two weeks after starting a regimen of dexfenfluramine 30mg/d who had not consumed alcohol or drugs. The patient, who reported to the emergency room became paranoid, delusional, combative, and had to be restrained after a violent episode at a federal building. Other symptoms included pressured speech, and further grandiose and paranoid delusions (Preval, 1997).

In animal studies, no potentiation of neurotoxicity of phentermine plus fenfluramine or fenfluramine alone has been indicated in a study analogous to that of patients treated with Phen-Fen therapy. Repeated administration of Fen as well as combined administration of Phen-Fen induces long-term depletion of axonal serotonin (5-HT) and loss of 5-HT transporters resulting in neurotoxicity (Halladay, 1998; Lew, 1997). Note that coadministration of phentermine and fenfluramine has been shown to reduce the craving for alcohol anJ cocaine (Baumann, 1996; Shoaib, 1997; Rothmann, 1998).

§ 1-8(b). Silicone Breast Implants.

Page 25. Replace "Scleradoma" with "Schleroderma" in fourth line of second paragraph of section.

Page 25. Delete comma after "systemic lupus" in fourth line of second paragraph of section.

Page 29. Add new § 1-10 after § 1-9(b):

§ 1-10. Material Safety Data Sheet (MSDS).

The Material Safety Data Sheet (MSDS) is a vital key to workplace controls. The author uses this document frequently. It is a technical document which must be provided by the manufacturer of a toxic product or chemical. It provides information on the safe handling and use of the product or chemical. The Right To Know Law requires the manufacturer to incorporate, at a minimum, the following sections into its MSDS:

1. *Identification:* The product's chemical name, common name, trade name, or trade secret registry number must be listed. The manufacturer's name, address, and emergency telephone number will also be listed.

2. *Physical Data:* The odor and appearance of the substance are described and the product's Boiling Point, Vapor Pressure, Evaporation Rate, Percent Volatility and Solubility in Water are listed.

3. *Hazardous Ingredients:* The names of all hazardous ingredients along with their percentages, TLVs, TELs, and other reference information are included.

4. *Fire and Explosion Hazard Data:* Flash Point, Flammable Limits, Auto-Ignition Temperature, and Decomposition Temperature are listed. The necessary type of fire extinguisher and any special fire-fighting procedures for the substance can be found under this heading.

5. *Health Hazard Data:* The symptoms and findings of overexposure to the substance are listed, along with emergency and first-aid procedures to be followed in the event of exposure.

6. *Reactivity Data:* This section refers to the stability of the substance.

7. *Spill or Leak Procedures:* This section designates specific methods to clean up a leak or spill, and also lists waste disposal methods.

8. *Special Protection Information:* This section lists the controls to be used when working with the substance. Controls may include ventilation, specific respiratory protection, glasses, gloves, and any other necessary protective equipment.

9. *Special Precautions:* This section provides details regarding special situations and precautions to be taken when handling and storing the substance.

10. *Date:* This section lists the date of preparation of the MSDS and the dates of any revisions.

References.

Page 30. Replace the reference beginning "Bernad, P.G., Ask Your Doctor ..." with the following reference:

Bernad, P.G., Ford, J.E., Kristal, S.B., *Lack of Causal Relationship Between Silicone Breast Implants and Neurological/ Rheumatological Diseases.* As presented to the 5th World Congress of the World Federation of Associations of Clinical Toxicology

Centers & Poison Control Centers, Taipei, Taiwan, R.O.C., November 8-11, 1994.

Anger, W.K., *Neurobehavioral testing of chemicals: impact on recommended standards.* Neurobehavioral Toxicology Teratology 1984; 6:147-153.

Anger, W.K., *Worksite behavioral research: results, sensitive method, test batteries, and the transition from laboratory data to human health.* Neurotoxicology 1990; 11:627-718.

Attention-Deficit Hyperactivity Disorder in Children. Well-Connected, Report No. 30, November 30, 1997.

Baumann, M.H., Schuster, C.R., Rothman, R.B., *Effects of phentermine and cocaine on fenfluramine-induced depletion of serotonin in mouse brain.* Drug & Alcohol Dependence 1996; 41(1):71-4.

Bowden, C.L., Dickson, J., *Mania from Dexfenfluramine, Letters to the Editor.* J. Clin. Psychiatry 1997; 58(12):548-49.

Brown, D., *Boundaries of "Gulf War Syndrome" Widen.* Washington Post, September 16, 1998; A4.

CFIDS Association of America, *CFIDS, Understanding CFIDS.* 1998.

DOD, *Case Narrative, 11th Marines.* Department of Defense, October 1998.

DOD, *Environmental Exposure Report, Depleted Uranium in the Gulf.* July 31, 1998.

DOD, *DOD Releases Second Environmental Exposure Report on Gulf War Illness — Effects of Oil Well Fires.* Press Release No. 572-98, November 5, 1998.

Environmental Protection Agency, *Guidelines for Ecological Risk Assessment.* Notice, Federal Register 63(93).

Environmental Protection Agency, *Guidelines for Ecological Risk Assessment.* Notice, Federal Register 63(93):26926-26954, 1998.

Furmento, M., *The Pesticides Are Not the Main Problem.* New York Times, June 30, 1998, A27.

Gadow, et al., *Long-term methyl phenidate therapy in children with comorbid attention-deficit hyperactivity disorder and chronic multiple tic disorder.* Archives of General Psychiatry 1999; 56(4):330-36.

Greenberg, D.B., *Neurasthenia in the 1980s: Chronic Mononucleosis, Chronic Fatigue Syndrome, and Anxiety and Depressive Disorders.* Psychosomatics Vol. 31(2), 1990.

Halladay. A.K., Fisher, H., Wagner, G.C., *Interaction of phentermine plus fenfluramine: neurochemical and neurotoxic effects.* Neurotoxicology 1998; 19(2):177-83.

Lew, R., Weisberg, B., Vosmer, G., Seiden, L.S., *Combined phentermine/fenfluramine administration enhances depletion of serotonin from central terminal fields.* Synapse 1998; 26(1):36-45.

McAllister, B., *Panel's Report Challenges Gulf War Syndrome Theory,* __________ 1998.

Medical Board of California, *Chronic Fatigue Syndrome: A Mystery and an Albatross.* Action Report 1999.

Neurometric Assessment Helps Subtype Attention Deficit Hyperactivity Disorder. BRAINTRAC Vol. 1(1), 1992.

Neurometrics Reveals Amantadine-Responsive Attention Deficit Subtype Disorder in Adolescent Referred for Depressive Disorder. BRAINTRAC Vol. 1(2), 1992.

NIH, *Chronic Fatigue Syndrome: Information for Physicians.* NIH Publication No. 97-484, December 18, 1998.

Preval, H. Pakyurek, A.M., *Psychotic Episode Associated with Dexfenfluramine.* Letters to the Editor, Am. J. Psychiatry 1997; 154(11):1624-25.

Raison, C.L., Klein, Haven M., *Psychotic Mania Associated with Fenfluramine and Phentermine use.* Letters to the Editor, Am. J. Psychiatry 1997; 154(5), 711.

Rothmann, R.B., Elmer, G.I., Shippenberg, T.S., Rea, W., Baumann, M.H., Annals of the NY Academy of Sciences 1998; 844:59-74.

Shoaib, M., Baumann, M.H., Rothman, R.B., Goldberg, S.R., Schindler, C.W., *Behavioural and neurochemical characteristics of phentermine and fenfluramine administered separately as a mixture in rats.* Psychopharmacology 1997; 131(3):296-306.

Stapleton, S., *Diet Drugs: Problems and Prospects.* American Medical News, November 9, 1998.

Chapter 4

LABORATORY ANALYSIS

§ 4-2. Sampling and Storage.

§ 4-2(e). Biopsy.

Page 65. Add at end of § 4-2(e):

The author uses a technique known as skin punch biopsy developed by Justin McArthur at Johns Hopkins University. A skin punch biopsy is taken from any site on the body where skin may be found. The usual presenting symptoms are complaints of numbness, tingling and burning sensation in an arm or leg. These symptoms may be distal or proximal. Even when routine nerve conduction velocities and electromyographic analyses are normal, the skin punch biopsy may reveal abnormal small unmyelinated sensory nerve fibers that innervate the skin. The skin punch biopsy procedure is done with great care. Pain is usually minimal. After the biopsy, the tissue is carefully placed in chemicals and prepared methodically. The small unmyelinated sensory fibers are identifiable after immunological fixation under the microscope. Abnormalities are identifiable both qualitatively and quantitatively depending on the shape, morphology, size and quantity of fibers. These abnormalities have been seen in various medical conditions associated with neurotoxicity, either from the disease itself or from its treatment.

Chapter 7

VOLATILE SOLVENTS

§ 7-5. Individual Solvents.

Page 216. Add new subsection after § 7-5(j)(1):

§ 7-5(k). Trichloroethene.

The preferred sampling technique for trichloroethene is exhaled human breath. Since organic constituents of breath are indicative of bloodborne concentrations through gas exchange in the blood/breath interface in the lungs, the presence of specific compounds such as volatile organic compounds (VOCs) can indicate recent exposure. Some researchers prefer sampling and analyzing breath over direct measurement from blood because the technique is noninvasive, potentially infectious waste is avoided, and the measurement of gas-phase analytes is much simpler in a gas matrix than a complex liquid phase such as blood. One study used a single breath canister (SBC), though others are available (Pleil, 1995). This method can actually predict actual blood levels using breath elimination curve calculations. The results indicated that 22% of inspired trichloroethene was excreted through exhalation with the first compartment of blood as 75% of that fraction. Note that the second and third compartments in this model were highly perfused tissues and lesser perfused tissues respectively. Thus, approximately 78% of all trichloroethene that enters the body during inhalation exposure is metabolized, stored, or excreted through pathways other than exhalation. It was determined that 66% of this activity occurs in the perfused tissue or deeper compartments.

References.

Pleil, J., Fisher, J., Lindstrom, A., *Trichloroethene Levels in Human Blood and Exhaled Breath from Controlled Inhalation Exposure*. Environmental Health Perspectives 1998; 106(9):573-80.

Pleil, J., Lindstrom, A.B., *Measurement of volatile organic compounds in exhaled breath as collected in evacuated electropolished canisters*. J. Chromatogr. B: Biomed. Appl. 1995; 665:271-79.

Chapter 8

METALS

§ 8-1. In General.

Page 235. Add at end of § 8-1:

A revolutionary technique has been developed by the Mobil Corporation to clean up toxic wastes. It has been used by the Pacific Northwest National Laboratory (PNL) of the Department of Energy in Richland, Washington. Ceramic beads clean up huge amounts of metals in soil and water through a molecular process that acts like a sponge. Called SAMMS, an acronym for "self-assembled monolayers on mesoporous supports," the beads have hexagonal shapes. Inside each bead is an embedded circular framework of oxygen, carbon, and hydrogen atoms that ends in a thiol group. The center of the molecule is the attachment cite. A spoonful of this ultimate pollution fighter is capable of absorbing surface area of toxic waste the size of a football field. In addition, the beads can be tailor-made for action on specific materials such as precious metals. The 3M Company is working on embedding the ceramic beads in conventional membrane filters.

§ 8-2. Lead.

Page 239. Add at end of § 8-2:

A large study of the lead-smelting industry has found that the lead dust mineralogy varies widely throughout the smelter, consisting of remnant sulfides and multimetal oxide phases. Lead dusts produced in the ore storage and sinter areas of the smelter have larger particle sizes and react later in the extraction steps than do the dusts produced in the blast and dross furnace areas. Near the furnace can be found high amounts of soluble lead oxide, lead sulfate, and soluble lead. Additionally, large particles emitted from the smelter settle out of the atmosphere fairly rapidly. However, the smaller particles emitted from the smelter are more bioavailable and can be transported many kilometers in the form of PbSO4, PbO, PbO4, and PbS. Thus, if lead bioavailability is related to its solubility as determined through sequential extraction, the health effects related to lead exposure are enhanced in the blast and dross furnace processes.

It is now possible to clean up toxic lead waste with SAMMS technology developed by the Mobil Corporation.

§ 8-3. Mercury.

Page 243. Add at end of § 8-3:

It is now possible to clean up toxic mercury waste with SAMMS technology developed by the Mobil Corporation.

§ 8-4. Arsenic.

Page 257. Replace "nitially" with "initially" in second line of first full paragraph.

Page 258. Add at end of § 8-4:

A case of a suicide attempt with water-dissolved arsenate has been reported. Symptoms of the poisoning included severe nausea, vomiting, hypotension, and diarrhea. Although nausea and vomiting subsided within 2 days, diarrhea lasted for a week. There were slight elevations of AST and ALT. The patient returned to the hospital 2-3 weeks later complaining of numbness in finger, toe, and foot sole bilaterally. Parethesias followed and progressed one month later, spreading to both legs and hands. The patient was treated with intravenous lipo-alprostadil but died.

Perhaps the greatest mass poisoning by arsenic occurred in the fall of 1998 in Bangladesh. Millions of people had been exposed through drinking water delivered by hand-operated pumps located in a vast system of tube wells. Most of the pumps were 10 to 20 years old and provided a vehicle for the naturally occurring arsenic to reach a level of carcinogenic solubility. Ironically, the crisis developed over the past 25 years as the government, with the help of UNICEF and other groups, urged villagers to abandon disease-carrying pond water in exchange for water sources contained in underground aquifers. Overlooked was the source of subterranean arsenic. The abnormal symptoms to this exposure has included skin ulcers. The legal limit in groundwater arsenic content in Bangladesh is 0.05 mg/l. However, over half of the country's districts report wells with levels exceeding the recommended amount. The World Health Organization has set a safety standard arsenic in water at 0.01 mg/l (NYT 11/10/98).

References.

Bearak, B., *New Bangladesh Disaster: Wells That Pump Poison.* New York Times, November 10, 1998, A1.

Researchers Draw A Bead in Toxic Waste. Business Week, September 14, 1998.

Spear, T.M., Svee, W., Vincent, J.H., Stanisich. N., *Chemical Speciation of Lead Dust Associated with Primary Lead Smelting.* Environ. Health Perspec. 1998; 106(9):565-571.

Watanabe, K., Yamamoto, K., Nakamura, T., *Delayed and Chronic Polyneuropathy Caused by Acute Arsenic Toxicity.* First Draft, Case Report 8437, Funayama Hospital, Yonezawa, Yamagata, Japan, 1997.

Chapter 9

ORGANOPHOSPHATE INSECTICIDES

§ 9-1. Overview.

Page 287. Add at end of § 9-1:

In April 29, 1999, a representative of the EPA's Neurotoxicology Division announced that there are no plans to remove organophosphates from the register of legal insecticides. It was stated that this was based, in part on their usefulness which outweighed their potential health risks (Hilson, 1999). Because of their worldwide distribution in agriculture and most household gardens, there has been a steady increase in accidental OPP poisoning. Since organophosphates cause irreversible cholinesterase inhibition, the most definitive measurement of OPP poisoning is to measure serum pseudcholinesterase activity (Bardin, 1994; Hayes, 1982; Jeyeratnam, 1990).

§ 9-4. Sensory Effects.

Page 292. Add at end of § 9-4:

Exposure to organophosphates (OPP) has been associated with the development of sensitivities to the odors of multiple chemicals that before exposure had been tolerated (Wilson, 1997).

References.

Bardin, P.G., et al., *Organophosphate and Carbamate Poisoning.* Arch. Intern. Med. 1994; 154:1433-41.

Hayes, W.J., *Organophosphate Insecticides.* In: Hayes, W.J., ed., Pesticides Studied in Man. Baltimore, Md.: Williams and Wilkins, 1982; 285-315.

Hilson, H.A., Personal Communication, April 29, 1999.

Jeyaratnam, J., *Acute Pesticide Poisoning: A Major Health Problem.* World Health Stat. Q. 1990; 43:139-45.

Wilson, C., *EPA Memorandum Links Chlorpyrifos Poisoning to MCS.* Our Toxic Times Vol. 8(3) 1997.

Chapter 11

THE ROLE OF NUTRIENTS

§ 11-5. Vitamin Deficiency and Excess.

§ 11-5(c). Vitamin B_1 (Thiamine).

Page 346. Add at end of § 11-5(c):

Thiamine is necessary for glucose metabolism. Morbidity, and even death in some rare cases, is a possible medical outcome in thiamine deficiency. A case report has been published of a young female receiving parenteral nutrition without a preparation of intravenous vitamins. She was diagnosed with lactic acidosis. Episodes of nausea, vomiting, diarrhea, and abdominal pain were symptoms of an earlier undiagnosed condition for three years. Administration of thiamine improved the condition. Requirements for thiamine escalate when a person has a fever, a high glucose load or experiences physical stress, or is pregnant. Thiamine needs may be increased by hemodialysis and peritoneal dialysis, diuretic therapy, and diarrhea (Romanski, 1990).

§ 11-5(e). Vitamin B_3 (Niacin).

Page 347. Add at end of § 11-5(e):

Lipid-lowering therapies (HMG-CoA reductase inhibitors) such as Niacin have been shown to potentiate peripheral neuropathy. The onset of neuropathy associated with lipid lowering varies between days to years after the start of therapy, and complete resolution can take from 3 to 12 months after discontinuation. A review of the literature shows 45 cases of peripheral neuropathy associated with simvastatin, lovastatin, and provastatin which all exacerbated the condition of peripheral neuropathy.

§ 11-5(j). Vitamin C (Ascorbic Acid).

Page 351. Replace title of § 11-5(j) with the following:

§ 11-5(j). Vitamin C (Ascorbic Acid, Ascorbate).

Page 351. Add at end of § 11-5(j):

The recommended daily allowance (RDA) for vitamin C is under revision by the Food and Nutrition Board of the National Academy of Sciences. The current RDA is 60 mg/d established in 1980 (based on scurvy prevention) and was not changed in 1989. The new proposal ranges from 200-280 mg/d or at least less than 1000 mg/d since more than that amount may pose adverse health effects in some individuals. The new recommendations have been based on extensive research that has been conducted on its biochemical, molecular, clinical, and epidemiological activity. Note that vitamin C has been demonstrated to reduce the effects of cancer.

Page 351. Add new subsection after § 11-5(j):

§ 11-5(j)(1). Grapefruit Juice.

Grapefruit juice has been shown to elicit a number of drug interactions. Given the increased number of prescriptions for the elderly, this is of particular interest to gerontologists and other physicians treating senior citizens. The metabolism of drugs is thought to be inhibited by grapefruit juice most likely through the cytochrome P450 system (CYP3A3, CP1A2, CYP2D6) (Progress Notes, Fall 1998).

Pages 355-356. Delete existing § 11-6 and all its subsections and replace with the following new § 11-6 and subsections:

§ 11-6. Dietary Supplements: The New "Miracle" Drugs and New Hope for the Millennium.

§ 11-6(a). General Nutrition.

Any discussion of dietary supplements or additives presupposes healthy nutrition. A popular (and recently revised) way to know what foods are best is the Food Guide Pyramid. The pyramid has four levels: at the base are breads, cereals, rice and pasta; then come the vegetables and fruits; next are meat, poultry, fish and dairy products; finally, there are the oils, fats and sweets. Information on nutrition abounds and may be enriched by what can be learned in a good health food store.

§ 11-6(b). Miracle Supplements.

American society has embraced with great optimism a multitude of dietary supplement products. These food additives and supplements are touted to have great potential to enhance health, promote youth, and generally improve "quality of life." Unfortunately, the realities are not that simple. The claims made for these products are often fraught with misconceptions, and consumption of these supplements may pose potentially dire health consequences for the consumer. The consumer needs to be aware.

Most dietary supplement products are not evaluated by the Food and Drug Administration (FDA). This simple fact is not known by many Americans. The FDA does not analyze these supplements for efficacy, quality or even safety. The law only provides that manufacturers of dietary supplements make sure that, as far as they know, the labeling is truthful and not misleading, or at least not intentionally misleading. It is obvious that the main goals of manufacturers are to promote and sell the products. Manufacturers, therefore, will present the products in the most positive light. Unfortunately, many food supplements, additives, and vitamins found in health food stores are promoted without even minimal scientific justification. Though manufacturers have an obligation and a responsibility for making certain that the dietary ingredients in the supplements are safe, and not harmful to the individuals who consume them, neither manufacturers or distributors need to register with the FDA prior to making supplements available. FDA approval is not needed before manufacturing, producing, marketing, or selling dietary supplements.

It has come to my attention as a clinical neurotoxicologist who has worked in the field of product liability that these issues become extremely important, not only for clinicians, but for health care providers and for attorneys. Dietary supplements frequently have no salutary effects and, worse, they may actually cause harm to those who consume them.

§ 11-6(b)(1). Melatonin.

As a neurologist and neurotoxicologist who has been interested in sleep medicine for a number of years, I am frequently asked about a product called melatonin, the principal hormone of the pineal gland. In 1958, Lerner isolated melatonin from bovine pineal glands. In 1965,

Wurtman and Axelrod characterized the pineal gland as a "neuroendocrine transducer," important in the conversion of neural signals from the external environment. Apparently, the pineal gland converts multiple stimuli into a neuroendocrine output affecting cerebral homeostasis. The pineal gland and melatonin have, since that time, been recognized as serving many functions, including that of a "regulator of regulators" or a primary clock in circadian rhythm, and also, potentially, that of a pacemaker. Though it weighs only 75 to 150 mg, the pineal gland exerts an influence on many biological functions. Through the secretion of melatonin, the pineal gland maintains the homeostasis of the organism and influences the temporal organization of metabolic, physiological, and behavioral processes. It has some effect on immunomodulation and, from a neurologist's point of view, it serves as a synchronizer of biological rhythms. It may have effects on regulation of cerebral blood flow, neuroprotective activity, regulation of sexual maturation and reproduction, and temperature control. It does have effects on regulation of sleep, mood and pain, modulation of cognitive functioning, and regulation of neurotransmitter functioning. The pineal gland is thought to be linked with the control of the hypothalamic-pituitary neuroendocrine system and may be considered a specialized functional part of the limbic system.

Melatonin, the main product of the pineal gland, probably has multiple effects, but one primary effect is the inducement of sleep. Primarily effective in older individuals, it allows a person to become sleepy and serves as a hypnotic and a fairly good sleeping medication. It can be bought over the counter in various dosages—frequently 3 to 5 mg—and is to be taken on a nightly basis to help with sleep. Some have suggested that it may be effective in reducing jet lag. At this time, there are not enough scientific data to make any further suggestions in terms of its utility, although some have suggested that the pineal gland itself may play a role in some degenerative neurologic diseases.

§ 11-6(b)(2). 5-hydroxy-L-tryptophan (5-HTP).

5-hydroxy-L-tryptophan (5-HTP) products are currently marketed and widely promoted as dietary supplements. These products have been touted and promoted as useful for treating insomnia (see melatonin), depression, obesity, and even children with attention deficit disorder. Unfortunately, Food and Drug Administration scientists have confirmed the presence of impurities in some of these products. One of these impurities is known as "peak X." Although the significance of finding peak X and other impurities in dietary supplements containing 5-HTP is unknown, previous experiences with these products suggests caution in their use. Many individuals who take these over-the-counter products are not aware of the potential hazards. Peak X was identified in one case of the illness called eosinophilia-myalgia syndrome (EMS) associated with 5-HTP in 1991. This became a major product liability medical/legal issue in the early 1990s. Impurities similar to peak X were also found in L-tryptophan that was associated with a 1989 epidemic of EMS. 5-HTP and L-tryptophan are related in that 5-HTP is synthesized from L-tryptophan in the body. The exact causes of the 1989 epidemic and of the cases of EMS associated with 5-HTP remain somewhat unclear, although at least one manufacturer was found to have some adulterants in its products, and it was these adulterants that were thought to be the primary cause of the EMS.

EMS is a serious systemic illness. It is characterized by elevation of certain white blood cells and by severe muscle pain. The Centers for Disease Control and Prevention (CDC) have identified more than 1,500 cases of EMS, including at least 38 deaths associated with the use of L-tryptophan. The medical literature reports ten previous cases of EMS worldwide associated with the use of products containing 5-HTP. It is not clear whether these cases of EMS were caused by L-tryptophan, by 5-HTP, by one or more other impurities, or even by other possible causes. At this time, the FDA is unaware of any recent illnesses associated with the 5-HTP products being sold as dietary supplements. The widespread promotion and use of these products began only recently. These products will require further monitoring by the FDA working in conjunction with the CDC and the National Institutes of Health (NIH).

§ 11-6(b)(3). L-tryptophan.

L-tryptophan is related to niacin, a water-soluble vitamin. The niacin requirements of humans and many animal species are normally met in part by the conversion of dietary tryptophan to niacin. In other words, one does not need to take supplements of niacin because tryptophan is converted into niacin. The conversion is to consider 60 mg of tryptophan as equivalent to 1 mg of niacin. Some foods, such as milk and eggs, contain little niacin but have sufficient tryptophan to more than offset the lack of niacin. Meat contains high levels of both preformed niacin and tryptophan. The need for tryptophan is unclear if one regularly consumes an adequate diet.

The term "niacin" is used in a generic sense for both nicotinic acid and nicotinamide (niacinamide). Nicotinamide functions in the body as a component of two coenzymes, nicotinamide adenine dinucleotide (NAD) and nicotinamide adenine dinucleotide phosphate (NADP). These coenzymes are present in all cells and participate in metabolic processes. They are very important in glycolysis (the breakdown of glycogen), fatty acid metabolism, and tissue respiration. Without these coenzymes, the cells cannot live.

Pellagra is a multiple deficiency disease associated with diets providing only low levels of niacin equivalents and low levels of other B vitamins. It flares up when the skin is subjected to strong sunlight and is characterized by dermatitis, diarrhea, inflammation of the mucous membranes, and, in severe cases, dementia. Pellagra was first well-described in 1941 by Harris. It was a widespread problem in the southern United States in the early part of this century and is still a significant problem in Africa and Asia.

A new study published in the February 1999 issue of the American Medical Association's Archives of General Psychiatry showed evidence that an eating disorder, bulimia nervosa, may be caused in part by a chemical malfunction in the brain and not merely by an excessive desire to be thin. Bulimics typically alternate between binge eating and starving or purging. The study involved ten recovered bulimics and twelve normal women. The subjects were given identical-looking fruit drinks and snacks, some with tryptophan and some without. The subjects were not told which was which. The recovered bulimics were more affected psychologically than the other subjects by being deprived of tryptophan. Tryptophan is an amino acid that occurs naturally in many foods and is used by the body to make serotonin, a mood- and appetite-regulating chemical. The study's findings suggested that lowered brain serotonin function can trigger some of the clinical features of bulimia in individuals vulnerable to the disorder. Bulimia is biologically rooted and seems to have something to do with the system's inability to regulate serotonin. Tryptophan like that used in the study is not available in the United States. L-tryptophan supplements were withdrawn from the market in 1990 after thirty-six people died and many others became ill. Tryptophan is licensed, however, in Britain for treatment of depression and other disorders.

It has been found and reported that there have been abnormal levels of a serotonin-related chemical in the spinal fluid of actively bulimic women. This is an example where tryptophan may be important as a dietary supplement, but it needs to be supervised by health care workers, researchers or doctors rather than taken over the counter.

§ 11-6(b)(4). Carnitine.

Carnitine-Sigma-Tau Pharmaceuticals has recently revised the adverse reaction section of the labeling for Carnitor (levocarnitine) tablets, oral solution and injection solution. The revision provides for the following statement regarding the occurrence of seizures in some patients receiving Carnitor: "Seizures have been reported to occur in patients with or without pre-existing seizure activity receiving either oral or intravenous level carnitine. In patients with pre-existing seizure activity, an increase in seizure frequency and/or severity has been reported. This is an important point regarding carnitine, which has been touted as safe and problem-free.

§ 11-6(b)(5). Erythropoietin (EPO).

Erythropoietin (EPO), an agent that increases the number of red blood cells, is a highly recommended medication for patients who are chronically anemic because of renal failure. It is used clinically to treat dialysis patients. It has also been used illicitly by athletes, both Olympic and non-Olympic, as an alternative to "blood doping." EPO is extremely difficult to detect because the extra blood cells are the athlete's own. However, athletes who take too much EPO can develop various syndromes, including stroke, hyperviscosity, myocardial infarction and clots such as thrombophlebitis or embolism.

§ 11-6(b)(6). Anabolic Steroids.

Athletes use steroids to combat breakdown in muscle fibers during exercise. The side effects of steroid use are well-documented. They include hepatic lesions, clotting disorders, lowered levels of high-density lipo-protein cholesterol, acne, baldness, breast growth in men, and smaller testicles. Other complications include coronary artery disease, thromboembolic complications, intraabdominal bleeding, hepatocellular neoplasms, and hepatic necrosis as a result of long-term steroid use. Psychological deficits, such as uncontrolled aggression and psychosis, have also been reported.

§ 11-6(b)(6)(i). Testosterone.

Testosterone is used by athletes and other body builders to build muscles. Muscle fiber cells are targets for testosterone. As it enters these cells, protein growth is stimulated, resulting in enlarged muscle cells. Testosterone decreases the amount of cortisone in the body, reducing the body's natural response against stress and inflammation. Excessive amounts of testosterone can cause heart disease and other problems, including impotence.

§ 11-6(b)(6)(ii). Androstenedione.

Androstenedione is a prehormone that becomes an anabolic steroid when it enters the body. It is converted into testosterone which results in increased muscle mass.

Manufacturers of androstenedione warn men with prostate problems and pregnant women not to take the supplement. Since testosterone use is prohibited, androstenedione and other steroids are taken by athletes to cover up increased levels of testosterone in their bodies. Professional Baseball permits the use of androstenedione, but other sports associations, including the National Football League and the International Olympic Committee, have prohibited it. Physiological possession of these substances may cause an athlete to be banned and stripped of medals by these organizations (New York Times, September 8, 1998).

§ 11-6(b)(6)(iii). Dihydroepiandrostene (DHEA).

The neurosteroid dihydroepiandrostene (DHEA) has been called "the elixir of youth," but recently this claim has suffered a setback. In a report from San Diego dated March 2, 1999, Neurocrine Biosciences, the company that makes this product, announced that in phase II and III clinical trials, DHEA showed no greater effectiveness in patients with Alzheimer's disease than did a placebo. Previous trial had suggested DHEA was helpful in patients with memory loss. Based on these recent results, Neurocrine Biosciences will no longer pursue further development of DHEA.

§ 11-6(b)(6)(iv). Human Growth Hormone.

Human Growth Hormone stimulates the intracellular breakdown of body fat, allowing more to be used for energy. It is a natural hormone so added amounts don't show up in blood or urine tests. For this reason, it has become a popular performance-enhancing substance among athletes. There are risks associated with consumption of human growth hormone, however, including muscle and bone disfigurement, jutting forehead, elongated jaw and general features of acromegaly. Heart and metabolic problems have also been described.

§ 11-6(b)(6)(v). Other Anabolic Steroids.

The April 8, 1999, issue of *The New England Journal of Medicine* reported the case of a large subcapsular hepatic hematoma and subsequent intraabdominal hemorrhage associated with the abuse of anabolic steroids by a 24-year-old male body builder. The patient was admitted to the hospital with right upper quadrant pain and multiple other medical problems. He had been taking daily mesterolone 50 mg, nandrolone 400 mg, clomiphene 50 mg, and chorionic gonadotropin 1250 International Units. He was found to have abnormal liver function tests, and an abdominal computed tomography (CT) showed a large subcapsular hematoma in the right liver lobe. The patient had to be observed in the intensive care unit. An abdominal sonogram showed more than 1.5 liters of free fluid in the abdominal cavity. Surgical exploration showed the affected hepatic region. A biopsy was done which showed extensive hepatic necrosis. Coronary artery disease, thromboembolic complications and abdominal bleeding caused by benign liver tumors are known complications of long-term abuse of anabolic steroids. Subcapsular hematoma is now added to that list.

§ 11-6(b)(7). Herbs.

Herbs are also used as food additives. There have been few reports of toxicity due to herbs.

§ 11-6(b)(7)(i). Ginseng.

Ginseng is commonly referred to as Panax quinquefolium L. or Panax Ginseng. The word panax is derived from a Greek word meaning "all healing." Panax Ginseng is also known as American ginseng, Chinese ginseng, and Korean ginseng. Ginseng is the most widely used plant in traditional medicine and now plays a major role in the herbal health care market. It has been used for more than two thousand years. The human-shape of the root of the ginseng plant actually led proponents of the Doctrine of Signatures to believe that the root could strengthen any part of the body. Through the ages, the root has been used to treat many diseases including hardening of the arteries, bleeding disorders, colitis, cancer, and aging. Today, ginseng is popular due to its "adaptogenic effect," a stress-protective effect of the saponin content. A wide range of ginseng products is available, ranging from fresh or dried roots to extract solutions, capsules, tablets, cosmetics, sodas and teas. The taste of these products may be disagreeable. Some products closely resemble the whole root in composition, but many contain little or no detectable ginsenoside concentration. Some preparations have been adulterated with phenylbutazone, aminopyrine or mandrake root.

Millions of Americans regularly use ginseng. It is widely used as a tonic to treat lack of stamina. The most common effects of ginseng are nervousness and excitation. There have been few reports of severe reactions. Health risks and side effects following the proper administration of designated therapeutic doses are not well-recorded. Overdoses can bring about Ginseng Abuse Syndrome, which is characterized by sleepiness, hypertonia, and edema. Patients have reported feelings of stimulation, well-being, and increased motor and cognitive efficiency, but have also suffered diarrhea, skin eruptions, nervousness, sleeplessness and hypertension. Ginseng has been reported to have an estrogen-like effect in women. The whole root has been reported to cause a hypoglycemic effect. Patients who must control their blood glucose levels should take ginseng with caution.

§ 11-6(b)(7)(ii). Ginkgo Biloba.

The ginkgo is the world's oldest living tree species. The sole survivor of the family Ginkgoaceae, it dates back more than two hundred million years to the Permian Period. Ginkgo trees may live as long as a thousand years and grow to a height of about one hundred and twenty-five feet. Ginkgoes have fan-shaped leaves. In China, the ginkgo was cultivated as a sacred tree, and it plays a significant role in traditional Chinese medicine.

Known for its antioxidant and neuroprotective effects, ginkgo has been recommended to treat cerebral insufficiency, dementia, circulatory disorders, and asthma. It is also used to treat tinnitus hearing disorder and as an anti-anxiety medication, a stress reducer, and a memory booster. The average daily dose is 120 mg of ginkgo biloba extract (GBE) in two or three doses orally. It may also be given in a parenteral dosage of 50 to 100 mg. In traditional Chinese medicine, the daily dose is three to six grams of leaves as an infusion. Ginkgo must be protected from light and moisture.

Research data on ginkgo biloba are incomplete. One study — a meta-analysis of eleven placebo-controlled, randomized double-blind studies — concluded that 150 mg per day of GBE was superior to placebo in treating patients with cerebrovascular insufficiency.

Ingestion of the ginkgo biloba extract has not been associated with severe side effects. The German literature lists ginkgo's possible side effects as headaches, dizziness, heart palpitations, and gastrointestinal and dermatological reactions. There is a toxic syndrome called Gin-Nan food poisoning that is recognized in the Orient in children who have ingested ginkgo seeds. Ingestion of fifty seeds produced tonic-clonic seizures and loss of consciousness. In one report, there was a spontaneous bilateral subdural hematoma. American patients taking ginkgo biloba have reported severe bleeding during surgery, especially when the herb has been combined with aspirin. Consumers of ginkgo biloba who are about to undergo elective surgery should alert their doctors and stop consumption of the herb well beforehand.

It is now recognized that ginkgo biloba has a potent inhibitory effect on the platelet activating factor known as PAF by displacing it from receptor-binding sites. Extracts of ginkgo biloba, therefore, have the potential to interact with antibody therapy.

As baby boomers age, a new growth industry promoting herbal and dietary supplements and designer drugs has developed. These products, promoted in books, advertisements, and television shows, are claimed to improve thinking, memory, attention span, and concentration and generally to keep a person young in both mind and body. An article in the Sunday, April 4, 1999, edition of *The New York Times* pointed out that new national companies have been started to promote these concepts (Meier, 1999). Hot new initial public offerings (IPOs) are being presented. It is estimated that by 2030 the number of Americans over age 65 will double. A new term of art to describe memory problems has even been established: "senior moment." The aging process itself, however, does not really damage memory. Aging does affect short-term memory, *i.e.*, the ability to recall recently learned information; but long-term memory is fairly stable and remains intact despite aging.

§ 11-6(b)(7)(iii). Echinacea.

Echinacea is a water-soluble immuno-stimulating polysaccharide with antibacterial effects. It is used to help patients suffering from common colds, cough, bronchitis, fevers, urinary tract infections, and inflammation of the mouth and pharynx. It may also be used to treat patients with wounds and burns. Echinacea is administered as expressed juice prepared in a concentration of 2.5:1. It is stabilized with 22% alcohol. When used internally, the recommended dosage is 6 to 9 milliliters of the expressed juice.

§ 11-6(b)(7)(iv). Phytoestrogen and Estrogen Substitutes.

Isoflavones such as phytoestrogens are estrogen-like substances derived from plants, especially soybeans, black cohosh root and red clover. They are used by women to reduce the incidence of hot flashes and other symptoms of menopause. An herb called dong quai (Chinese origin) has been reported by patients to be effective. Other remedies include primrose oil, vitamin B complex, Vitamin E, Progesterone cream and the progestin-type hormone progestrol (Megace). Health supplements are not regulated by the FDA. It is not known if these substances have actual physiological mechanisms or work by the placebo effect (*The Washington Post*, Health, 1998) Environmental xenoestrogens resulting from such sources as exposure to estrogenic industrial chemicals can have adverse effects on human populations, including developmental, oncological, and endocrinological problems. Note that this is in contrast to the beneficial effects of phytoestrogens such as genistein, diaidzein, and coumestrol.

§ 11-6(b)(7)(v). Ephedrine, Ephedra, and Ma Juang.

A number of herbal stimulants contain ephedrine, ephedra, or ma juang, a natal Chinese herb. Advertisers usually target young people for these products, claiming that they provide a safe and legal high. Herbal stimulants, sold under names such as Cloud Nine, Ultimate Xphoria, and Herbal Ecstasy, have become extremely popular among the "rave" culture. Herbal stimulants can have central nervous system effects, and may have adverse effects on the heart and blood pressure. Within normal dosages, they may cause psychosis, seizures, heart attacks, strokes, and other problems. The products are suspected to have contributed to the deaths of fifteen people nationally, resulting in a ban on the stimulants in Nassau County, New York. The FDA issued a warning about the dangers of herbal stimulant pills in April 1996, having received reports of approximately 400 adverse reactions to the pills. Most states have made the herbal stimulant ecstasy illegal as of May 1999, but it remains legal in Washington, D.C., due to a technicality (Lambert, 1996; Fox News, 1990).

§ 11-6(b)(8). Estrogen.

Estrogen Replacement Therapy (ERT) reduces the effects of Alzheimer's disease in some postmenopausal women. Apparently, estrogen produces increased activation in the inferior parietal lobule during tasks requiring storage of verbal material (Neurology Update, 1999).

§ 11-6(b)(9). Enzymes.

A nutritional supplement called Enada, promoted as an "energy-giving natural enzyme," has recently been marketed to treat chronic fatigue syndrome. Enada is the brand name of the company Menuco's version of a natural substance known as NADH, a coenzyme. It has apparently helped as many as 72% of patients with chronic fatigue syndrome. More than 500,000 Americans have been diagnosed with chronic fatigue syndrome, and it is estimated that two million people think they have it. The clinical diagnosis is difficult. No specific etiology has been found. Note that chronic fatigue syndrome is marked mainly by a lack of energy. How many of us have a lack of energy? Some doctors attribute chronic fatigue syndrome to psychological factors. It has also been associated with infections, possible viral infections, and autoimmune disorders.

§ 11-6(b)(10). Creatine.

A naturally occurring substance produced in the liver and kidneys and found in meat, creatine has been used for twenty years, including by British team members in the 1992 Olympics. Short studies have shown no negative side effects to creatine use but little is known about the long-term effects according to the American College of Sports Medicine. Anecdotal reports of potential side effects include gastrointestinal distress, nausea, muscle cramping, and increased blood pressure. Creatine appears to promote physical strength and power and to boost performance in sports activities requiring short-term maximum effort such as sprinting and throwing. Weight gain is also a by-product of taking creatine.

§ 11-6(b)(11). Gamma Butyrolactone (GBL).

In January 1999, the FDA ordered makers of the "health supplement" gamma butyrolactone (GBL) to recall the products. Supplements containing GBL have been promoted under many names and have been claimed to help build muscle, improve physical performance, reduce stress and induce sleep — kind of a magic bullet to cure all ills. The FDA warned that the supplements were dangerous and had already killed one person. Nineteen other people had become unconscious and had gone into comas after using the products. When taken orally, GBL is converted in the body to gamma hydroxybutyrate (GHB), a potent unapproved drug. GHB is being investigated under the supervision of doctors for the treatment of narcolepsy. Because it has serious side effects — including seizures, vomiting, slow breathing, slow heart rate, and coma — it should not be taken except in the context of an FDA-approved study.

References.

Basin, S., et al., *The effects of supraphysiologic doses of testosterone on muscle size and strength in normal men.* New England J. Medicine 1996; 335:1-7.

Correa, P., *Human Gastric Carcinogenesis.* Cancer Research 1992; 52:6735-6740.

Ishak, K.G., *Hepatic lesions caused by anabolic and contraceptive steroids.* Semin. Liver Dis. 1981; 1:116-28.

Krucoff, C., *Body of Evidence.* Washington Post, Health Section, July 7, 1998; A16.

Lambert, B., *Nassau to Ban Sale of Herbal Stimulant Linked to a Death.* New York Times, April 17, 1996; B1.

Levine, M., *New Concepts in the Biology and Biochemistry of Ascorbic Acid.* NEJM 1986; 314:892-902.

Levine, M., et al., *Criteria and Recommendations for Vitamin C Intake.* JAMA 1999; (15):145-1423.

Meier, Barry, *Industry's Next Growth Sector: Memory Lapses. The New York Times,* Sunday, April 4, 1999.

Neurology Reviews, *Statins, Niacin Linked to Peripheral Neuropathies.* Neurology Reviews, August, 1999; 36-37.

Noble, H.B., *Questions surround performance enhancers.* New York Times, September 8, 1998; D7.

Progress Notes, *Grapefruit Juice-Drug Interaction.* Pharmacy Committee News, Fall 1998.

Romanski, Susan A., McMahon, Molly M., *Metabolic Acidosis and Thiamine Deficiency.* Mayo Clin. Proc. 1999; 74:259-63.

Schumacher, J., Muller, G., Klotz, K.-F., *Large Hepatic Hematoma and Intraabdominal Hemorrhage Associated with Abuse of Anabolic Steroids* [Letter]. New England Journal of Medicine 1999; 340(14):1123-24.

Chapter 12

OTHER TOXIC AGENTS

§ 12-1. Gases.

§ 12-1(a). Carbon Monoxide.

Page 370. Add at end of § 12-1(a):

Delayed neuropsychological sequale (DNS) as a morbidity of CO poisoning can be reduced by treatment with hyperbaric oxygen (HBO). No sequale developed in patients treated with HBO as compared to 23% of patients treated with 100% ambient-pressure oxygen. DNS after CO poisoning cannot be predicted on the basis of clinical history of the patient or CO level (Thom, 1995).

Carbon monoxide has also been implicated as a neurotransmitter. It is the predominant neurotransmitter found in mature olfactory receptor neurons affecting both sensitization and desensitization responses via activation of guanylyl cyclase. Direct effects include neurotransmission, memory, regulation of blood vessel tone, and GI vascular tone, all of which are abnormal in MCS and Gulf War Syndrome (Verma, 1993).

§ 12-1(d). Hydrogen Sulfide.

Page 372. Add at end of first paragraph of § 12-1(d):

Hydrogen Sulfide has been identified as a toxic chemical to which soldiers were exposed in the Persian Gulf War (DOD, 1998).

§ 12-1(f). Methylene Chloride.

Page 373. Add after first paragraph of § 12-1(f):

Methylene Chloride can also be found in insecticides, fumigants, aerosols, fire extinguishers and Christmas tree bubble lights. The greatest occupational exposure is in the furniture industry where it is used in the following: foam blowing to make upholstery for new furniture; foam adhesive operations (i.e., putting upholstery on furniture frames); and in paint stripping for furniture refinishing after replacing 1,1,1,-trichloroethane due to its ozone effects. Halogenated solvents like methylene chloride are regulated on the basis of neurotoxicity.

Page 374. Add at end of § 12-1(f):

Acute exposure is known to produce dose-related changes in psychomotor performance and cognitive abilities. In 1992, OSHA proposed to revise the permissible exposure limits to methylene chloride — from 500 ppm to 25 ppm — based on carcinogenicity. This regulation is scheduled to protect 186,000 workers who handle methylene chloride in the furniture shopping industry (NMAS, Advisor, Spring 1994).

Page 387. Add new § 12-5 and new § 12-6:

§ 12-5. Chemotherapy Agents.

Chemotherapy agents have been used to treat cancer for many years. Extensive clinical research study shows effectiveness in some populations. Side effects include, nausea, vomiting and acute reactions. Platinum-based chemotherapy has a 4% relative risk of causing leukemia based on a cohort study of 28,971 women in North America and Europe who had received a diagnosis of ovarian cancer between 1980 and 1983. Combination therapy of cisplatin and carboplatin has a 6.5% risk. There is a dose-related response with relative risks reaching 7.6% at doses of 1000mg or more of platinum. Radiotherapy did not increase the risk for leukemia (Travis, 1999).

12% of patients on ifosfamide demonstrate signs of somnolence or confusion. If coma develops, stop the agent.

§ 12-6. Polychlorinated Biphenyls (PCBs).

Polychlorinated biphenyls (PCBs) were used in insulation for transformers and electrical capacitors from the 1930s to 1977. They were banned thereafter due to suspected carcinogenicity. Recently, a large study of occupational exposure to toxic levels of PCB chemicals has found no link to increased mortality from cancer (Cushman, 1999).

PCBs are global environmental contaminants. There are 209 related congeners that have a common biphenyl structure but have differences in the number and position of chlorine substitutions. PCBs are lipophilic and found in the food chain in measurable amounts as well as in the fat of all human populations. New Bedford harbor in southeastern Massachusetts is considered one of the most contaminated sites for PCBs in the United States. A study has shown breast milk concentrations of women residing in the area ranging from 1100 ng/g milk fat has concluded that the benefits of breast feeding with the contaminated milk outweighs the health risk to exposed infants. The FDA currently recommends PCB concentrations of no more than 1500 parts per billion in commercial milk. Conversely, the developing nervous system seems to be susceptible to PCB toxicity. Increased infant mortality, congenital syndrome of low birth weight, ectodermal effects, cognitive deficits and behavioral problems have been seen in children who ingested cooking oil contaminated with PCBs (Korrick, 1998).

References.

Cushman, J.H., *Study Finds Little Risks from PCBs.* The New York Times, March 10, 1999; A12.

DOD, *Case Narrative, 11th Marines.* Department of Defense, October 1998.

Korrick, S.A., Altshul, Larisa, *High Breast Milk Levels of Polychlorinated Biphenyls (PCBs) among Four Women Living Adjacent a PCB-Contaminated Waste Site.* 1998; 106(8):513-18.

NMAS, Advisor, National Medical Advisory Service, Spring 1994.

Thom, S.R., *Delayed Neuropsychologic Sequale After Carbon Monoxide Poisoning: Prevention by Treatment with Hyperbaric Oxygen.* Annals of Emergency Medicine 1995; 25(4):474-80.

Travis, L.B., *Risk of Leukemia After Platinum-Based Chemotherapy for Ovarian Cancer,* NEJM 1999; 340(5):351-57.

Verma, A., et al., *Carbon Monoxide: A Putative Neural Messenger.* Science 1993; 259:381-84.

Page 391. Add new Chapters 13 and 14 after end of Chapter 12:

Chapter 13

COMPLEMENTARY AND ALTERNATIVE MEDICINE (CAM)*

"Undress," as George Herbert says, "your soul at night, not by self-examination, but by shedding, as you do your garments, the daily sins whether of omission or commission and you will make a free man, with a new life."

—Sir William Osler, *Advice to Young Physicians*

§ 13-1. Complementary and Alternative Medicine: Mainstream and Fashionable Concepts.

Complementary medicine includes practices that are used concomitantly with conventional Western treatments, alternative medicine is limited to practices that replace Western medical treatments. A 1990 survey of approximately 1500 adults in the U.S. who were asked about practices that were generally defined as not being taught in American medical schools and were unavailable in U.S. hospitals, found that, projected from this sample, about 60

*Adapted from *Alternative Medicine: Expanding Medical Horizons,* a report prepared under the auspices of the Workshop on Alternative Medicine, held in Chantilly, Virginia, on September 14-16, 1992.

million Americans used alternative medical treatments in 1990 at an estimated cost of $13.7 billion. Two-thirds of these people did not inform their doctors of their alternative therapy treatments which included chiropractic, homeopathy, herbs, naturopathy, Chinese medicine, and acupuncture. In fact, it is thought that there were more visits to the offices of alternative healers than to primary care physicians. It is not impossible that as third party interests become more interested in paying for alternative medical practices, allopathic physicians will increase their referrals to these entities (Onopa, 1999). Note that in a study of physicians in which 28% of respondents referred actual patients to alternative medicine therapies, discontinuance of the doctor-patient relationship has been reported to be more common among specialists than among primary care physicians (Crock, 1999).

The realization that the public is interested in new forms of treatment, perhaps because of a certain frustration and the lack of effective treatment for many diseases has been striking and ground breaking. The Office of Alternative Medicine (OAM) was formed through congressional mandate under the 1992 National Institutes of Health (NIH) Appropriations Bill. The NIH is one of eight health agencies of the U.S. Public Health Service (PHS) and is part of the U.S. Department of Health and Human Services (DHHS). According to the official Congressional mandate which established the OAM, it was the stated purpose of the Office to "facilitate the evaluation of alternative medical treatment modalities" to determine their effectiveness. The current name for OAM is the National Center for Complementary and Alternative Medicine. It was established in 1998 under provisions of the Omnibus Appropriations Bill (P.L. 105-217, 11 Stat 2681). The Office is located on the NIH campus in Bethesda, Maryland. The creation of this office is a major breakthrough in terms of concepts of medical illness and their treatment.

§ 13-2. Nutritional and Food Supplements.

One approach to the subject of nutritional and food supplements is to break down the complementary and alternative medicine area into subsections. One section would be certain products used as nutritional and food supplements. These products are used for preventive or therapeutic purposes. Some are used in combination.

Single nutrient use includes the following: ascorbic acid, also known as vitamin C, carotene, tocopherols (vitamin E), Folic Acid, niacin, niacinamide, pantothenic acid, riboflavin, thiamine, the various fat-soluble vitamins including A, B and K, biotin, choline, the various minerals calcium, magnesium, selenium, electrolytes, potassium, iodine, iron manganese, carnitine, glutamine, phenylalanine, amino acids, melatonin, steroids, prehormones, androstenedione, phyto-estrogens, DHEA, inositol, and fatty acids. These would be considered nutritional and food supplements that are important.

§ 13-3. Mind-Body Medicine.

Another section would be an area that involves behavioral, social, spiritual and psychological approaches to health, sometimes termed Mind-Body Medicine. It is thought that there are four categories in the mind body medicine area. This would include mind-body systems, a subcategory involving the whole system of mind-body method, for example, hypnosis. It appears that patients are attracted to alternative medicine because they find that many of these practices are in agreement with their personal philosophy of health care delivery. Mind-Body medicine uses many important psychological features in medical treatment and prophylaxis (Astin, 1999).

Complementary and Alternative Medicine portions include yoga and Tai Chi. There is also behavioral medicine. This is conventional and certainly mainstream. It has been used for many years including hypnosis and biofeedback. The notion of support groups, psychotherapy, meditation and progressive muscle relaxation are important behavioral medicine components. These are frequently practiced in conventional medical settings. More extended and more atypical other forms of therapy including art therapy, music therapy, dance therapy and humor have received great attention in recent films and multiple articles in newspapers.

Religion and spirituality are important components of the whole Complementary and Alternative Medicine field, including spiritual healing, confession and prayer. Spirituality Constructs such as love, hope and faith are all part of the religion and spirituality. Studies have been done to scientifically assess the effectiveness of prayer in sick individuals (Springer and Eicher, 1999).

§ 13-4. Social and Contextual Alternative Intervention.

Another method of treatment would be social and contextual areas. This refers to social, cultural and symbolic intervention. Another important category would involve complete systems of theory and practice that are more Eastern or Oriental and cannot be explained by medical approaches. These systems have their own descriptive term, have their own hierarchy and analysis as well as terminology. These include acupuncture and Oriental medicine which is not only use of needles but also a way of life that includes diet and herbal formulas, and may include massage and manipulation.

There are nutritional indigenous systems which include Native American medicine, ayurvedic medicine and other traditional indigenous peoples medicine.

§ 13-5. Unconventional Western Medicine.

An additional system is so-called unconventional Western system which is alternative medical systems developed in the West. These include homeopathy, environmental medicine, and orthomolecular medicine, which refers to products used as nutritional and food supplements and not covered in other categories. These products are used for preventive or therapeutic purposes, and finally naturopathy which is an eclectic collection of natural systems and therapies that is very popular in the United States. Another system is lifestyle and disease prevention system designed to prevent the development of illness and identify and treat risk factors, support healing and recovery process. Some of these are unconventional approaches including electrodermal diagnostics. Another system is lifestyle therapy, behavioral changes, dietary changes, exercise, stress management and nutrient control. Health promotion is a part of this, as well.

§ 13-6. Biological and Pharmacological Therapies.

Biologically based therapeutics include herbal treatment — plant-derived preparations. These include the famous ginkgo biloba, garlic, ginseng, echinacea, saw palmetto, Kava, Aloe Vera, feverfew, green tea, yohimbine, valerian and many others. There are, of course, combinations of these individual herbs, as well. Part of the enthusiasm for the "New Medicine" is the aging of the baby boomers. The consumers of this New Medicine, many of them reaching 50 and older, have not only engaged but reported the development of alternative and complementary medicine, perhaps seeking everlasting life and high quality of life. These consumers have spent more than twelve billion dollars on natural supplements last year. Sales continue to grow at more than ten percent a year. The preparations made from herbs, for example aloe, for good bowel movements, and valerian for restless sleep are being used by millions of Americans on a daily basis. Mainstream journals such as the Journal of the American Medical Association (JAMA) released an issue devoted entirely to the study of herbs and alternative remedies. Americans spend as much out of pocket that is not reimbursed by health insurance on alternative medicines as in all unreimbursed physician services.

Special diet therapies should be mentioned including vegetarian diets, high fiber diets, the Pritikin diet and other diets named after individuals.

Pharmacological, biological and instrumental interventions are also unconventional medicines. These include such things as antineoplastons, shark cartilage, various chelation therapies such as with EDTA, ozone therapy, hydrogen peroxide therapy, hyperbaric oxygen treatment, enzyme therapy and bee pollen.

§ 13-7. Manipulative Healing.

Manipulative and body-base systems are based on manipulation or movement of the body, including chiropractic medicine, massage and body works, osteopathic manipulative therapy, craniosacral osteopathic manipulative therapy, Swedish massage, applied kinesiology, reflexology, rolfing, Pilates Method, Alexander Technique, Felden Kreis Technique, Acupressure, and Chinese Tui Na massage.

More unconventional physical therapies include high colonics and coffee enemas, various types of hydrotherapy, and light and color therapies.

§ 13-8. Biofield Medicine and Bioelectromagnetics.

Biofield medicine involves systems that use subtle energy fields in and around the body for medical purposes. This includes therapeutic touch, healing touch and others like Reiki.

Bioelectromagnetics refers to the unconventional use of electromagnetic fields for medical purposes and use of magnets for various types of treatment.

References.

Anonymous, *Open Learning. Complementary therapies and research.* Nt. Learning Curve 1999; 2(12):5-11.

Astin, J.A., Shapiro, S.L, Lee, R.A., Shapiro, D.H., Jr., *The construct of control in mind-body medicine: implications for healthcare.* Alternative Therapies in Health & Medicine 1999; 5(2):42-47.

Crock, R.D., Jarjoura D., Polen, A., Rutecki, G.W., Alternative Therapies in Health & Medicine 1999; 5(2):61-66.

Katzenbach, M.S., *"Voices" reader asserts her soul's individual destiny (letter).* Alternative Therapies in Health & Health 1999; 5(2):22.

Micozzi, M.S., *Historical aspects of complementary medicine [Review].* Clinics in Dermatology 1998; 16(6):651-58.

Muscat, M., *The Osher Center for Integrative Medicine at UCSF: healing the whole person with "relationship-centered" medicine.* Alternative Therapies in Health & Medicine 1999; 5(2):36-37.

Onopa, J., *Complementary and alternative medicine.* Hawaii Medical Journal 1999; 58(2):9-19.

Springer, S.C., Eicher, D.J., *Effects of a prayer circle on a moribund premature infant.* Alternative Therapies in Health & Medicine 1999; 5(2):22.

Chapter 14

FORENSICS

§ 14-1. Overview.

The twenty-first century will continue to advance the revolution in technology as it applies to evidence and information-gathering in criminal cases and injury lawsuits. The determination of cause and effect in injury claims will become increasingly arduous as workers are exposed to myriad potentially hazardous chemicals and products. A new accountability has emerged with the ruling in *Daubert v. Merrill Dow Pharmaceuticals* that is essentially slowing the pace of the "injury claimant business." The *Daubert* ruling was designed to ensure that only meaningful expert testimony be heard by a jury. Thus, many prominent injury experts have recently found themselves being dismissed by judges who are suspicious of persons purporting to be "experts in many cases." The Hippocratic oath taken by physicians is supposed to ensure ethical practice and to protect the public, and, in theory, physician expert witnesses should be cautioned by their oath. The ruling in *Daubert* seems to be a decision to protect industry, though its thrust is admirable. The ruling aims to reduce frivolous and unfounded trial litigation, but this is how the decision is described on an insurance company web site:

> In a 1993 ruling, *Daubert v. Merrill Dow Pharmaceuticals*, 509 U.S. 579 (1993) the U.S. Supreme Court established [a] criteria for trial judges to act as "gatekeepers" in determining whether certain expert testimony is admitted under the Federal Rules of Evidence. The court identified five non-exclusive factors for assessing the validity of scientific evidence:

1. Has the theory or technique on which the expert opinion is based been tested?
2. Has the theory or technique been published or subjected to review?
3. Are standards maintained controlling the theory or technique?
4. What is the error rate for the specific technique?
5. Has the scientific community generally accepted the theory or technique?

The court stressed that inquiring into these factors is to be a flexible process, with the trial judge determining "whether the testimony's underlying reasoning or methodology is scientifically valid and properly can be applied to the facts at issue."

The above ruling was tested in *General Electric Co. et al. v. Joiner et al.*, 118 S. Ct. 512 (1997). The case concerns the standard an appellate court should apply when reviewing a trial court decision to admit or exclude expert testimony.

The underlying case involved a plaintiff alleging he contracted small-cell lung cancer from occupational exposure to PCBs. The trial judge granted defendants summary judgment asserting that the plaintiff's expert failed to establish a link between PCB exposure and small-cell lung cancer. The court stated: "The expert's opinion of a causal link is not supported by the epidemiological and animal studies submitted by the plaintiffs."

The Eleventh Circuit Court ruled that the trial judge excluded the evidence because he had drawn different conclusions from the underlying research than did the experts. In reversing the trial judge, the Circuit Court adopted a "particularly stringent" standard for determining the validity of a trial court's exclusion of expert testimony.

The U.S. Supreme Court overruled the Eleventh Circuit, stating that the Federal Rules of Evidence did not alter the trial judge's "gatekeeper" role in screening scientific evidence. The Supreme Court concluded that the appellate court is to give deference to the evidentiary rulings of a trial judge and reverse only if there is a finding of abuse of discretion.

The ruling solidifies the role of the trial court in preventing expert testimony from influencing a jury where there is no reasonable scientific basis for the opinion. This is favorable to defense interests in situations where plaintiffs attempt to use unsubstantiated expert opinion to prove causation.[1]

§ 14-2. Manipulation.

The manipulation of parties for gain by litigation constructs is not a new phenomenon. For many years, experts have testified in cases over airplane parts, beer containers, ladders, playground equipment, winches, and, of course, tires.

Historically, attorneys have influenced the psychological data submitted as admissible evidence in forensic cases in a number of ways. They advise their clients on how to answer and prepare them for psychological evaluations, they inform patients not to disclose certain information important to psychologists, and they alter their clients' perceptions of what has actually happened in hazardous exposure or injury. Attorneys have been known to "doctor up" clinical history and fabricate misleading data regarding the impact of injury. It follows that this influencing of what juries see as evidence can ultimately influence the outcome of litigation.

Another way in which cases can be influenced is through *response bias,* or providing information in a systematic, erroneous fashion, for example, during medical, psychological, and neuropsychological evaluation. In particular, forensic situations can elicit behaviors that are influenced by the potential financial reward, the pressures of litigation, what may be perceived as expected for a particular injury, additional symptoms of physical or emotional distress, and cognitive

---

1. "The Gatekeeper," by Michael Mikitiuk, <http://www.zurichre-na.com>.

deficits that are causally disconnected from underlying physiological and psychological dysfunction.

§ 14-3. *Daubert.*

The thrust of *Daubert* is to get to the facts of litigation and to dismiss witnesses who are not directly involved personally with their expert testimony. OSHA is challenged by *Daubert*, on the other hand, because many employers continue to violate ergonomic guidelines at the workplace, such as those governing manual materials handling, intense keyboarding, and manufacturing. The Secretary of Labor was challenged by *Daubert* in a federal administrative law case alleging that thirteen different jobs at Dayton's Tire's Oklahoma City plant presented "ergonomic stressors." The Secretary failed to establish the first element that an activity presented a hazard. Even if the first element had been met, three others would have had to be addressed: the hazard must have been "recognized;" the hazard must have been likely to cause death or serious physical harm; and the hazard could have been feasibly abated. OSHA estimates that back and injury claims carried a $2.7 billion price tag from 1989 through 1996 in Washington state alone, and caused 24.5 million days off the job (WIM, 1998).

Daubert is not only a challenge to attorneys, psychologists, neurologists, neurotoxicologists, scientists, corporations, and plaintiffs, but also to judges. Judges must eliminate personal bias and admit lack of knowledge in some cases and seek expert witnesses for the bench. Although many are adhering to this concept, variance exists in the courts on this issue. Frivolous lawsuits, uninformed and non-expert witnesses are seriously threatened as judges determine the validity of expert witnesses and their testimony. Appeals courts must be vigilant to reexamine all cases where "abuse of discretion" has been exercised by a trial judge and must remedy all conditions whereby hazards and exposures result in injury to individuals.

§ 14-4. Liability for Vaccination Injury.

Patients may be injured following vaccination. Damages are collected under the National Childhood Vaccine Injury Act, 42 U.S.C.A. §§ 300aa-1 to 300aa-21(a). If a patient receives compensation for damages under this Act, the patient may not proceed with a civil action against the physician who administered the vaccine. *Harman ex rel. Harman v. Borah,* 720 A.2d 1058 (Pa. Super. Ct. 1998), *reargument denied,* Dec. 15, 1998, was a case of a child and his parents who brought suit against the physician who administered a measles, mumps, and rubella vaccine to the child. The vaccination resulted in encephalitis and permanent neurologic damage to the child. The parents and child had already received a judgment in the Federal Claims Court under the National Childhood Vaccine Injury Act. The trial court held that, under the provisions of the statute, injury from a vaccine can be compensated either by a civil action or through claims made under the remedy in the Federal Court of Claims as provided by the statute. Thus, the civil action against the physician who had administered the vaccine was precluded by the plaintiffs' acceptance of compensation through the Federal Court of Claims. This result is in accord with the opinions of most courts that have addressed this issue. However, physicians may be subject to suit if the plaintiffs elect not to seek the remedy provided by the National Childhood Vaccine Injury Act.

References.

Lees-Haley, P.R., *Attorneys Influence Expert Evidence in Forensic Psychological and Neuropsychological Cases.* Assessment 1997; 4:321-324.

Lees-Haley, P.R., *Manipulation of Perception in Mass Tort Litigation.* Natural Resources & Environment 1991; 12(1):64-68.

Lees-Haley, P.R., Zasler, N.D., Margulies, S., English, L.T., Stevens, K.B., *Response Bias in Plaintiffs' Histories.* Brain Injury 1997; 11:791-799.

Schmitt, R.B., *Who is an Expert? In Some Courtrooms, The Answer is Nobody.* Wall Street Journal, June 17, 1997; A8.

WIM, OSHA/Ergonomics. Briefs. Work Injury Management March 1998.

INDEX

H

L

M

N

O